John MURTAGH'S
practice tips

John MURTAGH'S
practice
tips

EIGHTH EDITION

John Murtagh AO

MBBS, MD, BSc, BEd, FRACGP, DipObstRCOG

Emeritus Professor in General Practice, School of Primary Health Care, Monash University, Melbourne, Victoria
Professorial Fellow, Department of General Practice, University of Melbourne, Melbourne, Victoria
Adjunct Clinical Professor, Graduate School of Medicine, University of Notre Dame, Fremantle, Western Australia

Justin Coleman

MBBS, FRACGP, MPH (Hons 1)

General Practitioner, Wurrumiyanga, Tiwi Islands NT
Senior Lecture, Flinders University
Editor, *Diabetes Management Journal*
Chair of Choosing Wisely working group, RACGP

McGraw Hill

This eighth edition published 2019
First edition 1991
Reprinted 1992 (twice), 1993 (twice), 1994 (twice)
Second edition 1995
Reprinted 1997, 1999, 2001
Third edition 2000
Reprinted 2002, 2004
Fourth edition 2004
Fifth edition 2008
Sixth edition 2013
Reprinted 2013
Seventh edition 2017

NATIONAL LIBRARY OF AUSTRALIA

A catalogue record for this book is available from the National Library of Australia

John Murtagh and Justin Coleman
Murtagh's Practice Tips 8e
ISBN: 9781743767429

Published in Australia by
McGraw-Hill Education (Australia) Pty Ltd
Level 33, 680 George Street, Sydney NSW 2000
Product Manager: Diane Gee-Clough
Content Producer: Genevieve MacDermott
Copyeditor: Julie Wicks
Proofreader: Rosemary Moore
Cover design: Christa Moffitt, Christabella Designs
Typeset in NimbusRomDOT 10/11 by SPi Global
Printed in Singapore on 80 gsm woodfree by Markono Print Media Pte Ltd

Foreword to the eighth edition

It is now 28 years since I had the honour of writing the foreword to the first edition of *Practice Tips*. Since then, the wisdom and practical skills of John Murtagh have spread throughout the medical world through his writings.

This eighth edition incorporates several new features, including an update on the management of emergencies, therapeutic plastic procedures, more injection techniques and the management of lumps and bumps. This edition includes a new chapter on technology, raising the awareness of the role of technology in improving access to information for everyday practice.

I have no doubt that this new edition of *Practice Tips* will find a place on the bookshelves of many practitioners in general practice and in emergency departments.

GEOFF QUAIL
Clinical Associate Professor
Department of Surgery
Monash University
Melbourne

Foreword to the first edition

In a recent survey of medical graduates appointed as interns to a major teaching hospital, the question was posed, 'What does the medical course least prepare you for?' Half the respondents selected practical procedures from seven choices.

While we are aware that university courses must have a sound academic basis, it is interesting to note that many newly graduating doctors are apprehensive about their basic practical skills. Fortunately, these inadequacies are usually corrected in the first few months of intern training.

Professor John Murtagh, who has been at the forefront of medical education in Australia for many years, sensed the need for ongoing practical instruction among doctors. When appointed Associate Medical Editor of *Australian Family Physician* in 1980 he was asked to give the journal a more practical orientation, with a wider appeal to general practitioners. He was able to draw on a collection of practical procedures from his 10 years as a country doctor that he had found useful, many of which were not described in journals or textbooks. He began publishing these tips regularly in *Australian Family Physician*, and this encouraged colleagues to contribute their own practical solutions to common problems. The column has been one of the most popular in the journal, and led to an invitation to Professor Murtagh to assemble these tips in one volume.

The interest in practical procedures is considerable—as witnessed by the popularity of practical skills courses, which are frequently fully booked. These have become a regular part of the Monash University Postgraduate Programme, and some of the material taught is incorporated in this book.

It is particularly pleasing to see doctors carrying out their own practical procedures. Not only is this cost-effective, in many cases obviating the need for referral, but it also broadens the expertise of the doctor and makes practice more enjoyable.

I congratulate Professor Murtagh and Dr Coleman on the compilation of this eighth edition, which I feel certain will find a prominent place on the general practitioner's bookshelf.

GEOFF QUAIL
Past Chairman
Medical Education Committee
Royal Australian College of General Practitioners
(Victorian Faculty)

Contents

Foreword to the eighth edition	v
Foreword to the first edition	v
Preface	xix
About the authors	xx
Acknowledgments	xxii
Sterilisation guidelines for office practice (RACGP)	xxiii

1 Skin repair and minor plastic surgery — **1**

Principles of repair of excisional wounds	1
Gloves	**1**
Wounds and suturing	**1**
Practising suturing	1
Taping wounds	1
Skin preparation antiseptic solutions	2
Standard precautions	2
Knot tying[3]	3
Holding the scalpel	5
Safe insertion and removal of scalpel blades	5
Debridement and dermabrasion for wound debris	5
Continuous sutures[4]	5
The pulley suture	6
The cross-stitch	7
The purse-string suture	7
Excisions	7
Planning excisions on the face	7
Elliptical excisions	8
Prevention and removal of 'dog ears'	8
The lazy s repair	9
M-plasty	9
The three-point (corner) suture	9
Inverted mattress suture for perineal skin	10
Skin grafts	**10**
Flaps	**10**
Triangular flap wounds on the lower leg	10
Excision of skin tumours with sliding flaps	11
Primary suture before excision of a small tumour	13
Multiple ragged lacerations	13
Avoiding skin tears	13
Vessel ligation[4]	13
The transposition flap[7]	14
The rotation flap	14
The rhomboid (limberg) flap	15

The 'crown' excision for facial skin lesions   15
Z-plasty   15
Repair of cut lip   16
Wedge excision and direct suture of lip   17
Wedge resection of ear   17
Repair of lacerated eyelid   18
Repair of tongue wound   19
Avascular field in digit   19
Removal of skin sutures   20
Pitfalls for excision of non-melanoma skin cancer   20
W-plasty for ragged lacerations   21
Bush suture   21
Split skin injuries   21
Debridement of traumatic wounds   21
Debridement of skin in a hairy area   22
Hair removal   22
Wound management tips[9]   22
When to remove non-absorbable sutures   23

References   **24**

2   Injection techniques   25

Basic injections   **25**
Painless injection technique   25
Intramuscular injections   26
Reducing the sting from an alcohol swab   26
Painless wound suturing   27
Simple topical anaesthesia for wound repair   27
Slower anaesthetic injection cuts pain   27
Local anaesthetic infiltration technique for wounds   27
Disposal of needles   27
Bubbles in the syringe   28
Rectal 'injection'   28
Finger lancing with less pain   29
Digital nerve block   29
Regional nerve wrist blocks to nerves to hand   30
Regional nerve blocks at elbow   31
Femoral nerve block   31
Lateral cutaneous nerve of the thigh (LCNT)   32
Tibial nerve block   32
Medial plantar nerve block via dorsum of the foot   33
Facial nerve blocks   33
Specific facial blocks for the external ear   34
Penile nerve block   35
Intravenous regional anaesthesia (bier block)   35
Haematoma block by local infiltration anaesthetic   36
The caudal (trans-sacral) injection   37
Local anaesthetic use   37
Hormone implants   38

Musculoskeletal injections   **39**
Musculoskeletal injection guidelines   39
Injection of trigger points in back   39
Injection for rotator cuff lesions   40

Injection for supraspinatus tendinopathy	41
Injection for bicipital tendinopathy	41
Injections for epicondylitis	41
Injection for trigger finger	42
Injection for trigger thumb	43
Injection for tenosynovitis of the wrist	43
Injection for plantar fasciitis	44
Injection for trochanteric bursalgia	44
Injection of the carpal tunnel	45
Injection near the carpal tunnel	46
Injection of the tarsal tunnel	46
Injection for achilles paratendinopathy	46
Injection for tibialis posterior tendinopathy	46
Injection or aspiration of joints	47
Acute gout in the great toe	50
References	**51**

3 Treatment of lumps and bumps 52

Removal of skin tags	52
Removal of epidermoid (sebaceous) cysts	52
The infected epidermoid cyst	54
Sebaceous hyperplasia	54
Dermoid cysts	54
Acne cysts	55
Biopsies	55
Treatment of ganglions	56
Olecranon and pre-patellar bursitis	57
Excision of lipomas	57
Keratoacanthoma	58
Basal cell carcinoma (BCC)	58
Squamous cell carcinoma (SCC)	58
Pyogenic granuloma	59
Seborrhoeic keratoses	59
Cherry angioma	59
Chondrodermatitis nodularis helicus	59
ORF	59
Milker's nodules	59
Haemangioma of the lip	60
Aspiration of baker cyst	60
Aspiration and injection of hydrocele	60
Epididymal cysts	61
Testicular tumours	61
Torsion of the testicle	61
Steroid injections into skin lesions	61
Steroid injections for plaques of psoriasis	61
Hypertrophic scars: multiple puncture method	62
Keloids	62
Dupuytren contracture	63
Drainage of breast abscess	63
Aspiration of breast lump	64
Marsupialisation technique for bartholin cyst	64
Cervical polyps	65
Liquid nitrogen therapy	65

Trichloroacetic acid   67
Simple removal of xanthoma/xanthelasmas   67
Warts and papillomas   67
Molluscum contagiosum   68

References   **69**

| **4** | **Basic practical medical procedures** | **70** |

Venepuncture and intravenous cannulation   70
Rapid intravenous infusion catheter (RIC)   71
Nasogastric tube insertion   71
Nasogastric tube insertion in children   72
Urethral catheterisation of males   72
Urethral catheterisation of females   73
Catheterisation in children   74
Lumbar puncture   74
Lumbar puncture in children   75
Tapping ascites   75
Inserting a chest drain   76
Aspiration of pleural effusion   76
Subcutaneous fluid infusions   77
Continuous subcutaneous infusion of morphine   77
Intravenous iron infusion   77

Therapeutic venesection   **78**

References   **78**

| **5** | **Leg veins and ulcers** | **79** |

Percutaneous ligation for the isolated vein   79
Avulsion of the isolated vein   79
Endovascular treatment of veins   80
Treatment of superficial thrombophlebitis   81
Management of deep venous thrombosis (DVT)   81
Ruptured varicose vein   82
Venous ulcers[2]   82
Applying a compression stocking   83

References   **83**

| **6** | **TREATMENT OF ANO-RECTAL PROBLEMS** | **84** |

Perianal haematoma   84
Perianal skin tags   85
Rubber band ligation of haemorrhoids   85
Injection of haemorrhoids   86
Anal fissure[1]   87
Proctalgia fugax   87
Perianal abscess[2]   88
Pilonidal cyst ± abscess   88
Anal fistula   88
Perianal warts   88
Anal fibro-epithelial polyps   88
Pruritus ani   89
Rectal prolapse   89
Cautionary points regarding ano-rectal disorders   89

References   **89**

7	**Foot problems**	**90**
	Calluses, corns and warts	90
	Treatment of plantar warts	90
	Treatment of calluses[2]	92
	Treatment of corns	92
	'Cracked' heels	93
	Plantar fasciitis	93
	Morton's interdigital neuroma	96
	References	**96**

8	**Nail problems**	**97**
	Splinters under nails	97
	Onychogryphosis	98
	Onychomycosis	98
	Myxoid pseudocyst	98
	Subungual haematoma	99
	Ingrowing toenails (onychocryptosis)	100
	Bloodless field in a digit	101
	Wedge resection	102
	The elliptical block dissection open method	103
	Tip for post-operative pain relief	103
	Paronychia	103
	Excision of nail bed	104
	Nail avulsion by chemolysis	105
	Traumatic avulsed toenail	105
	Longitudinal traumatic nail laceration	105
	References	**105**

9	**Common trauma**	**106**
	General	**106**
	Essential tips for dealing with trauma	106
	Other cautionary tips	106
	Finger trauma	**107**
	Finger tip loss	107
	Amputated finger	107
	Finger tip dressing	107
	Abrasions	**108**
	Management (see chapter 1)	108
	Haematomas	**108**
	Haematoma of the pinna ('cauliflower ear')	108
	Haematoma of the nasal septum	109
	Pretibial haematoma	109
	Roller injuries to limbs	109
	Fractures	**109**
	Testing for fractures	109
	Spatula test for fracture of mandible	110
	First aid management of fractured mandible	110
	Fractured clavicle	111
	Bandage for fractured clavicle	111
	Fractured rib	111
	Phalangeal fractures	111

Slings for fractures   112
Important principles for fractures   115

Other trauma   **115**
Primary repair of severed tendon   115
Burns and scalds   115
Rapid testing of the hand for nerve injury   118

References   **119**

10 Removal of foreign bodies   120

General   **120**
Cautionary note   120
Removal of maggots   120
Removal of subcutaneous fly larvae (cutaneous myiasis)   121
Removal of leeches   121
Embedded ticks   121
Removal of ring from finger   122
Splinters under the skin   122
Removing spines of prickly pear, cactus and similar
plants from the skin   123
Detecting fine skin splinters–the soft soap method   123
Detecting skin splinters   123
Removing the implanon rod   123
Detecting metal fragments   124
Embedded fishhooks   124
Penetrating gun injuries   125

Ear, nose and throat   **126**
Removal of various foreign bodies   126
General principles about a foreign body in the ear   130
Insects in ears   130
Cotton wool in the ear   131
Fish bones in the throat   131

Genital and anal   **131**
Extricating the penis from a zipper   131
Removal of impacted vaginal tampon   132
Faecal impaction   133
Removal of vibrator from vagina or rectum   133

References   **133**

11 Musculoskeletal medicine   134

Temporomandibular joint   **134**
Temporomandibular dysfunction   134
The tmj 'rest' program   135
Dislocated jaw   135

The spine   **136**
Recording spinal movements   136
Spinal mobilisation and manipulation   136

Cervical spine   **138**
Clinical problems of cervical origin   138
Locating tenderness in the neck   138

Acute torticollis[1] 139
A simple traction technique for the cervical spine 139
Neck rolls and stretches 140

Thoracic spine **141**
Anterior directed costovertebral gliding 141
Thoracic spinal manipulation 141
Thoracolumbar stretching and manipulation 142

Lumbar spine **143**
Reference points in the lumbar spine 143
Tests for non-organic back pain 143
Movements of the lumbar spine 144
Nerve roots of leg and level of prolapsed disc 145
The slump test 146
Rotation mobilisation for lumbar spine 146
Lumbar stretching and manipulation technique 1 147
Lumbar stretching and manipulation technique 2 147
Exercise for the lower back 149

Shoulder **149**
Dislocated shoulder 149
The mt beauty analgesia-free method 151
Recurrent dislocation of shoulder 152

Elbow **152**
Pulled elbow 152
Elbow fractures and dislocations in children 153
Dislocated elbow 153
Tennis elbow 154

Wrist and hand **155**
De quervain tenosynovitis and finkelstein test 155
Simple tests for carpal tunnel syndrome 155
Simple reduction of dislocated finger 156
Strapping a finger 157
Mallet finger 157
Boutonnière deformity 158
Tenpin bowler's thumb 158
Skier's thumb (gamekeeper's thumb) 159
Colles fracture 159
Scaphoid fracture 160
Metacarpal fractures 160

Hip **161**
Age relationship of hip disorders 161
The ortolani and barlow screening tests[11] 161
Pain referred to the knee 161
Diagnosis of early osteoarthritis of hip joint 162
Buttock pain 162
The 'hip pocket nerve' syndrome 162
Ischial bursitis 163
Patrick or fabere test 163
Snapping or clicking hip 163
Dislocated hip 164
Fractured femur 165

Knee   **165**
Common causes of knee pain   165
Diagnosis of meniscal injuries of the knee   166
Lachman test   167
Overuse syndromes   167
Patellar tendinopathy ('jumper's knee')   167
Anterior knee pain   168
Diagnosis and treatment of patellofemoral joint pain syndrome   168
Dislocated patella   169

Leg   **169**
Overuse syndromes in athletes   169
Torn 'monkey muscle'   169
Complete rupture of achilles tendon   171
Treatment of sprained ankle   172
Mobilisation of the subtalar joint   173
Wobble board (aeroplane) technique for ankle dysfunction   173
Tibialis posterior tendon rupture   174

Plastering tips   **174**
Plaster of paris   174
Preparing a volar arm plaster splint (front slab)   175
Leg support for plaster application   176
Waterproofing your plaster cast   176
A long-lasting plaster walking heel   176
Supporting shoe for a walking plaster   176
Use of silicone filler   176
Prescribing crutches   177
Walking stick advice   177

References   **177**

12 Orodental problems   **179**
Emergency dental kit   179
Knocked-out tooth   179
Loose or partially dislodged tooth   179
Chipped tooth   180
Lost filling   180
Lost crown   180
Child with a bleeding mouth   180
Impacted wisdom tooth   180
Infections—tooth abscess, wisdom tooth or root canal infection   180
Bleeding tooth socket   180
Dry tooth socket   180
A simple way of numbering teeth   181
Aphthous ulcers (canker sores)   182
Geographic tongue (erythema migrans)   182
Black, green or hairy tongue   182
Calculus in wharton duct   183
A 'natural' method of snaring a calculus   183
Simple removal of calculus from wharton duct   183
Release of tongue tie (frenulotomy)   183

References   **184**

13 Ear, nose and throat	**185**
URTIs and sinus problems	**185**
Diagnosing sinus tenderness	185
Diagnosis of unilateral sinusitis	185
Inhalations for urtis	186
Nasal polyps	187
The ear and hearing	**187**
A rapid test for significant hearing loss	187
Water- and soundproofing ears	188
Use of tissue 'spears' for otitis externa and media	188
Preventing swimmer's otitis externa	188
Chronic suppurative otitis media and externa	188
Tropical ear	188
Ear piercing	189
Ear wax and syringing	189
Recognising the 'unsafe' ear	191
Air pressure pain when flying	192
Excision of ear lobe cysts	192
Infected ear lobe	192
Embedded earring stud	192
Problems with cotton buds	193
The nose	**193**
Treatments for epistaxis	193
Instilling nose drops	195
Offensive smell from the nose	195
Stuffy, running nose	195
Nasal irrigation	195
Senile rhinorrhoea	195
Nasal factures	195
Miscellaneous ENT pearls	**196**
Hands-free headlight	196
Self-propelled antral and nasal washout	196
Use of flo sinus care	196
Hiccoughs (HICCUPS)	196
Snoring	196
Tinnitus	197
Swallowing with a sore throat	197
Eustachian tube dysfunction and glue ear	197
Auriscope as an alternative to nasal specula	197
Chronic anosmia following URTI	198
Ticklish throat	198
Doctor-assisted treatment for benign paroxysmal positional vertigo	198
References	**200**
14 The eyes	**201**
Basic kit for eye examination	201
Eversion of the eyelid	201
Blepharitis	202
Flash burns	202
Wood's light and fluorescein	202
Simple topical antiseptics for mild conjunctivitis	202

Removing 'glitter' from the eye 202
Dry eyes 202
Eyelash disorders 203
Removal of corneal foreign body 203
Corneal abrasion and ulceration 204
Eye examination in infants 204
Excision of meibomian cyst 205
Local anaesthetic for the eyelid 205
Non-surgical treatment for meibomian cysts 205
Padding the eye 206
Managing styes 206
Application of drops 206
Visual acuity 206
The pinhole test for blurred vision 206
Relief of ocular pain by heat 207
Chemical burns to the eye 208
Protective industrial spectacles 208
Effective topical treatment of eye infections 208
Hyphaema 208
Subconjunctival haemorrhage 208

15 Tips on treating children **209**

Making friends 209
Distracting children 209
Management of painful procedures 210
'Bite the bullet' strategy 210
Using pacifiers (dummies) to ease pain 210
Sweet solutions for procedural pain in infants 210
Deep breath with blowing distraction 210
Taking medicine 210
Swallowing a tablet 210
Administration of fluids 210
Weighing a child 210
How to open the mouth 211
Spatula sketches for children 211
Instilling nose drops 211
Instilling eye drops in children 211
Intravenous cannula insertion 212
Difficult vein access 212
Easier access to a child's arm 212
Swallowed foreign objects 212
Wound repair 213
Wound infiltration 215
Fractures 215
Splints for minor greenstick fractures 216
Removing plaster casts from children 216
The crying infant 216
Cleaning a child's 'snotty' nose 217
Test for lactose intolerance 217
Breath-holding attacks 217
Itching and swollen skin rashes 218

Traumatic forehead lump   218
Suprapubic aspiration of urine   218
Clean catch midstream specimen   218
The 'draw a dream' technique   218
Assessing anxious children and school refusal   219
Surgery   220
Cardiopulmonary resuscitation in children   220

References   **221**

16 The skin   222

Rules for prescribing creams and ointments   222
Sunburn   222
Skin exposure to the sun   222
ACNE   223
Nappy rash   224
Atopic dermatitis (eczema)   224
Psoriasis   225
Skin scrapings for dermatophyte diagnosis   225
Spider naevi   226
Wood's light examination   226
Applying topicals with a 'dish mop'   226
Enhancing topical efficacy with occlusion   226
Watch base allergy   226
Chilblains   226
Herpes simplex: treatment options   226
Herpes zoster (shingles)   227
Unusual causes of contact dermatitis   228

17 Emergency procedures   229

Normal values for vital signs   229
Pulse oximetry   229
Acute coronary syndromes   230
The electrocardiogram   230
Urgent intravenous cutdown   232
Intraosseous infusion   234
Acute paraphimosis   234
Diagnosing the hysterical 'unconscious' patient   235
Electric shock   235
Head injury   236
Assessing sexual assault   237
Migraine tips   238
Hyperventilation   239
Pneumothorax   239
Cricothyroidotomy   240
Choking   241
Supra ventricular tachycardia (SVT)   241
Bite wounds   241
Stings   243
Coral cuts   243
Use of the adrenaline autoinjector for anaphylaxis   243

Major trauma   244
Blood loss: Circulation and haemorrhage control   244
Serious injuries and clues from association   244
Roadside emergencies   245
References   246

18 Technology and basic equipment   **247**
Note of caution   247
Technology   247
Medical phone apps   249
Computer   250
Medical records   251
Basic equipment   251
Gadgets   252
References   254

19 Miscellaneous   **255**
Measurement of temperature   255
Measurement of weight   256
Obtaining reflexes   256
Restless legs syndrome   257
Nightmares   257
Nocturnal cramps   258
Special uses for vasodilators   258
Nocturnal bladder dysfunction   259
Facilitating a view of the cervix   259
Condom on the speculum   259
Priapism   259
Premature ejaculation   259
Indomethacin for renal/ureteric colic   259
Cool cabbages for hot breasts   259
Makeshift spacing chambers for asthmatics   260
Coping with and swallowing tablets   260
Patient education techniques in the consulting room   261
Improvised suppository inserter   261
Collecting urine specimens   262
Bunion 'donuts'   262
The many uses of petroleum jelly (vaseline)   262
The many uses of paper clips   262
The uses of fine crystalline sugar   262
Sea sickness   262
Snapping the top off a glass ampoule   263
Medico-legal tips   263
Tips for aged care   263
Holistic treatment of patients with minor problems   264
References   264

Index   265

Preface

Murtagh's Practice Tips is a collection of basic diagnostic and therapeutic skills that can be used in the offices of general practitioners throughout the world. The application of these simple skills makes the art of our profession more interesting and challenging, in addition to providing rapid relief and cost-effective therapy to our patients. It has been written with the relatively isolated practitioner, doctor or nurse practitioner in mind. This means that a broad range of more complex procedures involving some degree of improvisation will be covered.

The art of medicine appears to have been neglected in modern times and, with the advent of super-specialisation, general practice is gradually being deskilled. The authors have been very concerned about this process, and believe that the advice in this book could add an important dimension to the art of medicine and represent a practical strategy to reverse this trend. John Murtagh has been writing and collecting these tips for over 30 years; they have been compiled by drawing on his experience, often through improvisation, in coping with a country practice for many years, and by requesting contributions from my colleagues. Doctors from all over Australia have contributed freely to this collection, and sharing each other's expertise has been a learning experience for all of us.

John has travelled widely around Australia and overseas running workshops on practical procedures for the general practitioner. Many practitioners have proposed the tips that apparently work very well for them. These were included in the text if they seemed simple, safe and worth trying. The critical evidence base may be lacking but the strategy is to promote 'the art of medicine' by being resourceful and original and thinking laterally. Joining John as co-author is Justin Coleman, who likewise has a special interest in 'Handy Hints for GPs'. These were serialised in a column in *Medical Observer*

for many years and subsequently collated in small publications called 'GP Tips'.

Many of the tips have previously been published in *Australian Family Physician*, the official journal of the Royal Australian College of General Practitioners, over the past decade or so. *Practice Tips* has proved immensely popular with general practitioners, especially with younger graduates commencing practice. The tips are most suitable for doctors working in accident and emergency departments. There is an emphasis on minor surgical procedures for skin problems and musculoskeletal disorders. A key feature of these tips is that they are simple and safe to perform, requiring minimal equipment and technical know-how. Regular practice of such skills leads to more creativity in learning techniques to cope with new and unexpected problems in the surgery.

Several different methods to manage a particular problem, such as the treatment of ingrowing toenails and removal of fishhooks, have been submitted. These have been revised and some of the more appropriate methods have been selected. The reader thus has a choice of methods for some conditions. Some specific procedures are more complex and perhaps more relevant to practitioners such as those in remote areas who have acquired a wide variety of skills, often through necessity. This eighth edition continues the emphasis on emergency procedures, particularly for acute coronary syndromes and on wound management.

It must be emphasised that some of the procedures are unorthodox but have been found to work in an empirical sense by the author and other practitioners where other treatments failed. The book offers ideas, alternatives and encouragement when faced with the everyday nitty-gritty problems of family practice, particularly in rural and remote practice. Evidence based medicine has been included where appropriate with helpful input from the RACGP's HANDI project.

About the authors

John Murtagh AO

MBBS, MD, BSc, BEd, FRACGP, DipObstRCOG

Emeritus Professor in General Practice, School of Primary Health Care, Monash University, Melbourne, Victoria
Professorial Fellow, Department of General Practice, University of Melbourne, Melbourne, Victoria
Adjunct Clinical Professor, Graduate School of Medicine, University of Notre Dame, Fremantle, Western Australia

John Murtagh was a science master teaching chemistry, biology and physics in Victorian secondary schools when he was admitted to the first intake of the newly established Medical School at Monash University, graduating in 1966. Following a comprehensive postgraduate training program, which included surgical registrarship, he practised in partnership with his medical wife, Dr Jill Rosenblatt, for 10 years in the rural community of Neerim South, Victoria.

Dr Murtagh was appointed Senior Lecturer (part-time) in the Department of Community Medicine at Monash University and eventually returned to Melbourne as a full-time Senior Lecturer. He was appointed to a professorial chair in Community Medicine at Box Hill Hospital in 1988 and subsequently as chairman of the extended department and Professor of General Practice in 1993 until retirement from this position in 2000. He now holds teaching positions as Emeritus Professor in General Practice at Monash University, Adjunct Clinical Professor, University of Notre Dame and Professorial Fellow, University of Melbourne. He combines these positions with part-time general practice, including a special interest in musculoskeletal medicine. He achieved the Doctor of Medicine degree in 1988 for his thesis 'The management of back pain in general practice'.

Professor Murtagh was appointed Associate Medical Editor of *Australian Family Physician* in 1980 and Medical Editor in 1986, a position held until 1995. In 1995 he was awarded the Member of the Order of Australia for services to medicine, particularly in the areas of medical education, research and publishing.

Murtagh's Practice Tips, one of Professor Murtagh's numerous publications, was named as the British Medical Association's Best Primary Care Book Award in 2005. In the same year, he was named as one of the most influential people in general practice by the publication Australian Doctor. John Murtagh was awarded the inaugural David de Kretser medal from Monash University for his exceptional contribution to the Faculty of Medicine, Nursing and Health Sciences over a significant period of time. Members of the Royal Australian College of General Practitioners may know that he was bestowed the honour of the namesake of the College library.

Today John Murtagh continues to enjoy active participation with the diverse spectrum of general practitioners—whether they are students or experienced practitioners, rural- or urban-based, local or international medical graduates, clinicians or researchers. His vast experience with all of these groups has provided him with tremendous insights into their needs, which is reflected in the culminated experience and wisdom of *Murtagh's General Practice*.

Justin Coleman

MBBS, FRACGP, MPH (Hons 1)

General Practitioner, Wurrumiyanga, Tiwi Islands NT
Senior Lecture, Flinders University
Editor, *Diabetes Management Journal*
Chair of Choosing Wisely working group, RACGP

Justin Coleman graduated from Melbourne University in 1992 and has spent half his career as a rural GP in Victoria and the remote Northern Territory, and the other half in Brisbane, working in Aboriginal and Torres Strait Islander health.

Soon after graduating, Justin began writing for the GP newspaper *Medical Observer* and hasn't stopped since. One of his weekly columns, 'Handy Hints for GPs', ran for 13 years. He even wrote 50 humorous columns until the editors lost their sense of humour.

Justin is a prolific writer for medical and non-medical readerships; he has published well over 1000 medical articles in around 50 different newspapers, magazines, books and journals. For five years he served as President of the Australasian Medical Writers Association and he regularly runs writing workshops for medical writers and academics.

Since completing a Master of Public Health (UQ 2011, first class hons), Justin has dedicated much of his career to educating other GPs about how to improve various aspects of medical practice. His interests include evidence-based medicine, the rational use of medical tests and treatments, and dealing with uncertainty during a GP consultation. He represents the RACGP on matters pertaining to conflicts of interest and fiercely guards his own independence, never having accepted payment from a pharmaceutical or medical device company.

For the past quarter of a century, Justin has supervised hundreds of medical students and GP registrars. He has taught in the medical schools of four universities and for a dozen medical education organisations.

Justin edited his first medical book 20 years ago and has remained a medical editor ever since. He completed a Writing and Editing program in 2010 (UQ, first class hons). He currently edits *Diabetes Management Journal*, writes and does peer reviews for the *MJA*, *AJGP* and *BMJ*, and is a member of the Australasian Health and Medical journal Editors' Network (AHMEN).

Acknowledgments

I would like to acknowledge the many general practitioners throughout Australia who have contributed to this book, mainly in response to the invitation through the pages of *Australian Family Physician* to forward their various practice tips to share with colleagues. Many of these tips have appeared over the past decade as a regular series in the official publication of the Royal Australian College of General Practitioners. The RACGP has supported my efforts and this project over a long period, and continues to promote the concept of good-quality care and assurance in general practice. I am indebted to the RACGP for giving permission to publish the material that has appeared in the journal and more recently from the HANDI project.

My colleagues in the Department of Community Medicine at Monash University have provided invaluable assistance: Professor Neil Carson encouraged the concept some 30 years ago, and more recently my senior lecturers provided considerable input into skin repair and plastic surgery (Dr Michael Burke) and expertise with orodental problems and facial nerve blocks (Professor Geoff Quail). Special thanks go also to Dr John Colvin, Co-Director of Medical Education at the Victorian Eye and Ear Hospital, for advice on eye disorders; Dr Ed Brentnall, Director of Accident and Emergency Department, Box Hill Hospital; Dr Alfredo Mori, Emergency Physician, The Alfred Hospital (femoral nerve block); Dr Mike Moynihan, Dr Clare Murtagh, Dr Lucas Wheatley for curriculum content and procedural advice, and the editorial staff of *Australian Family Physician*; Mr Chris Sorrell, graphic designer with *Australian Family Physician*; and in particular to Dr Clive Kenna, co-author of *Back Pain and Spinal Manipulation* (Butterworths), for his considerable assistance with musculoskeletal medicine, especially on spinal disorders.

Medical practitioners who contributed to this book are: Lisa Amir, Tony Andrew, Philip Arber, Khin Maung Aye, Neville Babbage, Peter Barker, Royce Baxter, Andrew Beischer, Ashley Berry, Cherry Bain, Peter Bourke, Peter Bowles, Tony Boyd, James Breheny, Ed Brentnall, Charles Bridges-Webb, Norman Broadhurst, John Buckley, Michael Burke, Marg Campbell, Patrick Campisi, Hugh Carpenter, Peter Carroll, Ray Carroll, Neil Carson, Robert Carson, Alan Chapeski Charles pharmacy (Murrumbeena), John Colvin, Peter Crooke, Graham Cumming, Joan Curtis, Hal Day, Jim Dickinsen, Tony Dicker, Clarrie Dietman, Robert J. Douglas, Mary Doyle, Graeme Edwards, Humphrey Esser, Iain Esslemont, Howard Farrow, Peter Fox, Michael Freeman, John Gambrill, John Garner, Jack Gerschman, Colin Gleeson, Peter Graham, Neil Grayson, Attila Györy, John Hanrahan, Geoff Hansen, Warren Hastings, Clive Heath, Tim Hegarty, Chris Hogan, Ebrahim Hosseini, Damian Ireland, Anton Iseli, Rob James, Fred Jensen, Stuart Johnson, Dorothy Jones, Roderick Jones, Dennis Joyce, Max Kamien, Trevor Kay, Tim Kenealy, Clive Kenna, Peter Kennedy, Hilton Koppe, Rod Kruger, Sanaa Labib, Chris Lampel, Bray Lewis, Ralph Lewis, Greg Malcher, Karen Martens, Jim Marwood, John Masterton, Jim McDonald, Sally McDonald, Peter McKain, A. Breck McKay, Peter Mellor, Thomas Middlemiss, Philip Millard, Les Miller, Geoff Mitchell, Andrew Montanari, David Moore, Michael Moynihan, Clare Murtagh, Alister Neil, Rowland Noakes, Colin Officer, Helene Owzinsky, Michael Page, Dominic Pak, Geoff Pearce, Simon Pilbrow, Ebrahim Pishan, Alexander Pollack, Vernon Powell, Cameron Profitt, Andrew Protassow, Geoff Quail, Farooq Qureshi, Anthony Radford, Peter Radford, Suresh Rananavare, Peter Rankin, Felicity Rea, Jan Reddy, Sandy Reid, Jill Rosenblatt, David Ross, Harvey Rotstein, Jackie Rounsevell, Carl Rubis, Sharnee Rutherford, Avni Sali, Paul Scott, Adrian Sheen, Jack Shepherd, Clive Stack, Peter Stone, Helen Sutcliffe, Royston Taylor, Alex Thomson, Jim Thomson, John Togno, Bruce Tonge, John Trollor, Ian Tulloch, Talina Vizard, Peter Wallace, Olga Ward, Vilas Wavde, David White, David Wilson, Ian Wilson, John Wong, Ian Wood, Freda Wraight, David Young, Your Doctors (Linda Mann, Anna Greer, John Hughes), Mark Zagorski.

In reference to part of the text and figures in spinal disorders, permission from the copyright owners, Butterworths, of *Back Pain and Spinal Manipulation* (1989), by C. Kenna and J. Murtagh, is gratefully acknowledged.

Many of the images in this book are based on those from other publications. Acknowledgment is given to the World Health Organization, publishers of J. Cook et al., *General Surgery at the District Hospital*, for figures 1.9, 3.7, 3.19, 4.33, 4.37, 9.13 and 14.4b,c and to Dr Leveat Efe for figures 1.3, 3.39, 3.42, 15.4 and 15.5.

Permission to use many drawings from *Australian Family Physician* is also gratefully acknowledged.

McGraw-Hill Education would also like to thank the following doctors who participated in the research survey for the this and previous editions, and in particular Dr Rachel Claydon (University of Queensland), Dr Christopher Leow (Echuca Moama Family Medical Practice) and Dr Gwendolyn Liow (Goulburn Valley Health) who also gave helpful reviews: Dr Hayder Al-Aubaidy, University of Tasmania; Dr Penny Burns, Western Sydney University; Dr Jane Cooper, University of Tasmania; Dr Judi Errey, University of Tasmania; Dr Danijela Gnjidic, The University of Sydney; Dr David King, University of Queensland; Dr Jane Landers, Highbury Family Practice Unit SA; Professor Siaw-Teng Liaw, University of New South Wales; Dr Nicholas McLernon, University of Western Australia; Dr Jason Ong, The University of Melbourne; Dr Joel Jin-Oh Rhee, University of New South Wales; Dr Jon Young Teo; Dr Keren Witcombe, University of Western Australia.

Sterilisation guidelines for office practice (RACGP)

The strict control of infection, especially control of the lethal HIV virus and the hepatitis B and C viruses, is fundamental to the surgical procedures outlined in this book. Summarised guidelines include:

- All doctors and staff need to be taught and demonstrate competency in hand hygiene, dealing with blood and body fluid spills, standard precautions and the principles of environmental cleaning and reprocessing of medical equipment.
- Practices should appoint an infection prevention and control coordinator with responsibility for overseeing a comprehensive infection prevention and control program including implementation of practice cleaning policies.
- Practices should perform regular infection prevention and control risk assessments, and determine how best to manage any identified risks through a combination of education and training, as well as redesign of work practices.
- Use single-use pre-sterilised instruments and injections wherever possible.
- The use of single-use sterile equipment minimises the risk of cross-infection. Items such as suturing needles, injecting needles, syringes, scalpel blades and pins or needles used for neurological sensory testing should be single-use.
- Assume that any patient may be a carrier of hepatitis B and C, HIV and the human papilloma virus.
- Hand washing is the single most important element of any infection control policy: hands must be washed before and after direct contact with the patient. For non-high-risk procedures, disinfect by washing with soap under a running tap and dry with a paper towel, which is discarded.
- Antiseptic handwash (e.g. 2% chlorhexidine) or alcohol hand rubs or wipes have also proven to be effective in reducing the spread of infection.
- Alcohol-based hand rubs, used according to product directions, are appropriate where hand hygiene facilities are not available (e.g. home visits).
- Promote the '5 moments of 'hand hygiene'' as an important part of infection control and practice.
- Disposable auroscope tips should be used.
- Sterile gloves and goggles should be worn for any surgical procedure involving penetration of the skin, mucous membrane and/or other tissue.

- Avoid using multi-dose vials of local anaesthetic. The rule is 'one vial—one patient'.
- Safe disposal of sharp articles and instruments such as needles and scalpel blades is necessary. Needles must not be recapped.
- Instruments cannot be sterilised until they have been cleaned. They should be washed as soon after use as possible.
- Autoclaving is the most reliable and preferred way to sterilise instruments and equipment. Bench-top autoclaves should conform to Australian Standard AS 2182.
- Sterilisers without a printer or data logger are obsolete and should not be used.
- Chemical disinfection is not a reliable system for routine processing of instruments, although it may be necessary for heat-sensitive apparatus. It should definitely not be used for instruments categorised as high risk.
- Boiling is not reliable as it will not kill bacterial spores and, unless timing is strictly monitored, may not be effective against bacteria and viruses.
- All staff should be immunised according to standard immunisation recommendations.
- Masks may be used by unimmunised staff and also by patients to prevent the spread of disease (suspected or known) by droplets.
- Ensure the application and removal of personal protective equipment is consistent with the Australian Guidelines for the Prevention and Control of Infection in Healthcare.
- Include information stating the management of waste must conform to state or territory regulations.
- Goggles and face shields need to be used by staff where there is a risk of splashing or spraying of blood or body fluids such as during surgical procedures, venepuncture or cleaning of instruments.

Note: For skin antisepsis for surgical procedures, swab with povidone-iodine 10% solution in preference to alcoholic preparations.

Reference: RACGP Infection control standards for office based procedures (5th Edn). www.racgp.org.au/FSDEDEV/media/documents/Running a practice/Practice standards/Infection-prevention-and-control.pdf

Chapter 1

SKIN REPAIR AND MINOR PLASTIC SURGERY

PRINCIPLES OF REPAIR OF EXCISIONAL WOUNDS

It is important to keep the following in mind:[1]
1. Plan all excisions carefully.
2. Check previous scars for healing properties.
3. Aim to keep incision lines parallel to natural skin lines.
4. Take care in poor healing areas, such as backs, calves and knees; and in areas prone to hypertrophic scarring, such as over the sternum of the chest, and the shoulder.
5. Use atraumatic tissue-handling techniques.
6. Practise minimal handling of wound edges.
7. Use Steri-Strips™ after the sutures are removed.

Gloves

The use of gloves for these procedures is advisable; ideally sterile gloves but a landmark study (Heal et al.) demonstrated that sterile gloves have no advantage over non-sterile clean boxed gloves.[2]

Wounds and suturing

Suturing is a fundamental and important skill for which patients may judge the performance quality of their practitioner. This skill involves the appropriate method of treating a wound. Small superficial cuts heal well if debrided and cleaned with a suitable antiseptic such as chlorhexidine, and covered with a clean adhesive dressing.

PRACTISING SUTURING

Appropriate materials:
- peaches—skin mimics children's skin
- grapes—mimics delicate skin
- butcher's offerings—pig's trotters, chicken breast, beef tongue, chicken trachea.

TAPING WOUNDS

The use of wound closure tape (e.g. Steri-Strips) for smaller clean wounds is to be encouraged (Fig. 1.1). Children may not tolerate repair of wounds with local anaesthetic and suturing, so appropriate closure with tape after disinfection and drying is recommended—as is the use of their hair for scalp wounds (Chapter 15). Primary sutures should be avoided in contaminated or severely contused wounds, especially if there has been a delay of 4 hours or more before repair. Such wounds should be cleaned, trimmed and a dry dressing applied. They can then undergo primary suturing on the fifth day.

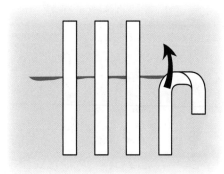

Fig. 1.1 Steri-Strip closure of a clean wound

Steri-Strips

These adhesive strips are ideal for smaller clean cut wounds, which should first be disinfected and dried.

Method

1. It is usual to start in the centre of the wound.
2. Render the strip taut and straight with a finger on either side of the strip as it is placed over the wound (Fig. 1.1).
3. Lock it in place then repeat with a series of strips at appropriate intervals. The strips can be bolstered by applying a cross-strip parallel to the wound.
   Steri-Strips can also be used to supplement a sutured wound.

How long

They are usually worn until they fall off or are removed in 5 to 7 days.

Removal

Soak in water. Remove any cross-strip. Then as you press down on skin, lift one end, then the opposite end and gently lift it off the wound, pulling towards the middle.

SKIN PREPARATION ANTISEPTIC SOLUTIONS

- Aqueous chlorhexidine gluconate
- Alcoholic chlorhexidine gluconate
- Chlorhexidine and cetrimide
- Povidone-iodine (aqueous)
- Povidone-iodine (alcohol base)

Rules:
- Blot dry any pools of preparation solutions.
- Alcohol-based preparations are flammable.
- Avoid alcohol on mucous membranes and on sensitive skin, e.g. eyelids, scrotum.
- Avoid chlorhexidine contact on eye or middle ear. It can cause conjunctivitis and severe corneal damage.

STANDARD PRECAUTIONS

Mandatory safety measures

- Goggles
- Gloves

Common mistakes for excisional surgery

- Skimping (inadequate margins)
- Tension on skin edges
- Suture material too thick
- Too large a bite
- Opposing edges inverted (due to needle entering skin at a shallow angle)
- Stitches left in too long
- Inadequate early compression

Minimising bleeding in the elderly

Stop anticoagulants (if possible) before a significant procedure. Examples:
- warfarin—3 days
- clopidogrel—10 days
- aspirin—7 days
- NSAIDs—2 to 5 days (check half life)
- NOACs—3 to 4 days.

Suture material (Table 1.1)

- Monofilament material includes silk (natural) and Ethilon and Vicryl® (artificial). Monofilament nylon sutures are generally preferred for skin repair. They produce less tissue reaction than silk.
- Use the smallest calibre compatible with required strains.
- The synthetic, absorbable polyglycolic acid or polyglactin sutures (Dexon™, Vicryl) are stronger than catgut of the same gauge, which is uncommonly used now. The monofilament absorbable sutures (Monocryl®, Maxon)[1] are most suitable for subcuticular suturing.

Table 1.1 Selection of suture material (guidelines)

Skin	nylon 6/0	face, eyelids
	nylon 5/0	elsewhere
	nylon 4/0	hands, forearms
	nylon 3/0	back, scalp
	nylon 2/0	knees
Deeper tissue (dead space)	Dexon/Vicryl 3/0 or 4/0	
Subcuticular	Monofilament absorbable (e.g. Monocryl 4/0)	
Vessel ligatures	Dexon/Vicryl	

Instruments

Examples of good-quality instruments:
- locking needle holder (e.g. Crile-Wood 12 cm)
- skin hooks
- iris scissors.

Holding the needle

The needle should be held in its middle because this will help to avoid breakage and distortion, which tends to occur if the needle is held near its end (Fig. 1.2a).

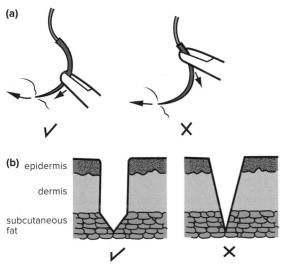

Fig. 1.2 Correct and incorrect methods of (**a**) holding the needle; (**b**) making incisions

Incisions

Incisions should be made perpendicular to the skin (not angled) (Fig. 1.2b).

Dead space

Dead space should be eliminated, to reduce tension on skin sutures. Use buried absorbable sutures to approximate underlying tissue. This is done by starting suture insertion from the fat to pick up the fat/dermis interface so as to bury the knot (Fig. 1.3).

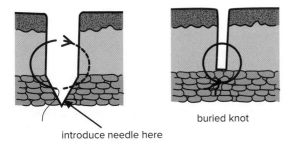

Fig. 1.3 Eliminating dead space

Everted wounds

Eversion is achieved by making the 'bite' in the dermis wider than the bite in the epidermis (skin surface) and making the suture deeper than it is wide. Shown is:
- a simple suture (Fig. 1.4a)
- a vertical mattress suture (Fig. 1.4b).

The mattress suture is the ideal way to evert a wound.

Number of sutures

Aim to use a minimum number of sutures to achieve closure without gaps, but sufficient sutures to avoid tension. Place the sutures as close to the wound edge as possible.

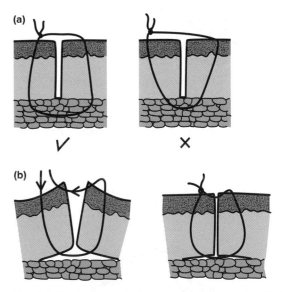

Fig. 1.4 Everted wounds: (**a**) correct and incorrect methods of making a simple suture; (**b**) making a vertical mattress

KNOT TYING[3]

Special techniques of knot tying are necessary to achieve a secure knot. Insecure knots leading to slippage of a tie may result in substantial blood loss or at least revisiting the surgery. The ability to tie a secure knot should be a reflex action based on practice for the proceduralist. The friction between threads of the suture material is also a factor in avoiding slippage of the knot. The monofilament braided synthetics, particularly nylon and polyesters, are more supple and easier to handle so that knots are easier to tie securely.

Reef knot

The traditional secure knot is the reef knot, which is a firm interlocking knot. The basic element is a half-hitch and it forms the basis of the surgeon's knot. In this knot, one thread is looped around the other and the knot is completed by a mirror image of the first throw. It is achieved by tying the first throw one way and then reversing it. The two free ends of one suture emerge from either above or below the loop created by the other suture (Fig. 1.5). It is basically two loops that pull against each other to interlock. Consider it as 'left over right' and then 'right over left'.

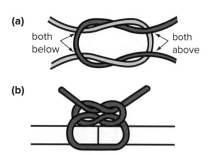

(a)

both below   both above

(b)

Fig. 1.5 Two views of tying a reef knot **(a)** and **(b)**

Granny knot

A granny knot is formed when the reverse of this mirror image throw is formed; that is, the throws go the same way. The free ends emerge one above and one below each loop (Fig. 1.6). It is best to avoid this knot in surgical practice as it tends to slip and is therefore dangerous for precise surgery as the wound will open.

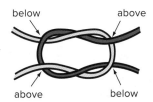

below   above

above   below

Fig. 1.6 The granny knot

The surgeon's knot

Also known as the square knot, it involves the same pattern as the reef knot, except that there are two throws on each side of the knot instead of one (Fig. 1.7). The ends of the thread should be pulled at 180° to each other.

The instrument knot

The instrument knot, which is the most common knot, uses the principle of the reef knot. Initially, the thread is wound twice around the needle holder (say in a clockwise direction) to create the double loop of a surgeon's knot and then firmly tied (Fig. 1.8a). On the reverse side, the thread is wound around the needle holder in the opposite direction (an anti-clockwise spiral), thus creating the double loop of a surgeon's knot. The knot is finally secured by pulling the ends at 180° to each other (Fig. 1.8b).

(a)

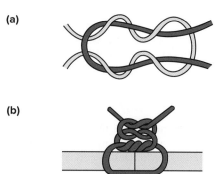

(b)

Fig. 1.7 Two views of tying a surgeon's knot **(a)** and **(b)**

(a)

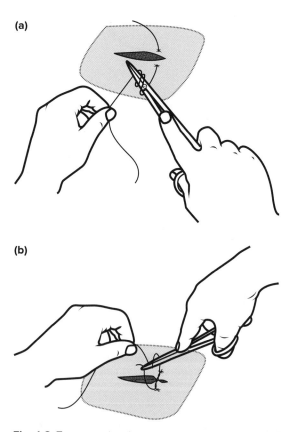

(b)

Fig. 1.8 Two steps in tying an instrument knot **(a)** and **(b)**

Ligatures on vessels

Every precaution must be undertaken to avoid the ligature slipping. The first tie should be very tight, and the second slacker than the first. For deep ties on vessels it is best to tie with the hands and keep the ties parallel to the wound. Do not pull upwards on the tie. Leave an adequate cuff of tissue past the tie (see Fig. 1.8).

HOLDING THE SCALPEL

The two common methods of holding a scalpel are:
- the pen grip, and
- the underhand grip.

The pen grip, which is the one most commonly used in minor surgery, is used for fine incisions or excisions and for dissection with the scalpel. Most of the movement imparted to the blade comes from the hand and fingers (Fig. 1.9). The underhand or table-knife grip (Fig. 1.10) is traditionally used for long incisions, such as in abdominal surgery. A larger handle and blade are used.

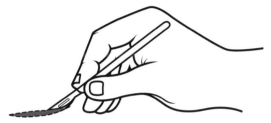

Fig. 1.9 The pen grip

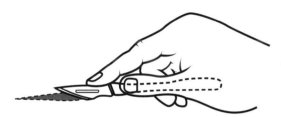

Fig. 1.10 The underhand grip

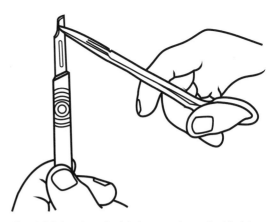

Fig. 1.11 Loading the blade onto the scalpel holder

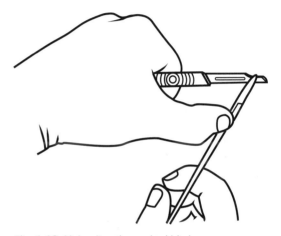

Fig. 1.12 Unloading the scalpel blade

SAFE INSERTION AND REMOVAL OF SCALPEL BLADES

While the majority of skin surgery is now performed using disposable scalpels, it is equally appropriate to use firm two-piece metal scalpel holders and blades. For safe handling it is important to become deft at using forceps to insert scalpel blades onto the scalpel handle (Fig. 1.11), and also to remove the blade. In the latter the thumb can be used to facilitate unloading by steadily pressing against the forceps (haemostat clamp) in an extension movement (Fig. 1.12). Another blade unloading method is to grasp the blade with the forceps and rotate the forceps to lift the end of the blade, which is then pushed off the handle.

DEBRIDEMENT AND DERMABRASION FOR WOUND DEBRIS

If grit and other foreign material such as oil is left in the wound, an unacceptable tattoo effect will occur in the healed wound. This can be avoided by meticulous exploration of the wound to remove debris, and dermabrasion for superficial grit.

CONTINUOUS SUTURES[4]

Continuous subcuticular (intradermal) running suture

This type of suture was developed to approximate skin edges with minimal scarring.

This is ideal for the repair of episiotomy wounds with an absorbable suture after the dead space has been closed. It has a limited place in skin repair where monofilament nylon material is best, especially for removal of the suture. The non-absorbable suture method requires meticulous placement without kinks or knots that may impede later removal. Both ends are left free but the total suture can be tied over the wound (Fig. 1.13(b)). Supplementary interrupted skin sutures or Steri-Strips may be necessary for accurate skin-edge apposition. A non-absorbable suture may be removed after 1 to 2 weeks by cutting one end of the suture and gently pulling, with countertraction from the other end.

Method

This suture picks up dermis only (picking up the epidermis and fat is not acceptable), and should be inserted uniformly at the same level without gaps in the linear direction (Fig. 1.13a).

'Over-and-over' suture

This is a useful time saver, especially where a meticulous cosmetic result is not required. One disadvantage is the tendency to bunch the wound up. The suturing should not be too tight nor too widely spaced (Fig. 1.13c).

Blanket stitch

The blanket or 'running lock' stitch does not tend to bunch up the wound. A double turn at each stitch converts it into a locked suture (Fig. 1.13d).

THE PULLEY SUTURE

The pulley suture, also called the 'near-far, far-near' suture, which is a modification of the vertical mattress suture, is a very useful technique for the closure of difficult wounds, especially those on the lower leg. It may be used as a temporary measure to reduce tension and approximate skin edges while placing interrupted sutures. It permits approximation of the wound when an extra 2-3 mm of space needs closing and the normal method falls short of adequate closure.

Method

1. Introduce the needle 3-4 mm from the edge of the wound.
2. Let the needle emerge about 8-10 mm from the wound edge on the opposite side.
3. Reintroduce the needle at 8-10 mm on the original side.
4. Finally, let the needle emerge at 3-4 mm on the opposite side (Fig. 1.13e).

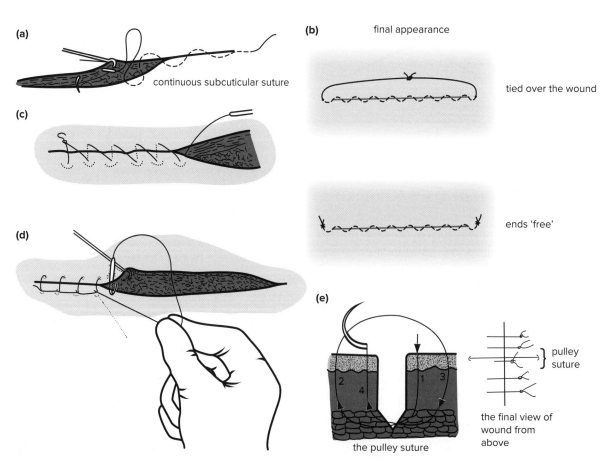

Fig. 1.13 (a) Subcuticular suture; **(b)** finishing a subcuticular suture (non-absorbable) **(c)** 'over-and-over' suture; **(d)** blanket stitch; **(e)** pulley suture

1.13 (a), (b) and (c) Reproduced from I. McGregor, *Fundamental Techniques of Plastic Surgery,* Churchill Livingstone, Edinburgh, 1989, with permission.

After the suture is in place, normal interrupted sutures can close the wound. However, the pulley suture may create too much tension and, if it does, it should be removed and replaced with a simple suture.

THE CROSS-STITCH

The cross-stitch, which is a type of pulley suture, is an excellent method for closing difficult wounds where there is likely to be some tension across the wound.

The cross-stitch is ideal for small circular wounds left after a 3–5 mm punch biopsy. It will shorten the scar and avoid the placement of two sutures. It gives a neater result than the vertical mattress or the horizontal mattress. Circular wounds up to 10 mm in diameter in areas of thicker skin can be closed with one such figure-of-eight suture.

Method

Consider a punch biopsy wound of 5 mm in diameter. Using a 5/0 or 6/0 nylon atraumatic suture, insert the needle from right of centre across the wound to left of centre, then from left of centre to right of centre on the next pass (or the other way, i.e. from left to right and back). Thus, four strands cross the wound and when tied create a pulley effect (Fig. 1.14).

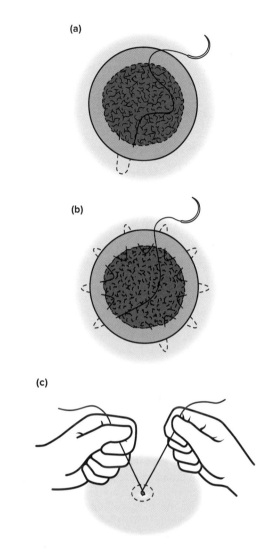

(a)

(b)

(c)

Fig. 1.15 Overview of purse-string suture

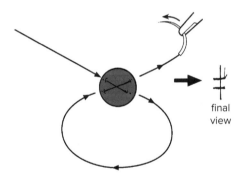

final view

Fig. 1.14 The cross-stitch: a type of pulley suture

THE PURSE-STRING SUTURE

This surgical suture is passed as a running stitch in and out of a circular wound so that when the ends of the suture—which finish up apposed—are drawn tight, the wound is closed like a purse (Fig 1.15). The needle passes through the deep dermis about 3–6 mm from the epidermal edge and eventually exits close to the entry point. The suture is most suitable to close the end of a hollow viscus or fixing tissue around a tube such as a catheter.

EXCISIONS

Incisions should be made perpendicular to the skin with symmetric edges and no angulation. The suture loop should be at least as wide at the base as it is at the skin surface. Poor technique may jeopardise healing. Best results are obtained with an ellipse where the length is 3 to 4 times the width. If a pigmented lesion has a problematic appearance, complete excision is recommended. The ABCDE mnemonic can be used to recognise lesions of most concern: A. asymmetry; B. border irregularity; C. more than one colour; D. diameter greater than 6 mm; E. increased elevation or enlargement. An excisional biopsy should be considered if a lesion has one or more of these concerns.

PLANNING EXCISIONS ON THE FACE

It is important to select optimal sites for elliptical excisions of tumours of the face. As a rule, it is best

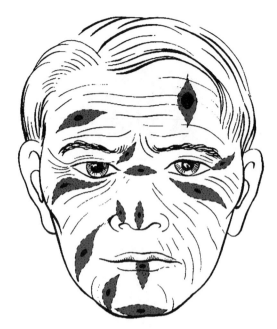

Fig. 1.16 Recommended lines for excisions on the face

Adapted from J.S. Brown, *Minor Surgery, a Text and Atlas*, Chapman and Hall, London, 1986.

for incisions to follow wrinkle lines and the direction of hair follicles in the beard area. Therefore, follow the natural wrinkles in the glabella area, the 'crow's feet' around the eye, and the nasolabial folds (Fig. 1.16). To determine non-obvious wrinkles, gently compress the relaxed skin in different directions to demonstrate the lines.

For tumours of the forehead, make horizontal incisions, although vertical incisions may be used for large tumours of the forehead. Ensure that you keep your incisions in the temporal area quite superficial, as the frontal branch of the facial nerve is easily cut.

ELLIPTICAL EXCISIONS

Small lesions are best excised as an ellipse. Generally, the long axis of the ellipse should be along the skin tension lines identified by natural wrinkles.

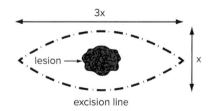

Fig. 1.17 Elliptical excision

The intended ellipse should be drawn on the skin (Fig. 1.17). The placement will depend on such factors as the size and shape of the lesion, the margin required (usually 2–3 mm) and the skin tension lines.

Note: The scalpel should be held at right angles to the skin.

Excision margin rules[5]

- 1–2 mm: moles and benign lesions
- 3 mm: BCCs
- 4 mm: SCCs
- Invasive malignant melanoma
  Breslow < 1 mm–1 cm margin; 1–4 mm–1–2 cm margin; > 4 mm–2 cm margin

General points

- The length of the ellipse should be 3 times the width (usual for head and neck).
- This length should be increased (say, to 4 times) in areas with little subcutaneous tissue (dorsum of hand) and high skin tension (upper back).
- Incisions should meet, rather than overlap, at the ends of the ellipse.
- A good rule is to obtain an angle at the end of 30° or less.
- These rules should achieve closure without 'dog ears'.

PREVENTION AND REMOVAL OF 'DOG EARS'

'Dog ears' are best avoided by using a long axis (at least 3 to 1) for an elliptical excision.

The fish-tail cut

However, if this axis turns out too short after excision, performing a fish-tail cut (Fig. 1.18a) will avoid the necessity of later correction.

Correction of a 'dog ear'

If a 'dog ear' results in the suture line after elliptical defect closure, it can be dealt with immediately by limited further excision and closure.

Method

1. Place a hook in the end of the wound, and elevate it; this defines the extent of the 'dog ear' (Fig. 1.18b).
2. Incise the skin around the base (1).
3. Stretch the resultant flap across the wound so that excess skin is defined and removed (2).
4. Complete the suturing of the wound, which will have a slight curve (3).

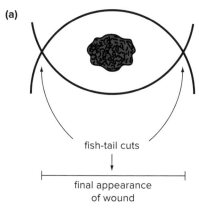

fish-tail cuts

final appearance
of wound

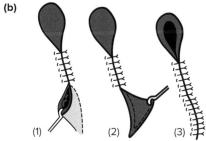

Fig. 1.18 Prevention of 'dog ears': **(a)** the fish-tail cut;
(b) correction of defect

1.18b Reproduced from I. McGregor, *Fundamental Techniques of Plastic Surgery*,
Churchill Livingstone, Edinburgh, 1989, with permission.[4]

THE LAZY S REPAIR

The lazy S excision is indicated when closing lesions
over convex surfaces. It elongates the actual length of
the scar so that the resulting scar will avoid buckling or
puckering in the middle (Fig 1.19).

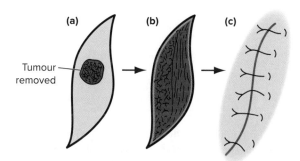

Fig. 1.19 Lazy S repair

M-PLASTY

This is an excisional technique to remove standing
cutaneous deformities (e.g. dog ears) and to shorten the
expected final length (Fig. 1.20).

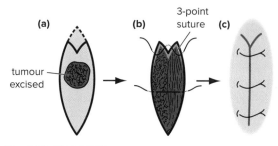

Fig. 1.20 M-PLASTY

THE THREE-POINT (CORNER) SUTURE

In wounds with a triangular flap component, it is often
difficult to place the apex of the flap accurately. The
three-point suture is the best way to achieve this while
minimising the chance of strangulation necrosis at the
tip of the flap.

Method

1. Pass the needle through the skin of the non-flap side
   of the wound.
2. Pass it then through the subcuticular layer of the
   flap tip at exactly the same level as the reception side.
3. Finally, pass the needle back through the reception
   side so that it emerges well back from the V flap
   (Fig. 1.21).

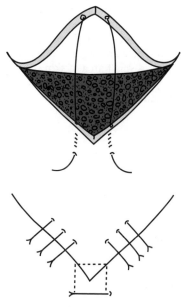

Fig. 1.21 The three-point suture

INVERTED MATTRESS SUTURE FOR PERINEAL SKIN

This method of repair of the perineum is suitable either for an episiotomy or a simple tear, and uses a technique of inverted vertical mattress sutures.

It is a simple method that provides a sound and comfortable repair. Because it is an interrupted suture wound, drainage is not sacrificed for the sake of comfort.

Method

1. Suture the vaginal tissue with a normal, continuous absorbable suture tied subcutaneously.
2. If the wound is very deep, a second internal layer of sutures should be inserted initially.
3. Close the perineal skin with the inverted mattress sutures (Fig. 1.22) using an absorbable suture. It is preferable to commence anteriorly, as this provides accurate opposition of the skin edges.

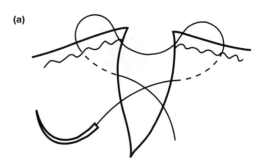

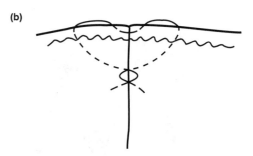

Fig. 1.22 Inverted mattress suture

Skin grafts

Skin grafting may be performed in the general practice setting to treat small areas of skin loss following accidents such as flap wounds on the lower leg and the tips of fingers (the most common reason). If the defect on the fingertip is small, grafting is not necessary since healing is usually good. There are two possible grafts:

- full thickness: a small area of skin is carefully taken with a sharp knife; all fat is debrided until only the dermis remains

- split skin: usually 0.25–0.5 mm thick using a silver razor dermatome (e.g. Aesculap).

The skin is then placed on paraffin gauge correctly orientated. The surface of the graft is then applied to the defect site after trimming the unit to fit the site. Then apply a firm Kaltostat (or similar) dressing.

Flaps

The basic types of flaps are:
- advancement
- rotation
- transposition.

TRIANGULAR FLAP WOUNDS ON THE LOWER LEG

Triangular flap wounds below the knee are a common injury and are often treated incorrectly. Similar wounds in the upper limb heal rapidly when sutured properly, but lower limb injury usually will not heal by first intention unless the apex of the flap is excised and a small donor graft implanted. Also think twice about suturing a pretibial laceration in an elderly person.

Proximally based flap

A fall through a gap in flooring boards will produce a proximally based flap; a heavy object (such as the tailboard of a trailer) striking the shin will result in a distally based flap.

Usually the apex of the flap is crushed and poorly vascularised; it will not survive to heal after suture.

Treatment method

1. Infiltrate a wide area around the wound with local anaesthetic (LA).
2. Excise the apex of the skin flap back to healthy tissue.
3. Loosely suture the angles at the base of the flap.
4. With a no. 24 scalpel, shave a small, split-thickness graft from the anaesthetised area proximal to the wound; place it on the raw area (Fig. 1.23).
5. Cover both the wound and donor site with petroleum jelly gauze, a non-stick dressing and a combine pad; strap firmly with a crepe bandage.

The patient should rest with the leg elevated for 3 days. Re-dress the wound on the fourth day.

Alternative (preferred) method

It may be possible to save the distal avascular flap, especially in younger patients, by scraping away the subcutaneous tissue on the flap and using it as a full-thickness graft.

Distally based flap

This flap, which is quite avascular, has a poorer prognosis. The same methods as for the proximally based flap can be used (Fig. 1.24).

EXCISION OF SKIN TUMOURS WITH SLIDING FLAPS

General practitioners, in both city and country, not uncommonly excise small skin tumours under local anaesthesia using an elliptical incision. Where the skin is tight, as on the trunk or thigh, suture of an elliptical wound creates tension at the centre. A split skin graft or Wolfe graft will solve the problem but all too often

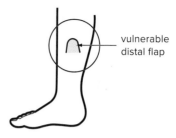

Fig. 1.24 Triangular flap wound repair: distally based flap

leaves a depressed, unsightly scar. A rotation flap will cover the deficiency nicely but requires the undermining of a large area of skin and time-consuming suturing. However, flaps require skill and practice, and it is the responsibility of the operator to ensure the intended procedure lies within their scope.

Double Y on V advancement flap method[6]

Tumours up to 2.5 cm in diameter can be excised and the deficiency repaired without tension by means of a double advancement flap fashioned from the 'wings' of the ellipse after the lesion has been excised. As the viability of the flaps relies on a blood supply from the subcutaneous tissue, do not undermine the flaps. Incise the skin and subcutaneous tissue vertically to the fascia. The elasticity of the subcutaneous tissues will permit the flaps to be advanced to the midline to be united by sutures (Fig. 1.25).

Alternative flap technique

More flexibility of the flaps can be obtained by undermining the flaps above and below the incision lines (Fig. 1.26). Viability of the flaps is not a problem.

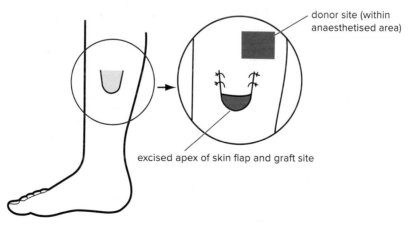

donor site (within anaesthetised area)

excised apex of skin flap and graft site

Fig. 1.23 Triangular flap wound suture

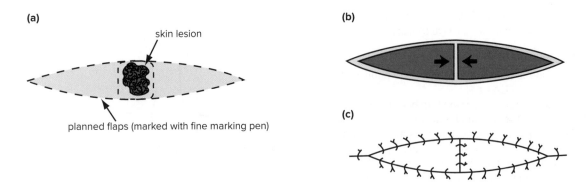

Fig. 1.25 Methods of excising skin tumour: **(a)** planned flaps marked; **(b)** triangular flaps advanced to midline; **(c)** flaps sutured to repair defect

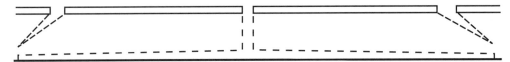

Fig. 1.26 Undermining of subcutaneous tissue (alternative variation)

The Y on V (or Island) advancement flap

This flap, which maintains a good blood supply, is ideal to close the end of an amputated fingertip in a child, or to use as an excision procedure on the face in the area of the nasolabial fold and lip where it conforms to skin creases.

Method

1. Mark the excision lines carefully before excising (Fig. 1.27a).
2. Excise the lesion as a square or rectangle.
3. Fashion the flap as a triangle about 2 to 2½ times the length of the defect. Carefully free the flap so that the skin remains on its subcutaneous tissue pedicle. This flap is referred to as an 'island'.
4. Using skin hooks, advance the base of the flap to the far edge of the defect with the help of blunt dissection and avoiding excessive tension (Fig. 1.27b).
5. Use three-point sutures at the two edges and at the apex.
6. Suture the sides of the wound (Fig. 1.27c).
7. Thus the V 'island' is converted to a Y-shaped scar.

H double advancement flap[6]

Like the double Y on V flap, this is suitable for areas with a good pad of subcutaneous tissue (e.g. re-excision of a melanoma on the arm). It is useful in places such as the forehead where the scars conform to skin creases. It is used where skin closure is impossible for a large ellipse. It can be tested, aborted or grafted.

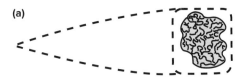

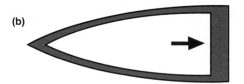

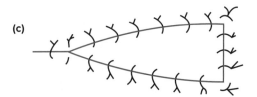

Fig. 1.27 The single Y on V method: **(a)** planned flaps marked; **(b)** 'Island' flap advanced to midline; **(c)** flaps sutured to repair defect

Method

1. Excise the tumour with a square excision.
2. Extend the excision lines to about 1½ times the length of the defect (Fig. 1.28a).
3. Excise the skin and subcutaneous tissue with care vertically to the fascia.
4. Dissect the skin flaps from the subcutaneous tissue and advance them towards each other (preferably with skin hooks) to meet in the middle (Fig. 1.28b).
5. Use three-point sutures to anchor the corners of the flaps and then suture the wound as shown in Figure 1.28c.

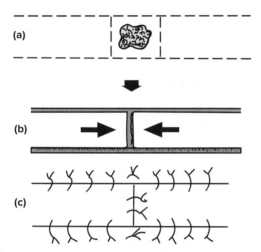

Fig. 1.28 The H double advancement flap: **(a)** excision of tumour with planned flaps; **(b)** pulling the flaps together; **(c)** flaps sutured to repair defect

PRIMARY SUTURE BEFORE EXCISION OF A SMALL TUMOUR

Before excising a small tumour, such as a dermatofibroma, skin tag or similar benign tumour, a primary suture can be inserted.

The advantages include better initial haemostasis and ability to operate singlehandedly.

Method

1. Infiltrate around the lesion with local anaesthetic.
2. Insert an appropriate suture (you may choose to insert more than one) to straddle the tumour (Fig. 1.29).
3. Excise the tumour. (Take care not to cut the suture.)
4. Secure the suture.
5. Add more sutures if necessary.

MULTIPLE RAGGED LACERATIONS

Lacerations in a cosmetically important place, such as the face, that have ragged edges or multiple components

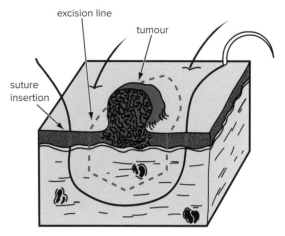

Fig. 1.29 Insertion of primary suture before excision of small tumour

should be trimmed and/or excised (Fig. 1.30). This will provide vertical edges and an organised wound, which can then be sutured meticulously. For the face, use 6/0 nylon. Sacrifice of small amounts of facial skin is justified in the interest of a linear and less obvious scar. Sometimes Z-plasty is required.

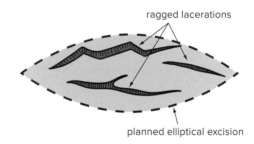

Fig. 1.30 Example of managing a group of multiple lacerations

AVOIDING SKIN TEARS

Avoid using adhesive tapes on friable skin or dehydrated skin. Instead, use a cohesive bandage such as Easifix or Tubigrip.

When a flap moves laterally into the primary defect it is called a transposition flap, and when rotated into the defect it is called a rotation flap. With these flaps, be careful to avoid a vascular disaster.

VESSEL LIGATION[4]

It is imperative to pay close attention to safe ligation of any bleeding vessels in the wound by clamping and using a properly placed ligature. A ligature applied too close to the cut end may subsequently slip and cause unexpected bleeding (Fig. 1.31).

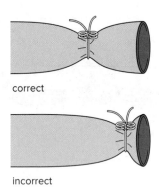

correct

incorrect

Fig. 1.31 Method of ligating a vessel to avoid slippage of the tie

THE TRANSPOSITION FLAP[7]

In the transposition flap, the flap moves sideways into the primary defect. The flap has a donor site that usually runs radial to the defect. The flap crosses over intervening normal skin to slot into the defect. The point at the base of the flap opposite the defect does not move, and this is the pivot point that is marked with an asterisk in Figure 1.32. The distance from the pivot point to the top of the flap should be the same as the distance from the pivot point to the far side of the defect. The donor site is closed directly. The transposition flap has widespread use, especially on the face and scalp.

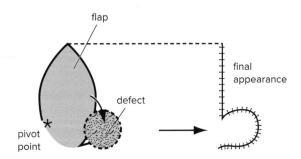

flap

final appearance

defect

pivot point

Fig. 1.32 The transposition flap

Adapted from A. Pennington, *Local Flap Reconstruction*, McGraw-Hill, with permission.[6]

THE ROTATION FLAP

The local rotation flap is a most useful procedure in general practice for the excision of skin lesions such as basal cell carcinomas (BCCs). The excision is semicircular and the pivot point is at the end of the releasing incision. The larger the flap, the more skin becomes available. This method is favoured for the excision of BCCs greater than 12 to 20 mm and other tumours, especially on shoulders and backs.

Method

1. Excise the tumour using a triangular excision, which, ideally, should be equilateral. Extend the excision beyond subcutaneous fat to the deep fascia-covering muscle (Fig. 1.33a).

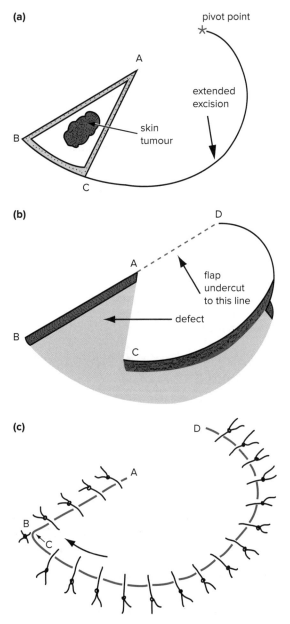

(a) pivot point

A

extended excision

skin tumour

B

C

(b) D

A

flap undercut to this line

defect

B

C

(c) D

A

B

C

Fig. 1.33 Rotation flap: **(a)** triangular area of excision with extended excision; **(b)** resultant skin defect; **(c)** appearance after suturing

2. Extend the excision in a curve to a length about 3 times that of the length of a side of the original triangular excision.
3. Now undercut the skin flap to the line AD (Fig. 1.33b).
4. Rotate this flap so that AC corresponds to AB without excessive tension.
5. Use simple sutures to close the wound (Fig. 1.33c).

Note: Blood is supplied to the skin on the back by the lateral cutaneous branch of each posterior intercostal artery and hence follows the line of the ribs. Make sure that the extended incision allows a blood supply to the flap—that is, that AD faces medially and not laterally.

THE RHOMBOID (LIMBERG) FLAP

The rhomboid flap is very useful for repairing defects that are difficult to suture directly or where the tension is in the wrong direction. It is most useful for removing lesions on the forehead, temple and scalp.

Method

1. Draw out the rhomboid and the relief extensions, making sure that the angles, lengths and directions are correct. The short diagonal of the rhomboid equals the length of the sides, giving the appearance of two equilateral triangles placed side by side. The direction of the relief extensions (theoretically four options) depends on the availability of skin.
2. Extend the diagonal for an equal distance in the desired direction and then draw a back line parallel to one of the sides of the rhomboid (Fig. 1.34a).
3. Remove the lesion and free the flaps by back-cutting.
4. Ensure that the 'x' lengths are equal.
5. Rotate the flap so that A moves to A1, B to B1 and C to B. This should fill the defect perfectly (Fig. 1.34b).
6. Care is required in suturing the corners—especially A and B, where subcutaneous three-point sutures are appropriate (Fig. 1.34c).
7. The resultant tension from the example illustrated is transverse (← →). This contrasts with longitudinal tension if sutured directly.

THE 'CROWN' EXCISION FOR FACIAL SKIN LESIONS

When the standard elliptical skin excision is unworkable or inappropriate, a crown-shaped excision provides an excellent alternative. This applies particularly to skin lesions adjacent to key facial structures such as the nose, lips, ears and eyes. The shape of the crown excision can vary—it does not always have to be curved.

Method

(Using a basal cell carcinoma adjacent to the nose as an example.)

1. Mark out the lines of excision around the lesion in a circle.

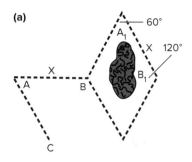

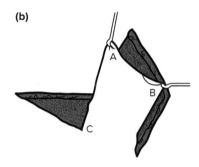

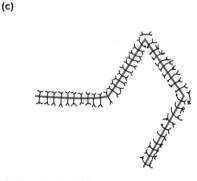

Fig. 1.34 The rhomboid flap

Reproduced from I. McGregor, *Fundamental Techniques of Plastic Surgery*, Churchill Livingstone, Edinburgh, 1989, with permission.

2. Extend the axis of the excision in the free skin (Fig. 1.35a).
3. On the 'obstacle' side, excise two small curved flaps as illustrated.
4. Suture the defect so that a Y-shaped wound is eventually produced (Fig. 1.35b).

Z-PLASTY

The Z-plasty is a procedure that redistributes wound tension by transposing two interdigitating triangular flaps. It brings in tissue from the sides to lengthen the wound and break up the tension across it. It therefore enhances the alignment of the direction of the scar. All arms of the Z are equal in length.[7]

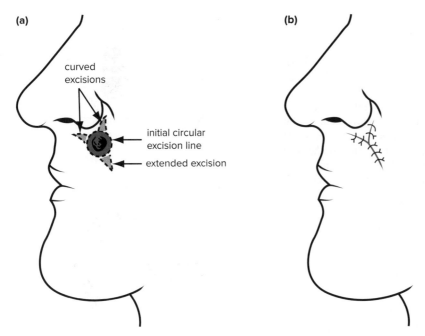

Fig. 1.35 (a) The 'crown' excision; **(b)** final appearance

Method (scheme for a longitudinal contracture)

1. Mark out the Z so that the angles are 60° and the arms are of equal length.
2. Incise along the lines to produce two flaps and free the flaps by dissection.
3. Transpose the flaps, then suture (Fig. 1.36).

Indications

- Treatment of contractures especially over joints (to lengthen)
- Facial scars (to change direction)

REPAIR OF CUT LIP

While small lacerations of the buccal mucosa of the lip can be left safely, more extensive cuts require careful repair. Meticulous cleansing is required, involving copious irrigation and removal of necrotic tissue with a scalpel or small scissors. Trim the wound edges. Carefully note the white roll and vermilion border before injecting. Local anaesthetic infiltration may be adequate, although a mental nerve block is ideal for larger lacerations of the lower lip.

For wounds that cross the vermilion border, meticulous alignment is essential. It may be advisable to premark the vermilion border with gentian violet or a marker pen. It is desirable to have an assistant.

Method

1. Close the deeper muscular layer (orbicularis oris) of the wound using 4/0 absorbable suture such as Vicryl. The first suture should carefully appose the mucosal area of the lip, followed by one or two sutures in the remaining layer (Fig. 1.37).
2. Next, insert a 6/0 monofilament nylon suture to bring both ends of the vermilion border together. The slightest step is unacceptable.
3. Close the inner buccal mucosa with interrupted 4/0 absorbable sutures.
4. Close the outer skin of the lip (above and below the vermilion border) with interrupted nylon sutures.

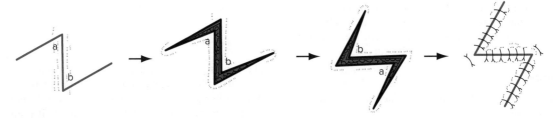

Fig. 1.36 Classic equilateral triangle 60° Z-plasty

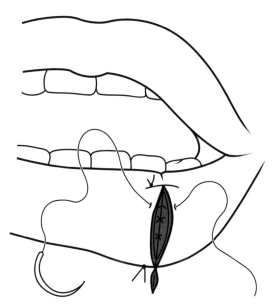

Fig. 1.37 Repair of cut lip

Post-repair

1. Apply a moisturising lotion along the lines of the wound.
2. Remove nylon sutures in 3 to 4 days (in a young person) and 5 to 6 days (in an older person).

WEDGE EXCISION AND DIRECT SUTURE OF LIP

Indications

- Small, invasive squamous cell carcinomas leading to a defect on less than one-third of the lip.

  Alternative procedures are required for larger defects and for tumours close to the angles of the mouth.

  An assistant is necessary to help achieve haemostasis, due to the copious bleeding from the inferior labial artery in the posterior third of the lip.

Method

1. Provide anaesthesia with a mental nerve block.
2. Carefully mark the excision outline, with special attention to the vermilion border (allow a 2–3 mm margin from the lesion). A small marker 'nick' or a stay suture at the border can be used as a guide.
3. Have the assistant hold the lip firmly on either side of the excision lines with gauze for a good grip, and slightly evert the lip.
4. Excise a clean, full-thickness wedge, with the apex extending almost to the mental fold (Fig. 1.38a).
5. Identify the labial arteries and either use diathermy or clamp and tie these bleeders.

6. Close the dead space of the muscular layer with interrupted 4/0 absorbable sutures, starting with accurate apposition of the main lip area (Fig. 1.38b).
7. Insert a 6/0 nylon suture precisely at the vermilion border (the slightest step is unacceptable) and one at the apex of the wound.
8. Close the buccal mucosa with interrupted absorbable sutures.
9. Finally, insert nylon sutures to the vermilion border and skin.

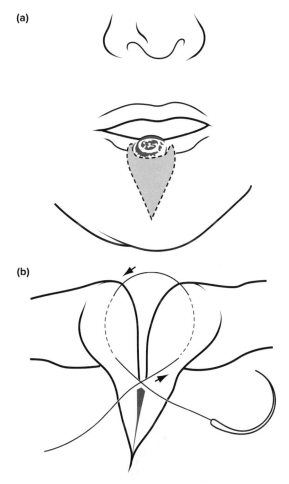

Fig. 1.38 Wedge excision of lip: **(a)** wedge of lip removed; **(b)** precise initial suture

WEDGE RESECTION OF EAR

This procedure is ideal for small tumours on the superior surface of the helix. The requirements are the same as for wedge excision of the lip.

Method

1. Provide LA by infiltrating subcutaneously around the appropriate margin of the ear. The area for infiltration

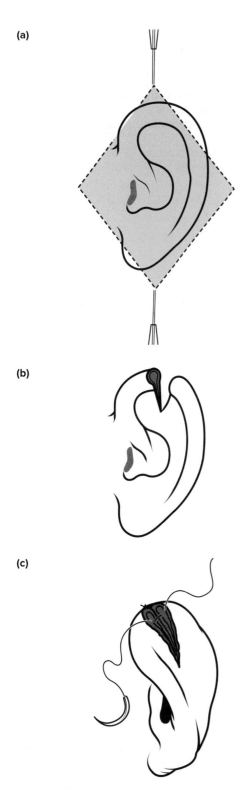

(a)

(b)

(c)

Fig. 1.39 Wedge resection of ear: **(a)** method of ear block with local anaesthesia infiltrated subcutaneously; **(b)** wedge of ear removed; **(c)** suturing in layers

(to cover all the ear) is shown in Figure 1.39a. This V infiltration method is the simplest way to block the ear completely. Specific nerve blocks are outlined in Chapter 2.

2. Cleanse with antiseptic.
3. Mark an outline of the area of excision with the back of the scalpel and, with a marker, the margins for the first suture (e.g. the rim of the helix).
4. With tension applied by the assistant, excise a wedge, cutting cleanly through the skin and cartilage (Fig. 1.39b). The anterior skin is incised with a scalpel and then surgical scissors or the scalpel cuts through the cartilage and posterior ear skin so that the posterior and anterior aspects of the wedge are an exact match.
5. Brisk bleeding should soon cease with direct pressure.
6. Place the first suture to achieve meticulous alignment. Place a non-absorbable mattress suture to ensure hypereversion.
7. Suture the skin on the anterior surface with 6/0 nylon.
8. When the assistant folds the ear over, place and bury a few interrupted absorbable sutures in the cartilage (Fig. 1.39c). This step is optional, as granuloma formation may complicate buried sutures.
9. Suture the skin of the posterior surface with nylon.

The dressing

A single layer of paraffin gauze is used, then a double layer of gauze folded around the ear, so that it sits back in its normal position. The dressing is firmly fastened with tape.

The dressing is changed in 3 days and the sutures removed in 6 days.

REPAIR OF LACERATED EYELID

General points

- Ensure that the tear duct is not involved.
- Preserve as much tissue as possible.
- Do not shave the eyebrow.
- Do not invert hair-bearing skin into the wound.
- Ensure precise alignment of the wound margins.
- Tie suture knots away from the eyeball.

Method

1. Place an intermarginal suture behind the eyelashes if the margin is involved (Fig. 1.40a).
2. Repair conjunctiva and tarsus with 6/0 absorbable sutures (Fig. 1.40b).
3. Then repair the skin and muscle (orbicularis oculi) with 6/0 nylon (Fig. 1.40c).
4. If suture ends threaten to touch the eyeball, cut ends long and tape down to skin.

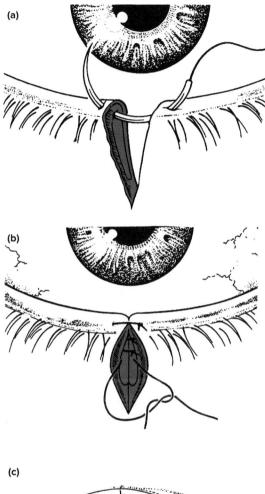

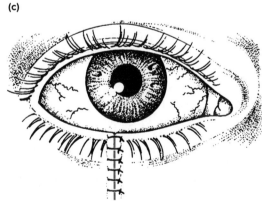

Fig. 1.40 Repair of lacerated eyelid: **(a)** initial suture; **(b)** repair of deeper layer; **(c)** outer skin sutured last

REPAIR OF TONGUE WOUND

Wherever possible, it is best to avoid repair to wounds of the tongue because these heal rapidly. However, large flap wounds to the tongue on the dorsum or the lateral border may require suturing. The best method is to use buried absorbable sutures.

Method

1. Infiltrate with 1% lidocaine LA and leave for 5 to 10 minutes. (Sucking ice may provide adequate analgesia.)
2. Use 4/0 or 3/0 absorbable sutures to suture the flap to its bed, and bury the sutures (Fig. 1.41).

It should not be necessary to use surface sutures. If it is, 4/0 silk sutures will suffice.

The patient should be instructed to rinse the mouth regularly with salt water until healing is satisfactory.

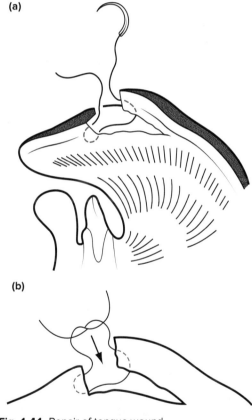

Fig. 1.41 Repair of tongue wound

AVASCULAR FIELD IN DIGIT

A bloodless field in the anaesthetised digit (after a digital block) can be achieved by using a rubber band as a simple tourniquet.

Method

1. Elevate the hand vertically (or the leg) for 2 minutes and wrap tape from the tip of the digit to its base.
2. Wrap a rubber band around the base of the digit to block circulation, and unwrap the tape.

3. Now place the limb on the table and complete the procedure (e.g. removing a foreign body or repairing a wound).
4. When completed, apply a dressing and snip the rubber band with a scalpel or scissors.

Alternative 'glove' method

1. Snip the tip off one finger of a sterile glove.
2. Put the glove on the finger or toe and roll the remaining latex down to the base of the digit.

REMOVAL OF SKIN SUTURES

Suture marks are related to the time of retention of the suture, its tension and position. The objective is to remove the sutures as early as possible, as soon as their purpose is achieved. The timing of removal is based on commonsense and individual cases. Nylon sutures are less reactive and can be left for longer periods. After suture removal it is advisable to support the wound with skin tape (e.g. Steri-Strips) for 1 to 2 weeks, especially in areas of skin tension.

Method

1. Use good light and have the patient lying comfortably.
2. Use fine, sharp scissors that cut to the point or a suture removal blade, and a pair of fine, non-toothed dissecting forceps that grip firmly.
3. Cut the suture close to the skin below the knot (Fig. 1.42a).
4. Gently pull the suture out towards the side on which it was divided—that is, always towards the wound (Fig. 1.42b).
   Note: In children, cut all sutures before removal.
5. If sutures are buried in dry scab, pre-soak the area in lubricant gel.

PITFALLS FOR EXCISION OF NON-MELANOMA SKIN CANCER

There are several anatomical pitfalls awaiting surgical excision. The following summarises potential problem areas.
- The face—for cosmetic reasons.
- The face—for potential nerve damage, especially the temporal branch of facial nerve (Fig. 1.43) and other branches of the facial nerve: zygomatic, buccal, marginal mandibular, cervical.
- The lips and helix of the ear—because of malignant potential.
- The eyelids.
- The inner-canthus of the eye with close proximity to the nasolacrimal duct.
- Mid-sternomastoid muscle area where the accessory nerve is superficial.

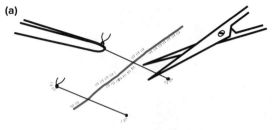

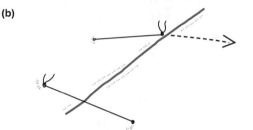

Fig. 1.42 Removal of skin sutures: **(a)** cutting suture; **(b)** removal by pulling towards wound

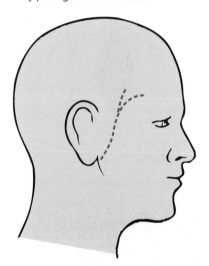

Fig. 1.43 The course of the temporal branch of the facial nerve

- Fingers where functional impairment may be a concern.
- Lower limb below the knee where healing, especially in the elderly, will be a problem.

Referral to a specialist

Referral should be considered when one or more of the following is involved:
- uncertainty of diagnosis
- any doubts about appropriate treatment
- tumours larger than 1 cm (depending on location)
- multiple tumours
- recurrent tumours, despite treatment

- incompletely excised tumours, especially when complete excision may be difficult
- recommended treatment beyond the skills of the practitioner
- anticipation of difficulty with technique or anatomy
- squamous cell carcinomas on the lips and ears
- infiltrating or scar-like morphoeic BCCs—particularly those on the nose or around the nasal labial fold, as there may be a problem in determining the tumour's extent and depth
- cosmetic concerns such as lesions of the upper chest and upper arms where keloid scarring is a potential problem
- areas where palpable regional lymph nodes suggest possible metastatic spread of squamous cell carcinoma: namely head and neck, axilla and groin.

W-PLASTY FOR RAGGED LACERATIONS

Jagged lacerations are usually best debrided with a small elliptical excision following wrinkle lines, when possible.

As a rule it is better to close a ragged wound without tension than to trim it and close it with considerable tension.

There is no rule that dictates that a laceration has to be closed as a straight line.

One procedure that debrides the sides of a ragged wound (too large for simple elliptical debridement) in a saw-toothed fashion is W-plasty. The sides of the wound have to match each other (Fig. 1.44a). With W-plasty, care should be taken to ensure that adequate blood supply is maintained. Select the pattern of debridement and make the initial incisions through the dermis, avoiding full-length incisions, which tend to result in rolled skin edges.

Apply simple sutures using three-point sutures at the apices of the triangular components (Fig. 1.44b).

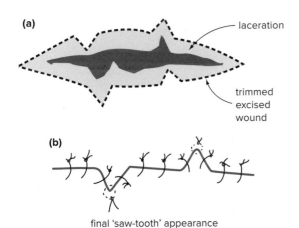

(a)

laceration

trimmed excised wound

(b)

final 'saw-tooth' appearance

Fig. 1.44 Technique of W-plasty

BUSH SUTURE

Campers rarely bring suturing tools for emergency laceration repair, but if the first aid kit has an ordinary straight needle and fishing line (or better, out-of-date suture material) a temporary bush repair solution becomes possible. Simply push the needle through both skin edges and, while in place, thread the suture material through; counter intuitively, start at the sharp end. Remove the needle out of the skin and off the thread, then tie the suture. Spare suture material also comes in handy for removing fish hooks using the 'fisherman's yank' (Chapter 10).

SPLIT SKIN INJURIES

These common injuries usually present after a blow to skin that is tightly stretched over bone such as the skull, face and knee. The splits are commonly linear or star-shaped (Fig. 1.45) A careful history of the nature of the injury is important, especially to determine if a closed high kinetic injury is involved such as hitting the head on the windscreen in an accident. As a rule, foreign material is rarely introduced so they can be treated as a clean wound after compulsory basic cleaning and inspection. Small islands of tissue that are well connected to deeper structures can be left and incorporated into the wound for the purpose of primary repair. If in doubt, it should be dissected out. In particular in high kinetic injuries, spicules of underlying bone may be present in the wound, necessitating removal prior to further inspection for fractures and other consequences.

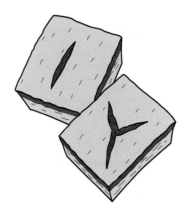

Fig. 1.45 Examples of split skin injuries

DEBRIDEMENT OF TRAUMATIC WOUNDS

The fundamental principle of debridement is to prevent infection and facilitate healing of open wounds by the manual removal of foreign, dead and contaminated material. Comprehensive wound assessment is needed before deciding whether to debride or not. Debridement may vary from simple irrigation with saline to a major clean up under general anaesthetic.

Basic equipment will include (sterilised) scrubbing brush, saline solution, scalpel and tissue forceps, artery forceps and a 20 mL syringe for irrigation.

The principles and process are summarised in Table 1.2.

Table 1.2 Principles of traumatic wound debridement

1.	Remove foreign bodies and gross contamination.
2.	Irrigate and scrub to remove surface debris.
3.	Wide prep and drape.
4.	Avoid tourniquets unless vital.
5.	Excise all dead tissue.
6.	Excise crushed or dubiously viable tissue if primary closure is planned or leave it to declare itself and plan a second-look debridement.
7.	Cut skin edges and deep surfaces back to bleeding tissue. Debride in the line of any longitudinal structures (e.g. limb arteries, veins or nerves) to avoid transection or damage.
8.	Further irrigate the wound to wash out bacteria, residual foreign bodies and small non-viable tissue fragments. Use normal saline, not povidone-iodine solution, antibiotics or other antiseptics as they may be tissue-toxic.
9.	Obtain haemostasis prior to completing the debridement.
10.	Decide whether a second-look debridement or formal closure is required.

Reproduced from Royal Australasian College of Surgeons, *Fundamental Skills for Surgery*, McGraw-Hill, Sydney, 2008, with permission.

One large US study showed that frequent debridement, e.g. at least once a week, accelerates the healing process.[8]

DEBRIDEMENT OF SKIN IN A HAIRY AREA

When debriding skin in a hairy area, it is important to realise that hair shafts grow obliquely to the skin. In order to avoid creating a hairless path along the length of the scar, try to debride the skin edges at the same angle as the hair shafts (Fig. 1.46). This avoids damage to the hair follicles.

Natural lacerations (such as from a blunt blow) to hairy areas such as the eyebrow do not leave a hairless patch of scar when sutured correctly. However, never shave eyebrows because regrowth is unpredictable.

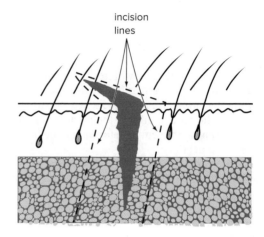

Fig. 1.46 Direction of trimmed incision lines in a hair-bearing area

HAIR REMOVAL

Removal is only necessary if hair will interfere with the incision site or if there is risk of wound contamination.

Keeping hairs out of wounds for suturing

While suturing in a hair-bearing area such as the scalp, it is important to keep hair out of the wound. This can be done by smoothing the hair down with K-Y gel, hair gel such as Brylcreem or adhesive tape.

Clearing shaved areas

An effective way to clean up a shaved area such as a scalp prior to surgical repair is to use strips of adhesive tape such as Micropore to pick up loose hairs.

WOUND MANAGEMENT TIPS[9]

Traumatic wounds

Primary wound closure rules

- Traditional rule—within 4 to 6 hours
- Facial wounds (uncontaminated)—within 12 to 24 hours
- Other wounds (uncontaminated)—8 to 12 hours

Delayed primary closure

- Wounds too old
- Heavy contamination
  Rule: Observe 3.5 days then repair if not infected.

Dressings

Table 1.3 indicates examples of the most appropriate dressing materials for the exudate level of the wound being treated.

Table 1.3 Appropriate dressing materials for various exudate levels

Dressing type	Exudate level
Film dressings (e.g. Tegaderm™)	Nil/minimal
Hydrocolloid (e.g. Duoderm®)	Low/moderate
Alginate (e.g. Algisite®)	Moderate/high
Foam (e.g. Allevyn®)	Moderate/high
Hydrogel (e.g. Solosite®)	Dry/sloughy

Post-operative wound care

Useful guidelines are:
- Use non-adherent dressings over excision wounds. Leave for 24 to 48 hours. Place an occlusive dressing over this for protection and when showering.
- After removal of dressing, clean daily with saline to remove crusting and to minimise infection.
- If concerned about infection, use thin application of chloramphenicol (or similar ointment).

For healing by secondary intention (such as after curette or diathermy):
- Use hydrocolloidal dressings (e.g. Intrasite, Duoderm, Rapid Healing Band Aids).
- Leave in situ for up to 7 days.

Healing cavities of incised cysts and abscesses

This practice tip outlines a simple method of promoting the healing of cavities resulting from drained abscesses or removed sebaceous cysts, especially infected cysts. The concept originally came from veterinary management of cysts in animals.

Method

1. For deep cavities resulting from surgical incision it is best to pack them first with sterile non-adherent gauze while the patient is anaesthetised. This controls haemostasis and maintains drainage.
2. The following day, remove the gauze and infiltrate the cavity with a hydrogel (e.g. Intrasite).
3. Cover the wound with appropriate waterproof dressing.
4. Change this every day or every second day until the wound heals.

Advantages

- The gel infuses to all recesses of the cavity that packing cannot reach.
- Patients can continue management themselves.
- More convenient for patients who have a considerable distance to travel.
- Less pain and discomfort compared with other dressings.
- Rapid healing.

WHEN TO REMOVE NON-ABSORBABLE SUTURES

For removal of sutures after non-complicated wound closure in adults, see Table 1.4.

Note: Individualise according to the nature of the wound and health of the patient and healing. In general, remove sutures as soon as possible. One way of achieving

Table 1.4 Time after insertion for removal of sutures

Area	Days later
Scalp	7–10
Face	3–5 (or alternate at 3, rest 4–5)
Ear	5–7
Neck	4 (or alternate at 3, rest 4)
Chest	8
Arm (including hand and fingers)	8–10
Abdomen	8–10 (tension 12–14)
Back	12–14
Inguinal and scrotal	7
Perineum	2
Legs	10
Knees and calf	12–14
Foot (including toes)	10–14

this is to remove alternate sutures a day or two earlier and remove the rest at the usual time. Steri-Strips can then be used to maintain closure and healing.

Additional aspects

In children, usually remove 1 to 2 days earlier. Allow additional time for backs and legs, especially the calf.

Nylon sutures can be left longer because they are less reactive. Alternate sutures may be removed earlier (e.g. from the face in women).

References

1. Perry R (Ed.). *Fundamental skills for surgery.* Sydney: McGraw-Hill Australia, 2008: 104–11.
2. Heal C, Sriharan S, Buttner P et al. Comparing non-sterile to sterile gloves for minor surgery: a prospective randomised controlled non-inferiority trial. Med J Aust, 2015; 202(1): 27–31.
3. Perry R (Ed.). *Fundamental skills for surgery.* Sydney: McGraw-Hill Australia, 2008: 148–69.
4. McGregor I. *Fundamental techniques of plastic surgery.* Edinburgh: Churchill Livingstone, 1989.
5. Expert group for Dermatology Guidelines. Skin cancer. eTG complete. Melbourne: Therapeutic Guidelines Ltd. Available from: www.tg.org.au. Accessed May 2019; Sladden M, Nieweg O, Howle J, Coventry B, Cancer Council Australia Melanoma Guidelines Working Party. Excision margins for melanoma *in situ.* Clinical practice guidelines for the diagnosis and management of melanoma. Cancer Guidelines Wiki, Cancer Council Australia. Accessed June 2019. (https://wiki.cancer.org.au/australia/Clinical_question: What_are_the_recommended_safety_margins_ for_radical_excision_of_primary_melanoma%3F/ In_situ)
6. Pennington A. *Local flap reconstruction.* Sydney: McGraw-Hill Australia, 2007.
7. Hayes M. *Practical skin cancer surgery.* Sydney: Churchill Livingstone–Elsevier, 2014.
8. Wilcox JR, Carter MJ, Covington S. Frequency of debridement of wounds: A retrospective and time to heal cohort study of 312,744 wounds. JAMA (Dermatology), 2013; 149(9):1050–58.
9. Rakel RE, Rakel DP. *Textbook of Family Medicine 9th edition.* Philadelphia: Elsevier Saunders, 2016; 562.

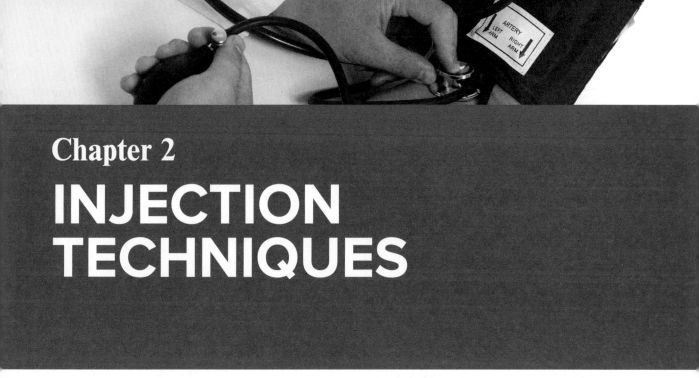

Chapter 2
INJECTION TECHNIQUES

Basic injections

PAINLESS INJECTION TECHNIQUE

Method 1

The essence of this technique is to ensure good muscle relaxation. The patient should be as comfortable as possible. For injections into the deltoid region, the patient should be sitting down with hand on the hip and with the muscle as relaxed as possible. For deep intramuscular injections the buttock is preferred, but care must be taken to inject in the upper outer quadrant. These patients should be lying face down. The buttock should be exposed and the patient encouraged to relax.

1. *Massage for muscular relaxation:* In this traditional method the injection site is well massaged for 20 seconds with an alcohol swab; probably more important for achieving relaxation than for ensuring that the skin is cleaned. Distract with conversation. It is easy to ensure that the underlying muscle is fully relaxed if firm, gentle pressure is applied with the non-injecting hand. When the muscle is relaxed, hold the syringe like a dart between the thumb and forefinger of the injecting hand.
2. *Sharp tap over site:* Before giving the injection, use the side of the back of the right (or dominant) hand to give a smart tap over the injection site (Fig. 2.1). A sharp flick with a finger or squeeze of the muscle can also be effective.
3. *The injection:* Follow this immediately by injecting the needle using the dart technique.
   Note: These steps follow in very rapid succession.

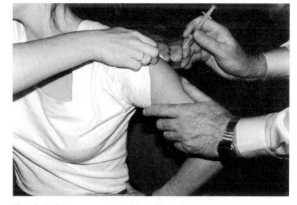

Fig. 2.1 Sharp tap with side of hand

Many patients will tell you with surprise that they did not feel the needle but were conscious of the sting of the injection material going into the tissues.

Method 2: Almost painless injections

A subcutaneous (SC) or intramuscular (IM) injection is almost always painless if the skin is stretched firmly before inserting the needle. If injecting the arm, for example, the third, fourth and fifth fingers should go medial to the arm while the thumb and index finger stretch the skin on the lateral surface (Fig. 2.2). The needle should be inserted quickly into the stretched skin.

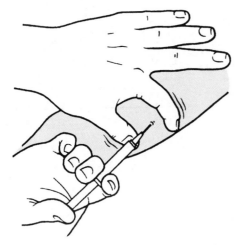

Fig. 2.2 Stretching the skin with thumb and index finger

Method 3: Muscle contraction–relaxation method

Use the muscle energy method by asking the patient to push their elbow against their hip as an isometric contraction for 7 seconds. Then quickly give the injection into the deltoid muscle (now relaxed).

Method 4: Needle gauge

The discomfort from an IM or SC injection can be minimised by using a smaller gauge needle, e.g. 30-gauge, especially for vaccinations in children.

INTRAMUSCULAR INJECTIONS

Deltoid injection

A good site to inject but avoid striking the humerus as injury can occur to the anterior branch of the axillary (circumflex) nerve. This nerve winds posteriorly around the surgical neck of the humerus, below the capsule of the joint, approximately 6–8 cm below the bony prominence of the acromion.

Thigh injection

The safest area for injection is into the anterolateral aspect of the thigh, into the vastus lateralis or rectus femoris (two of the four components of quadriceps femoris).

Buttock (ventrogluteal) injection

The sciatic nerve may be readily injured in a poorly placed deep intramuscular injection. The only safe area is the true upper outer quadrant (Fig. 2.3). The landmarks are the iliac crest superiorly, posterior superior iliac spine (PSIS) superomedially, the ischial tuberosity inferomedially, and the greater trochanter laterally. The sciatic nerve lies inferior to an imaginary line from PSIS to the greater

trochanter. After emerging from the pelvis, it follows a quarter circle course to a point halfway along the line drawn from the ischial tuberosity to the greater trochanter.

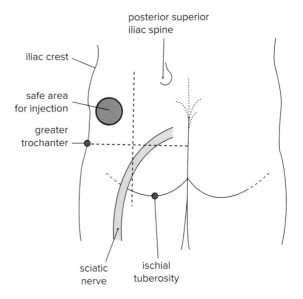

Fig. 2.3 Safest site for intramuscular injection into the left buttock

Ventrogluteal area—suitable for IM vaccination of infants and toddlers

This site has lower reactogenicity and similar immunogenicity to the two other recommended paediatric vaccination sites—deltoid and anterolateral thigh. It has practical implications for mass vaccination, especially in third world countries. The infant has to be suitably restrained.

Method

The tip of the index finger is placed on the anterior superior iliac spine, while the tip of the thumb is held against the index finger and placed on the greater trochanter. The injection site is in the middle of the triangle formed by the index and middle fingers spread apart (Fig. 2.4)

It is recommended to use a 25-gauge 25 mm needle, inserted at 90° to the stretched skin.

REDUCING THE STING FROM AN ALCOHOL SWAB

The sting from alcohol on the skin can be reduced by drying the skin with a piece of sterile gauze or cotton wool after swabbing. Alternatively, one can blow onto the preparation site or rapidly wave one's hand over it to achieve drying.

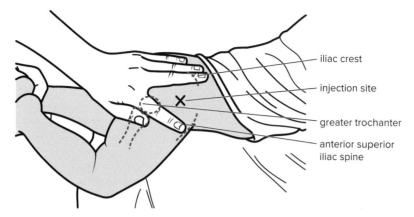

iliac crest

injection site

greater trochanter

anterior superior
iliac spine

Fig. 2.4 Ventrogluteal area suitable for injection of infants and toddlers

PAINLESS WOUND SUTURING

The objective is to administer local anaesthetic (LA) as painlessly as possible when treating a wound that requires suturing. The method applies to non-contaminated wounds only.

Method

1. Irrigate the wound with a small volume of LA.
2. Rather than inserting the needle into the skin, insert it into the subcutaneous tissue through the open wound (Fig. 2.5).
3. Infiltrate for the length of the wound on both sides. This method is relatively painless.

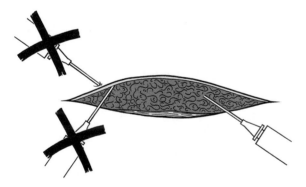

Fig. 2.5 A relatively painless method of administering local anaesthetic at a wound site requiring suturing

SIMPLE TOPICAL ANAESTHESIA FOR WOUND REPAIR

Drip a few drops of lignocaine or other local anaesthetic solution onto the wound and wait about five minutes. This provides suitable surface anaesthesia for infiltration or even simple suturing.

SLOWER ANAESTHETIC INJECTION CUTS PAIN

A study has shown that subcutaneous infiltration of local anaesthetic causes only half the pain if injected slowly over 30 seconds rather than rapidly over five seconds.

LOCAL ANAESTHETIC INFILTRATION TECHNIQUE FOR WOUNDS

This technique is applicable to larger wounds, contaminated wounds and planned excision of lumps. The anaesthetic should allow for adequate debridement and skin excision and suturing. Marking the boundaries and injection entry points will facilitate the procedure. Infiltrate both the dermis and underlying subcutaneous tissue. Figure 2.6 indicates the four entry points and eight needle positions required to cover the operative area. When changing needle direction, withdraw nearly all the needle but leave the tip in the dermis to avoid re-piercing the skin.

DISPOSAL OF NEEDLES

Recapping of used needles should be avoided, to eliminate as far as possible the risk of accidental puncture of the medical practitioner or practice nurse. The risk of contracting such infections as hepatitis B, C and HIV from a sharps injury is ever-present. Needles should be disposed of directly into a sharps container, which should be above child height and attached to the wall. Many types of sharps containers are available for use in the surgery and even in the doctor's bag.

The 'take it with you' needle disposal unit consists of a plastic bottle 2.5 cm in diameter and 8 cm in depth. The lid has an opening with a plastic flap on the underside. This opening is designed to allow introduction of the needle attached to its syringe and then withdrawal of the syringe to 'trap' the needle in the container. After

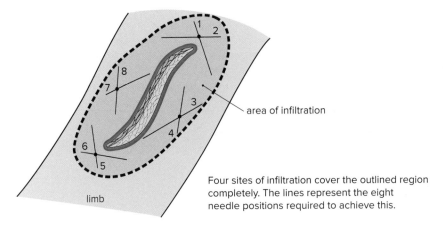

area of infiltration

Four sites of infiltration cover the outlined region completely. The lines represent the eight needle positions required to achieve this.

limb

Fig. 2.6 Wide multiple infiltration to completely cover the outlined region

the needle is introduced into the centre of the opening, it is tilted to the side. The syringe is then pulled sharply upwards to disconnect the needle (Fig. 2.7).

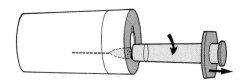

Fig. 2.7 The doctor's bag needle disposal bottle

Recapping of needles

Although the recapping of needles should be avoided, probably the safest way, if it really must be done, is to scoop up the needle guard with the used needle and syringe unit, using the dominant hand only. This reinforces the principle of always staying 'behind the needle', and keeps the thumb and forefinger of the non-dominant hand out of danger.

'Hole in one' method

This is a common method in developing countries where more sophisticated disposal methods are unavailable. Holes that are slightly larger than the size of the needle guard but smaller than the collar of it are drilled at an angle of 15° through the edge of the injection preparation table. The needle guard is placed into the hole while you give the injection. After the injection, the needle with used syringe is simply inserted into the guard. The whole unit is then placed in an old used drinking bottle.

Needle disposal in an emergency

When there is no sharps container available (during an emergency or an under-prepared home visit),

temporarily store the needle in a urine specimen container or a rigid soft drink bottle until a sharps bin is found. An alternative is to remove the plunger from a syringe, put the needle inside the barrel and replace the plunger.

BUBBLES IN THE SYRINGE

Some particularly viscous fluids (e.g. containing testosterone or antipsychotics) form multiple air bubbles in the syringe. To remove the bubbles, draw even more air into the syringe, tip upwards and expel the one large bubble, which will drag all the small air pockets with it.

Note that some pre-loaded syringes, such as the influenza vaccine, deliberately have some air in the syringe. This does not need to be expelled prior to injection.

RECTAL 'INJECTION'

When no veins can readily be found for intravenous injections, in some emergency situations the use of the rectal route is effective.

Diabetic hypoglycaemia

In some unconscious patients it may not be possible to administer the 'difficult' intravenous injection of 50% glucose, due to such factors as vasoconstriction and obesity.

However, the glucose can be given simply by pressing the nozzle of the syringe (usually a 20 mL syringe) gently but firmly into the rectum and slowly injecting the solution.

Convulsions

In children with a persistent febrile convulsion or in patients with status epilepticus, the rectal route can be used for administering a diazepam or midazolam solution with amazing success.

Example

Consider a 2-year-old child (weight 12 kg) with a persistent febrile convulsion. The dose of diazepam injectable is 0.4 mg/kg, so 5 mg (1 mL) of diazepam is diluted with isotonic saline (up to 5–10 mL of solution) and introduced into the rectum, preferably with a plastic fluid-drawing-up nozzle attached to the syringe.

Midazolam can also be administered rectally.

FINGER LANCING WITH LESS PAIN

A method of minimising the pain of lancing fingers for blood samples, especially for diabetics, is outlined.

Theory

The sides of the fingers are less painful than the pad or the base of the nail bed of the thumb or index finger (as traditionally used for bleeding). The thumb and index finger have heightened sensitivity, as presented in Penfield and Boldrey's homunculus.[1,2]

Method

1. Insert the lancet into the medial or lateral aspect of the third or fourth finger of either hand.
2. Provide firm pressure on the pad of the lanced finger with the opposing thumb on the pad of the finger. This ensures an adequate blood flow for the test strips.

Other viewpoints

Side of thumb

According to a randomised controlled trial published in *The Lancet* (1999, 354, pp. 921–2), the least painful area to lance for blood sugar testing was the side of the thumb. It would be worth conducting our own trial—the side of the thumb or the third or fourth finger![3]

Earlobe

A UK study of people with diabetes in 2003 found that the average pain score for finger pricking was 4 to 5 times higher than pricking the earlobe.

DIGITAL NERVE BLOCK

The digital nerve block is indicated for simple procedures on the fingers and toes. (A more proximal block, such as the brachial plexus block, is indicated for extensive injury.)

Each digit is supplied by four nerve branches: two dorsal and two palmar (or plantar). These nerves run forward adjacent to the respective metacarpal or metatarsal bone. The nerves to the fingers and toes are blocked at the base of the digit. The digital nerves lie

3–5 mm below the dorsal skin surface and at the 2, 4, 8 and 10 o'clock positions around the digit (Fig. 2.8).

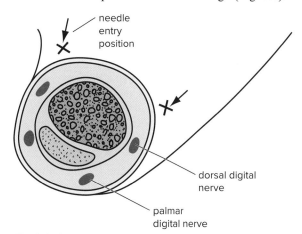

Fig. 2.8 Cross-section of finger showing position of digital nerves

Method

1. Lay the palm down to stabilise the site. The dorsal approach is less painful than the palmar.
2. Perform the block at the level of the respective metacarpal or metatarsal from the dorsal aspect.
3. Introduce the 25- or 23-gauge needle distal or adjacent to the metacarpal head (for the hand) immediately alongside the bone (at the level where a ring would be worn).
4. Insert at right angles to the skin and proceed as far as the palmar or plantar skin.
5. Inject 1–1.5 mL of LA without adrenaline (plain LA) on each side of the digit as the needle is slowly being withdrawn, so that the solution is spread evenly superficially and deeply (Fig. 2.9).

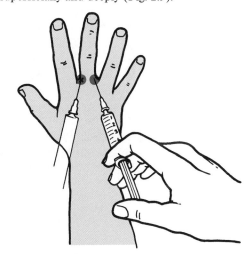

Fig. 2.9 The digital nerve block blocks both palmar (or plantar) and dorsal nerve branches

Alternatively, a wheal can be raised on the dorsal surface and the needle advanced as the injection is given.

Dosage

This is 2–3 mL of lidocaine or prilocaine 1%. Ring blocks usually provide anaesthesia for 60 minutes.

Note: Although adrenaline (epinephrine) was traditionally avoided in digital nerve blocks, a number of studies have demonstrated that it is safe in those without peripheral vascular compromise.[3,4]

Allow sufficient time for anaesthesia (5 to 20 minutes).

The thumb

The thumb requires only one injection in the midline of the palmar surface at the base of the thumb.

REGIONAL NERVE WRIST BLOCKS TO NERVES TO HAND

Partial or complete wrist block is very valuable for minor surgery or wound repair of the hand. The distribution of the cutaneous nerves to both surfaces of the hand is shown in Figure 2.10.

Median nerve block

Area supplied

- Palmar surface on radial (lateral) side involving fingers 1, 2, 3 and the radial half of 4.
- Dorsal distal aspect of same fingers.

Technique

- Identify palmaris longus (PL) tendon (flex wrist against resistance).
- Insert a 25-gauge needle between tendons flexor carpi radialis (FCR) and just lateral to PL.
- The point is almost exactly in the middle of the anterior surface of the wrist or a few millimetres to the radial site of the midline.
- Insert at level of proximal skin crease.
- Inject 1 mL 1% lidocaine superficially and 1–2 mL deep, angling the needle at about 60°.
- Cease the injection if median nerve symptoms such as tingling or pain develop.

Note: If PL is absent, inject midway between the flexor tendons and FCR.

Ulnar nerve block

Area supplied

- Ulnar (medial) aspect of hand (fingers 5 and half 4).

Technique

- Identify flexor carpi ulnaris (FCU) tendon and styloid process of ulna.
- Insert a 25-gauge needle between FCU and the ulnar artery on radial side FCU just medial to the artery at the level of the styloid process of ulna (similar level as for median nerve block). Beware of entering the ulnar artery.
- Inject 4 mL 1% lidocaine, preferably when paraesthesia has been induced by the needle.

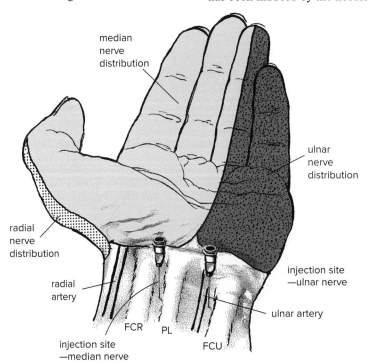

Fig. 2.10 Illustration of median and ulnar nerve blocks

Radial nerve block

Area supplied

- Radial half of dorsal aspect of hand.
- Base of thenar eminence.

Technique

Because of the anatomical variations in the divisions of the radial nerve near the wrist joint, it is preferable to raise a subcutaneous ring of 10 mL 1% lidocaine radially (from level with the FCR tendons), then around the radial border of the wrist dorsally (about 4 cm proximal to the wrist) to just lateral to the styloid process of the ulna.

REGIONAL NERVE BLOCKS AT ELBOW

Median nerve block

Extend the elbow and draw a line between the medial and lateral epicondyles, which is about 3 cm proximal to the flexion crease. Palpate the brachial artery and insert a 25-gauge 38 mm needle on the epicondylar line, about 0.5 cm medial to the artery, and elicit paraesthesia deep to the artery. Inject 5 mL of plain LA.

Ulnar nerve block

Flex the elbow to 30° and identify the ulnar nerve in the sulcus (groove) behind the medial epicondyle ('funny bone'). Inject 2 mL of lidocaine 1% with adrenaline 1–2 cm proximal to this position and elicit paraesthesia. The nerve can also be blocked with the needle outside the nerve using 5–10 mL plain LA.

Radial nerve block

Extend the elbow and draw a line between the two condyles (as above). Insert a 25-gauge 38 mm needle just lateral to the biceps tendon in the groove between it and the brachioradialis muscle on the epicondylar line. Direct the needle slightly cephalad and medial to contact the lateral epicondyle. Inject 2–4 mL of plain LA while the needle is withdrawn.

FEMORAL NERVE BLOCK

In a general practice setting, and especially in rural and remote areas, a femoral nerve block may prove useful in providing emergency analgesia for the transported patient with a fractured neck of femur or shaft of femur and in reducing the need for systemic opioids.

It is indicated in the analgesia of a fractured femur, especially the femoral shaft. Occasionally it may be used for anaesthesia of the anterior thigh for exploration of soft tissue injuries. Patients with effective blocks cannot mobilise since the quadriceps is weakened, so all patients must be appropriately splinted for transfer. Femoral nerve block is a safe, easy to learn and minimally invasive

procedure that can be repeated. Specific training with nerve stimulator guidance or ultrasound will reduce the incidence of arterial puncture.

Anatomy of the femoral nerve

The femoral nerve (L2, L3, L4) enters the anterior thigh about one finger's breadth lateral to the femoral artery immediately below the inguinal ligament. The femoral artery lies at the midpoint of the symphysis pubis and anterior superior iliac spine (ASIS). The femoral nerve lies at the midpoint of the pubic tubercle and the ASIS. The nerve is covered by two layers of fascia, the fascia lata and iliopectineal fascia (Fig. 2.11). Two 'pops' are therefore felt when piercing each of these layers.

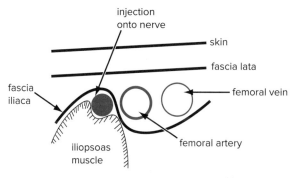

Fig. 2.11 Anatomical position of the femoral nerve in the femoral triangle with illustration of the position of the needle during nerve blockade

Materials

Alcohol swab, an appropriate needle is a 2.5 to 4 or 5 cm 22- or 21-gauge. A St Vincent's needle is ideal as it ends in a point. When introduced up to the hilt, a depth of 2.5–3 cm should be sufficient to reach the appropriate area. Otherwise, especially in obese subjects, a 4–5 cm needle can be used.

An appropriate local anaesthetic is 20 mL of 1% lidocaine, or 10 mL ropivacaine or 0.5% bupivacaine (preferred if available because it lasts up to 8 hours).

Method

Identify and mark the site for injection, which should be adjacent to (one finger breadth away) the femoral artery and over the femoral nerve at the level of the inguinal crease (Fig. 2.12). This crease is a skin fold 2 to 3 cm below, and parallel to, the inguinal ligament.

Insert the needle and aim it slightly rostral or headwards at about 35° to the skin. As you slowly inject, aspirate for blood and check for pain and paraesthesia. If paraesthesia is elicited, withdraw the needle by 1–2 mm and try again. If no blood is aspirated, fan out all the local anaesthetic as you move in and out, e.g. ¼ of dose medial, ¼ lateral, ¼ over nerve and ¼ during withdrawal. It should take

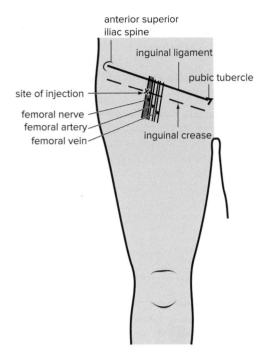

Fig. 2.12 Femoral nerve block (right side)

about 5 minutes for the anaesthesia to start developing. You should be about 3–4 cm deep to the skin surface.

If attempting to provide anaesthesia for a fractured neck of femur, massage the anaesthetic upwards towards the groin.

Precautions

The only real complication is striking the femoral artery or some small vessel, causing either systemic absorption or false aneurysm formation and local bleeding. Note time of procedure and doses of anaesthetic. The block is contraindicated in patients with severe scarring, infection or necrosis over the femoral triangle.

In children

Raise a bleb of LA just lateral to the femoral artery, below the inguinal ligament. Introduce a 23-gauge or lumbar puncture needle and advance it perpendicular to the skin. Fascia insertion 'pops' will then be heard.

LATERAL CUTANEOUS NERVE OF THE THIGH (LCNT)

A trapped LCNT causes meralgia paraesthetica of the thigh. The nerve lies just below the lateral end of the inguinal ligament and 1.5 cm medial to the anterior superior iliac spine (ASIS). The discomfort can be relieved by an infusion of 1 mL long-acting corticosteroid with 1 mL of LA immediately below the inguinal ligament and about 1.5 cm medial to the ASIS.

TIBIAL NERVE BLOCK

The tibial (posterior tibial) nerve can be blocked as it passes behind the medial malleolus, in front of the Achilles tendon, usually midway between these structures. It innervates most of the sole of the foot (Fig. 2.13).

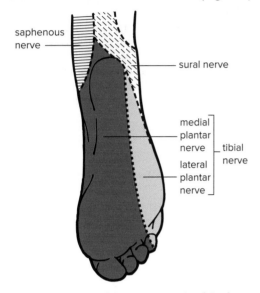

Fig. 2.13 Innervation of the heel and sole of the foot

Indications

- Operations on the foot
- Removal of plantar warts
- Injecting the plantar fascia
- Foreign bodies in sole

Method

1. Palpate the posterior tibial artery behind the medial malleolus. The tibial nerve lies immediately behind the artery.
2. Insert a fine-gauge needle just posterior to the artery, either at the level of the medial malleolus or just below it, pointing in an anterolateral direction (Fig. 2.14). Alternatively, insert the needle anterior to the artery.

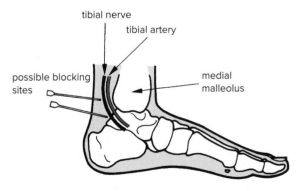

Fig. 2.14 Tibial nerve block

3. At about a depth of 1 cm, paraesthesia may be elicited, indicating the ideal location for injection. The depth of injection varies from 0.5 to 2 cm.
4. Inject 6–10 mL of 1% plain lidocaine, taking care not to puncture a blood vessel.

The block should induce an area of anaesthesia around the sole of the foot, making it ideal for the procedures listed. It usually does not anaesthetise the most proximal and lateral parts. The anaesthesia develops over 10 minutes and lasts for up to 2 hours.

Note: Avoid bilateral nerve blocks at the same visit. Bilateral anaesthesia may cause falls due to loss of balance. To obtain almost full anaesthesia of the plantar aspect of the foot a sural nerve block is necessary, as well as the tibial block.

Caution: Ensure that the injection is not given into the nerve.

MEDIAL PLANTAR NERVE BLOCK VIA DORSUM OF THE FOOT

The medial plantar nerve can be selectively blocked by an infiltration of 2–3 mL of 1% lidocaine on either side of the dorsalis pedis artery at the mid foot at approximately the level of the middle of the second metatarsal. Aim to puncture the skin only once by withdrawing slightly after the first infiltration to the side of the artery and repositioning on the other side.

Sural nerve block

The sural nerve, which runs behind the lateral malleolus, innervates most of the back of the heel and the lateral border of the sole. It is blocked by a subcutaneous infiltration of up to 5 mL of 1% plain lidocaine in a fanwise fashion from the Achilles tendon to the outer and upper border of the lateral malleolus (Fig. 2.15). Another landmark is

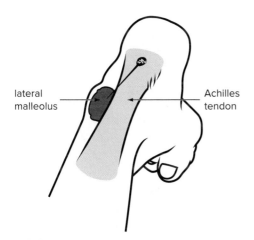

lateral malleolus

Achilles tendon

Fig. 2.15 Sural nerve block (infiltrate between the Achilles tendon and lateral malleolus)

the groove midway between the posterior border of the lateral malleolus and the calcaneus bone. You can inject LA between the skin and malleolar surface 1 cm behind and proximal to the tip of the lateral malleolus. This procedure anaesthetises the most proximal and lateral aspects of the sole of the foot. If combined with a tibial nerve block, most of the heel and sole of the foot will be covered.

FACIAL NERVE BLOCKS

Regional nerve blocks have advantages over infiltration for facial and oral anaesthesia because there is less tissue swelling at the operative site, a wider area is anaesthetised, and they are less painful.

General points

- Use 2% lidocaine with adrenaline. 1:2 000 000 for facial injections and 1:80 000 for intra-oral injections.
- Allow 5 to 10 minutes before commencing the procedure.
- Always aspirate to check for blood before injecting.
- Infiltrate around the nerve and not into it.
- Do not enter the foramina.

Supraorbital nerve block

Indications

Surgery to forehead, upper eyelids and scalp to vertex.

Method

1. Instruct the patient to look straight ahead.
2. Insert a 23- or 25-gauge 2.5 cm needle in a horizontal plane over the supraorbital foramen, at the upper border of the orbit, under the eyebrow, 2.5 cm from the midline (Fig. 2.16).
3. Inject 3–4 mL of LA.

Infraorbital nerve block

Indications

Surgery to:
- lower eyelid
- cheek
- side of nose and upper lip
- gingival tissues from midline to first molar.

Method 1: Intraoral approach (preferred to the extraoral route)

The infraorbital foramen lies above and in line with the second premolar, 1 cm below the infraorbital margin.
1. Elevate the upper lip and align the syringe along the long axis of the tooth.
2. Enter the mucosa at its reflection from the gum and advance a 23- or 25-gauge needle to just short of the foramen (until the bone is just contacted).
3. Inject 2–3 mL of LA.

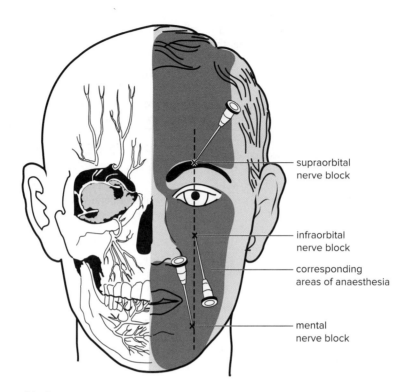

Fig. 2.16 Facial nerve blocks

Method 2: Extraoral approach

1. Instruct the patient to look straight ahead.
2. Insert the needle 1 cm below the infraorbital margin in line with the pupil, directing the needle towards the infraorbital foramen. Do not attempt to enter it.
3. Inject 2 mL of LA.

Mental nerve block

Indications

- Excision of oral and skin lesions
- Suturing lacerations: from midline to lower border of mandible (Fig. 2.16) to include lower lip and chin

Method (intraoral approach)

1. Palpate the mental foramen, which lies at the apex of the lower second premolar tooth.
2. Lift the lip forward and align the syringe with the long axis of this tooth.
3. Penetrate the mucosa and advance the needle to just short of the foramen. This is about halfway between the gum margin and the lower border of the mandible, about 2.5 cm from the midline.
4. Aspirate and inject 2 mL of LA.

   If the patient is edentulous, use as a reference a vertical line from the midpoint of the pupil.

SPECIFIC FACIAL BLOCKS FOR THE EXTERNAL EAR

For minor surgery and repair of lesions of the external ear, widespread infiltration can be used (Fig. 2.17). However,

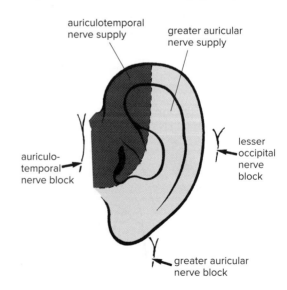

Fig. 2.17 Nerve supply to the ear and sites for the three nerve blocks

more specific blocks using 3 mL of 1% plain lidocaine for each nerve can be used. Care should be taken because of the proximity of branches of the carotid artery. The skin of the external ear is mainly supplied by three branches of the trigeminal nerve, namely:

- **Auriculotemporal nerve**—innervates upper anterior quadrant of lateral surface including tragus, crux of helix and adjacent helix.
  Blockage: Insert needle immediately posterior–inferior to temporomandibular joint.
- **Greater auricular nerve**—innervates remainder of lateral surface, including anti-helix and earlobe and most of medial (cranial) surface.
  Blockage: Insert needle just behind and inferior to the earlobe at the anterior border of the sternomastoid muscle.
- **Lesser occipital nerve**—innervates upper part of medial (cranial) surface.
  Blockage: Insert needle about 1 cm posterior to the ear at its midpoint.

PENILE NERVE BLOCK

The penis can be anaesthetised for procedures such as circumcision, wound repair and paraphimosis reduction by injecting local anaesthetic (without adrenaline) into the dorsal and ventral surfaces.

Method

1. Inject a ring of 5 mL of plain LA subcutaneously around the base of the penis, with the needle resting against the corpus cavernosum (Fig. 2.18a).
2. Inject 2 mL of LA into each of the grooves on the ventral surface (between the corpus cavernosum and spongiosum) (Fig. 2.18b).

INTRAVENOUS REGIONAL ANAESTHESIA (BIER BLOCK)

This technique uses an intravenous injection of local anaesthetic into an arm or leg that is isolated from the circulation by an arterial tourniquet. It produces excellent anaesthesia, muscle relaxation and (if desired) a bloodless operating field. Ideally, two doctors are required. It is also used in children over 5 years of age.

Indications

- Minor surgery, especially to upper arm (e.g. release of trigger finger, removal of foreign bodies)
- Reduction of limb fractures (e.g. Colles fracture)

Precautions

- The patient should be fasted as for a GA.
- Exclude patients with unstable epilepsy, second- or third-degree heart block, liver disease, severe vascular disease, allergy to LA agents or a condition precluding the use of a tourniquet.
- Obtain informed consent.

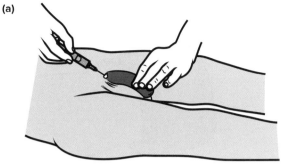

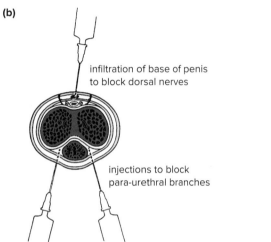

infiltration of base of penis to block dorsal nerves

injections to block para-urethral branches

Fig. 2.18 Penile nerve block: **(a)** infiltration of base of penis; **(b)** three injection approaches

- Ensure patient fasting—at least 4 hours.
- Avoid sudden release of LA (e.g. escaping beneath tourniquet).
- Maintain IV access with a needle in the vein of the opposite arm.
- Check the pressure of the tourniquet throughout.
- Have resuscitation equipment available, including a positive pressure oxygen system.
- Ideally, monitor with an ECG and SaO_2 (pulse oximetry).
- Maintain inflation for at least 20 minutes.
- Maximum inflation 45 minutes.

Method (for arm)

1. Cannulate vein (e.g. plastic 22-gauge IV cannula of IV set) and tape on.
2. Drain blood by simple elevation for 3 minutes or (for bloodless field) by an Esmarch bandage. This exsanguination is very important.
3. Apply a sphygmomanometer cuff or (better still) arterial pneumatic tourniquet.
4. Inflate to 100 mmHg above the patient's systolic blood pressure (50 mmHg above in children). Check for absence of the brachial or radial pulse. Remove the Esmarch and lower the arm.

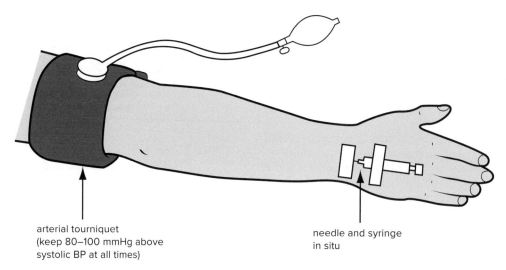

arterial tourniquet
(keep 80–100 mmHg above
systolic BP at all times)

needle and syringe
in situ

Fig. 2.19 Intravenous regional anaesthesia

5. Slowly inject 2.5 mg/kg of 0.5% plain lidocaine or prilocaine (preferred) (*without* adrenaline) into the indwelling needle (Fig. 2.19).

    Note: Usual adult dose is 30 mL of 0.5% prilocaine (maximum 40 mL).

6. The onset of anaesthesia is reasonably rapid (5 to 10 minutes). Confirm its adequacy. Remove the cannula in the arm being treated.

7. Watch carefully for side effects, e.g. restlessness, dizziness, tinnitus, seizures, bradycardia or hypotension.

8. Use a second doctor (if available) to perform the operative procedure.

9. On completion, ensure very slow release of the tourniquet. As soon as it is deflated, pump it up again rapidly, then slowly deflate. (Repeat this three times at the rate of once per minute if inflated for only 20 to 25 minutes. Serial deflation/inflation is considered to reinforce safety. Some do not use it.) Ideally, the tourniquet should not be released before 20 minutes after the infusion and left on no longer than 40 minutes.

10. Observe the patient carefully for at least 15 minutes.

    Note: More sophisticated double cuff tourniquets are available.

HAEMATOMA BLOCK BY LOCAL INFILTRATION ANAESTHETIC

In this procedure, local anaesthetic is injected directly into the haematoma surrounding the fracture. It usually employs the barbotage method of alternately injecting small amounts of anaesthetic and withdrawing small amounts of haematoma. A full aseptic technique is essential and caution is required for possible complications including infection. Ideally, ECG monitoring is recommended. Its use is not favoured because of the potential for adverse effects but it remains an option when no other anaesthetic methods, including the preferred Bier block, are available or practical.

Indications

This method has a place in the emergency reduction of fractures of the distal radius (notably Colles fracture), sometimes for distal ankle fractures and fractures of the upper extremity in children.

Method

- Use sterile gloves and prepare the overlying skin with a bactericidal agent.
- Use a 21-gauge needle and 1% plain lidocaine with a volume less than 10 mL.
- Localise the haematoma by aspirating blood into the syringe.
- Slowly inject the anaesthetic (up to no more than half the quantity) into the haematoma (Fig. 2.20).
- Withdraw an equivalent amount of the bloody fluid.
- Repeat injection and aspiration until the anaesthetic is dispersed.
- Wait 10 to 15 minutes and gently manipulate the displaced fracture to achieve satisfactory reduction.

Complications

- Infection, since a closed wound is converted to an open wound.
- For the distal radius—compartment syndrome, temporary paralysis of the interosseous nerve and carpal tunnel syndrome.
- Introduction of anaesthetic agent into the circulation with potential arrhythmias and seizures.

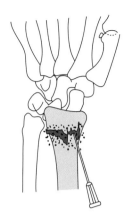

Fig. 2.20 Haematoma block: Illustration of injecting anaesthetic into the site of a Colles fracture

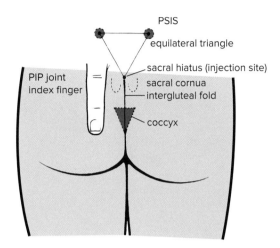

Fig. 2.21 Identify the sacral hiatus by four methods:
1. Palpating the sacral cornua.
2. Noting the upper limit of the intergluteal fold.
3. Measuring the tip of the coccyx to the PIP of the index finger.
4. Drawing an equilateral triangle with the base being the line between the postero-superior iliac spines.[5]

Reproduced from C. Kenna & J. Murtagh, *Back Pain and Spinal Manipulation*, Butterworths, Sydney, 1989, with permission.

THE CAUDAL (TRANS-SACRAL) INJECTION

An epidural injection is the appropriate way to treat persistent painful sciatica without neurological signs in a patient who is not a candidate for surgery but is making slow progress.

The lumbar epidural is technically more difficult than the caudal epidural and requires hospital day care. The caudal epidural is safer and within the skill of any medical practitioner. It can be performed in a general practice procedure treatment room with resuscitation facilities. The key to success is to identify the sacral hiatus and insert a needle (usually a 21- or 22-gauge, 36 mm needle is sufficient for most patients) at the appropriate angle in a cranial direction.

Identifying the sacral hiatus

The sacral hiatus can be identified in the following ways:
- Palpate the two sacral cornua and mark the hiatus at the top end of the hollow formed by the cornua.
- It lies directly beneath the upper limit of the intergluteal fold.
- It tends to correspond to the proximal interphalangeal (PIP) joint with the tip of the index finger resting on the tip of the coccyx.
- It lies at the caudal apex of an equilateral triangle drawn with the horizontal base between the posterior superior iliac spines (PSIS) (opposite S2). This apex is usually situated over the sacral hiatus (Fig. 2.21).

LOCAL ANAESTHETIC USE

Use 15–20 mL of half-strength solution (without adrenaline) of any of the local anaesthetics, such as plain lidocaine, procaine or bupivacaine. Corticosteroid is not necessary.

Injection procedure

Method

1. Inform the patient that the procedure is surprisingly comfortable but that some heaviness will be felt in the back of the legs and that pain may be initially exacerbated.
2. Mark the sacral hiatus after its identification.
3. Lie the patient prone with a pillow under the symphysis pubis to slightly flex the hips (or with the operating table 'broken').
4. Relax the glutei by inversion of the ankles (feet in pigeon-toe position).
5. Clean and drape the area, avoiding spirit running onto the anus. Using a 23- or 25-gauge needle, anaesthetise the skin and subcutaneous tissue.
6. Select a spinal tap cannula: 21-, 22- or 23-gauge 50 mm or a 21-gauge 38 mm standard single-use needle (preferred).
7. Insert the needle upwards (cranially) keeping strictly to the midline. The angle to the skin should be about 25–30° (Fig. 2.22); if too superficial, the needle will pass above the hiatus. When the ligament is pierced there is a sensation of 'giving'.
8. Angle the needle slightly downwards as you insert it for about 2 cm. Avoid proceeding any further because of the risk of piercing the dura.
9. Rotate the needle through 90° twice—check for a back flow of cerebrospinal fluid (CSF) or blood. If blood is obtained, partly withdraw the needle and reinsert

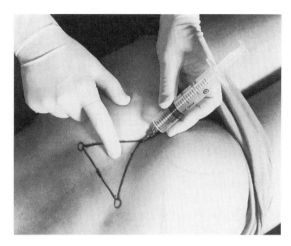

Fig. 2.22 The caudal epidural: the appearance of the procedure

it, keeping as far posterior as possible to avoid the greater concentration of veins anteriorly. If CSF is withdrawn, abandon the procedure.

10. Inject the fluid carefully and slowly over a 5-minute period (at least) with at least three aspiration checks for blood. The plunger of the syringe should move with relative ease.

11. Ask the patient to report any unusual symptoms such as giddiness or light-headedness, which is reasonably common but indicates a need for caution. Monitor the pulse and blood pressure during the procedure and stop the injection if an adverse reaction develops.

The injection can be repeated if the patient experiences a good, albeit temporary, result.

HORMONE IMPLANTS

Suitable sites for the subcutaneous insertion of crystalline pellets of the hormones, such as testosterone into the abdominal wall, are shown in Figure 2.23a. The preferred sites are in the anterior abdominal wall above and parallel to the inguinal ligament. A site just superolateral to the pubic hair is ideal.

The procedure is performed under local anaesthesia using a wide-bore trocar and cannula. It is simple and effective, and takes a few minutes only.

Equipment

You will need:

- 2–5 mL of 1% lidocaine with syringe
- povidone-iodine 10% antiseptic
- wide-bore trocar and cannula (use an expellor if available)
- scalpel with no. 11 (or similar) blade
- crystalline pellets (that will fit into the cannula)
- sterile gauze or suitable container, for 'catching' a dropped pellet
- sterile adhesive strips.

Method

To insert the hormone implants:

1. Choose the implantation site.
2. Infiltrate the sterilised skin with LA so that a small bleb is raised.
3. Make a small incision 5–10 mm long with the scalpel blade.
4. Insert the trocar and cannula through the incised skin at a shallow angle (Fig. 2.23b) for at least 2 cm. The end of the cannula now rests in a pocket in the subcutaneous tissue (care should be taken to avoid the rectus sheath).
5. Remove the trocar.
6. Grasp a pellet with sterile forceps and place it in the cannula.

Note: This part of the procedure is the most delicate because the pellet is likely to be accidentally dropped. Have an assistant standing by with a sterile receptacle or gauze to catch it.

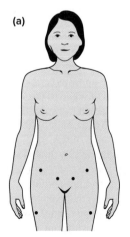

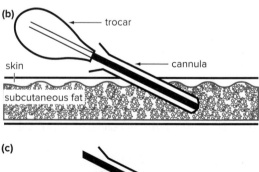

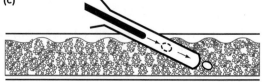

Fig. 2.23 **(a)** Suitable sites for insertion of pellets; **(b)** trocar and cannula are angulated into subcutaneous tissue after initial, more upright entry; **(c)** shows pellet in cannula pushed gently into place with expellor

7. Reinsert the trocar or expellor (ideally the expellor should extend 5 mm beyond the end of the cannula) and push the pellet into the subcutaneous 'pocket' (Fig. 2.23c).
8. The cannula and trocar (or expellor) are removed while maintaining pressure over the site for 1 minute to minimise bruising.
9. Apply sterile adhesive strips (or a suture) over the wound and then a light dressing.

Precaution: Ensure that you have the correct hormone for the correct patient and record the batch number.

Implanon®

Note: Implanon is usually inserted in the inside and middle of the arm about 8–10 cm above the medial epicondyle of the humerus. It is important that training in insertion is undertaken in this method. For removal, see Chapter 10.

Musculoskeletal injections

MUSCULOSKELETAL INJECTION GUIDELINES

Conditions that are considerably relieved by injections include:
- rotator cuff tendinopathy, especially supraspinatus tendinopathy
- subacromial bursitis
- bicipital tendinopathy
- lateral and medial epicondylitis
- trigger finger and thumb
- trochanteric bursalgia and gluteus medius tendinopathy
- tendinopathy around the wrist, e.g. de Quervain tenosynovitis
- plantar fasciitis
- knee conditions—anserinus tendinopathy/bursitis, biceps femoris tendinopathy.

Rules and guidelines

- Use any one of the depot (long acting) corticosteroid formulations: betamethasone (Celestone Chronodose), triamcinolone (Kenocort–A10 or A40) or methylprednisolone (Depo-Medrol, Depo-Nisolone).
- Use the more soluble formulation (Celestone Chrondose) for tendon sheath injection.
- Use a mixture of 1 mL of long-acting corticosteroid (CS) with 1% lidocaine (0.5–8 mL) for most injections.
- Conditions not very responsive and best avoided include patellar tendinopathy and Achilles tendinopathy.
- Conditions responsive for about 3 weeks only include epicondylitis and plantar fasciitis.
- Trochanteric bursalgia or gluteus medius tendinopathy is common, misdiagnosed often and responds exceptionally well to 1 mL CS + 8 mL lidocaine 1%.
- All injections of local anaesthetic use plain preparations (without adrenaline) unless otherwise specified.
- Corticosteroids are not very effective for trigger spots of the back.
- A subacromial space injection will be effective for most rotator cuff problems.
- Use corticosteroid without local anaesthetic for carpal tunnel injections and small joints.
- Intra-articular injections for arthritic joints have limited use: perhaps 2 to 3 times for osteoarthritis—best for monarticular rheumatoid arthritis.

- For soft tissue injections, avoid repeating under 6 weeks and use a maximum of four in 12 months.
- Tendons should never be injected; inject tendon sheaths but with caution because of the danger of rupture.
- Always aspirate before injecting into soft tissue to avoid injecting into a blood vessel.
- Contraindications include local and systemic infection, bleeding disorders and lack of informed consent.
- Warn the patient about potential adverse effects of corticosteroids, including tendon rupture and skin atrophy.
- Maintain a strict aseptic technique.
- An alternative to marking the injection point with a pen (which may wash off after wiping) is to press firmly with the tip of a sterile plastic needle cap to indent the skin for a couple of minutes.

INJECTION OF TRIGGER POINTS IN BACK

The injection of painful myofascial trigger points of the back and neck (Fig. 2.24) is relatively easy and may give excellent results. A trigger point is one characterised by:
- circumscribed local tenderness
- localised twitching with stimulation of juxtaposed muscle
- pain referred elsewhere when subjected to pressure.

Don't: use large volumes of LA; use corticosteroids; cause bleeding.

Do: use a moderate amount of LA (only).

Method

1. Identify and mark the trigger point, which must be the maximal point of pain.
2. Select a 21-, 22- or 23-gauge needle of a length compatible with the injection site. (A 38 mm needle will cover most areas of the back and neck.)
3. Insert the needle into the point until the patient complains of reproduction of pain, which may be referred distally.
4. At this point, introduce 5–8 mL of plain LA of your choice. (Lidocaine, procaine or bupivacaine 1% or 0.5% can be used.)
5. Recommend post-injection exercises and local massage for the affected segment.

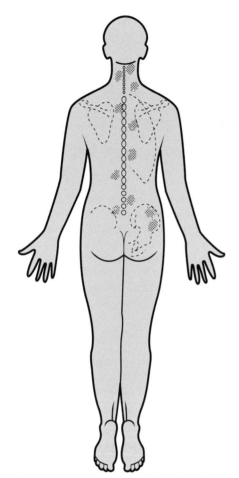

Fig. 2.24 Typical trigger points of the back[5]

Reproduced from C. Kenna & J. Murtagh, *Back Pain and Spinal Manipulation*, Butterworths, Sydney, 1989, with permission.

INJECTION FOR ROTATOR CUFF LESIONS

Injections of local anaesthetic and corticosteroid produce excellent results for inflammatory disorders around the shoulder joint, especially for supraspinatus tendinopathy. The best results are obtained with precise localisation of the area of inflammation, although injections into the subacromial space are all that is necessary to reach inflammatory lesions of the tendons comprising the rotator cuff and the subacromial bursa. Preliminary ultrasound diagnosis for shoulder lesions is recommended, but ultrasound is not required during the procedure.

The subacromial space injection for rotator cuff lesions (especially with impingement)

The recommended approach is from the posterolateral aspect of the shoulder, with the patient sitting upright.

Method

1. Draw up 1 mL of corticosteroid and 5–6 mL of 1% lidocaine.
2. Sit the patient upright and explain the procedure in general terms.
3. Identify the soft gap between the acromion and the humeral head with the palpating finger or thumb.
4. Mark this spot, about 2 cm below the edge of the acromion.
5. Swab the area with antiseptic.
6. Place the needle (23-gauge, 32 or 38 mm long) into this gap, 2 cm inferior to the acromion (Fig. 2.25).
7. Aim the needle so that it is felt passing beneath the acromion.
8. Insert for a distance of about 30 mm. The solution should flow into the subacromial space without resistance.

Tip: Place a weight (0.5–1 kg) in the hand nearest to the affected side to facilitate opening the subacromial space. It also distracts the patient!

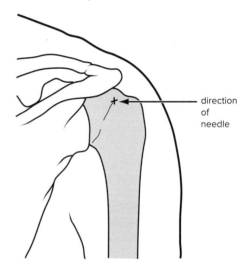

direction of needle

Fig. 2.25 Posterior view of the subacromial bursa injection site

The subacromial space injection for subacromial bursitis

The lateral approach is used for localised bursitis when there is localised tenderness over the subacromial space. It is important to angle the needle into the appropriate anatomical plane.

Method

1. Identify the lateral edge of the acromion and select the midpoint.
2. Insert the needle 10 mm below the edge of the acromion and angle it upwards at about 10° between the head of the humerus and the acromion.
3. Inject 1 mL of corticosteroid and 5–6 mL of 1% LA.

INJECTION FOR SUPRASPINATUS TENDINOPATHY

An injection directed onto the inflamed tendon of supraspinatus is so effective that it is preferable to administer a specific injection rather than a general infiltration into the subacromial space.

The tendon can be readily palpated as a tender cord anterolaterally as it emerges from beneath the acromion to attach to the greater tuberosity of the humerus. This identification is assisted by depressing the shoulder via a downward pull on the arm and then externally and internally rotating the humerus. This manoeuvre allows the examiner to locate the tendon readily.

Method

1. Identify and mark the tendon.
2. Place the patient's arm behind the back, with the back of the hand touching the far waistline. This locates the arm in the desired internal rotation and forces the humeral head anteriorly.
3. Insert a 23-gauge 32 mm needle under the acromion along the line of the tendon, and inject around the tendon just under the acromion (Fig. 2.26). If the gritty resistance of the tendon is encountered, slightly withdraw the needle to ensure that it lies in the tendon sheath and not the tendon.
4. The recommended injection is 1 mL of long-acting corticosteroid with 2 mL of LA.

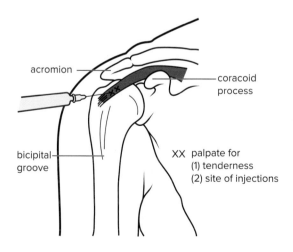

Fig. 2.26 Injection placement for supraspinatus tendinopathy

INJECTION FOR BICIPITAL TENDINOPATHY

Bicipital tendinopathy is diagnosed by finding an abnormal tenderness over the tendon when the arm is externally rotated. The usual site is the bicipital groove of the humeral head.

Method

1. The patient sits with the arm hanging by the side and the palm facing forwards.
2. Find and mark the site of maximal tenderness. This is usually in the bicipital groove and more proximal than expected.
3. Insert a 23-gauge needle at the proximal end of the bicipital groove above the tender area.
4. Slide the needle down the groove to reach the tender area (Fig. 2.27).
5. Inject 1 mL of long-acting corticosteroid and 2 mL of LA around this site.

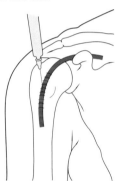

Fig. 2.27 Injection placement for bicipital tendinopathy

INJECTIONS FOR EPICONDYLITIS
Lateral epicondylitis (tennis elbow)

The key to successful injections is to have the tender lesion pinpointed precisely. The point of maximal tenderness is usually on or just distal to the lateral epicondyle, which coincides with 1–2 square cm of degenerate tendon. Warn the patient about the risk of skin thinning.

Equipment

You will need:
- an antiseptic swab
- a 25- or 23-gauge needle
- 1 mL of long-acting corticosteroid and 2 mL of LA (e.g. 1% lidocaine). Use a mixed solution (LA drawn last) in a 5 mL syringe.

Method

1. The patient sits with the elbow resting on a table, flexed to a right angle and fully supinated.

2. Using an anterior approach, palpate the tender area and mark it with a pen.
3. With the thumb (of the non-dominant hand) over the patient's lateral epicondyle and the fingers spread out around the elbow to steady it, insert the needle vertically downward to touch the periosteum of the tender point (Fig. 2.28).
4. After introducing about 0.5 mL of the mixed solution, partly withdraw the needle and reinsert it to ensure that the tender area is covered both deeply and superficially. Inject over at least two sites. A deeper injection minimises the risk of skin atrophy.

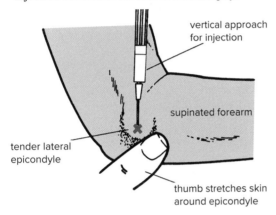

Fig. 2.28 Injection technique for tennis elbow

Post-injection

1. Ask the patient to 'work it in' during the next few hours with repeated extensions of the elbow joint and pronation of the wrist.
2. Warn the patient that the area will be painful for the next 24 hours and recommend moderately strong analgesics.
3. Repeat the injection in 2 to 4 weeks unless all the symptoms have been abolished.
4. A maximum of two injections only is recommended.

Medial epicondylitis (golfer's elbow)

A similar method is used to that for lateral epicondylitis. The elbow is flexed to about 45° and supinated with full external rotation of the shoulder of the affected arm. The anterior approach is used, and the tender area of the medial epicondyle injected as for lateral epicondylitis. Take care not to inject the ulnar nerve, which lies posterior and close to the medial epicondyle. It can be felt to move with flexion and extension of the elbow. Keep your finger over the nerve as you inject the usual 3 mL of mixed solution.

INJECTION FOR TRIGGER FINGER

Treatment of trigger finger or thumb by injection is often very successful, and usually relieves symptoms for a considerable period of time. The injection is made under the tendon sheath and not into the tendon or its nodular swelling. The fourth (ring) and middle fingers are most commonly affected.

There are three possible injection approaches: proximal, distal and mid-lateral. Distal is preferred.

Method (distal palmar approach)

1. The patient sits facing the doctor with the palm of the affected hand facing upward.
2. Draw 1 mL of long-acting corticosteroid solution and 0.5–1 mL LA into a syringe and attach a 23- or 25-gauge needle for the injection.
3. Insert the needle at an angle distal to the nodule and direct it proximally within the tendon sheath (Fig. 2.29). This requires tension on the skin with free fingers. To avoid injecting into the tendon, flex and extend the finger and ensure that the needle does not move.
4. By palpating the tendon sheath, you can (usually) feel when the fluid has entered the tendon sheath.
5. Inject 0.5–1 mL of the solution, withdraw the needle and ask the patient to exercise the fingers for 1 minute.

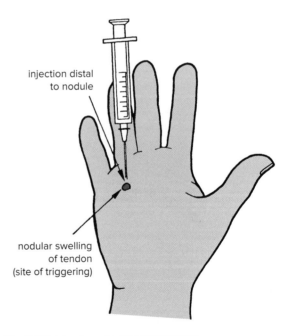

Fig. 2.29 Injection site for trigger finger

Method (proximal palmar approach)

Insert the needle about 1 cm proximal to the nodule and angle it to lie in the tendon sheath over the nodule. Flex the finger to confirm that it is the correct position. If the needle is in the tendon, withdraw it a fraction before injecting the solution.

Method (mid-lateral approach)

This approach uses a lateral approach at the level of the proximal phalanx and about 1 cm lateral to the anterior surface of the finger. Direct the needle towards the nodule and inject over the tendon. The fourth and fifth fingers are approached from the ulnar side and the second and third fingers from the radial side.

Post-injection

Improvement usually occurs after 48 hours and may be permanent. The injection can be repeated after 6 to 8 weeks if the triggering is not completely relieved.

If triggering recurs, surgery is indicated. This involves division of the thickened tendon sheath only.

INJECTION FOR TRIGGER THUMB

The injection for the trigger thumb follows a similar principle to the trigger finger but it is more difficult. With the hand rotated radially and the thumb extended, approach the nodule from the palmar (volar) aspect and inject into the tendon sheath just proximal to the nodule (Fig. 2.30).

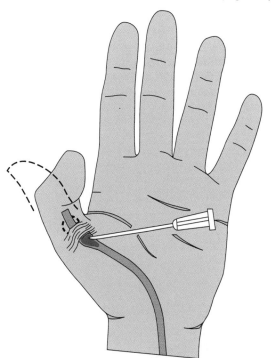

Fig. 2.30 Trigger thumb showing site of injection

INJECTION FOR TENOSYNOVITIS OF THE WRIST

Tenosynovitis of the wrist, especially that of the thumb abductors (de Quervain stenosing tenosynovitis), is a common problem that can readily be identified by tenderness, swelling and palpable crepitus over the tendon. It may respond to an injection of a long-acting corticosteroid, but care should be taken to inject the suspension into the tendon sheath rather than into the tendon. Warn the patient about the risk of skin atrophy.

Method for de Quervain tenosynovitis

1. Identify and mark the most tender site of the tendon and the line of the tendon. Draw up 1 mL each of LA and corticosteroid.
2. Thoroughly cleanse the skin with an antiseptic, such as povidone-iodine 10% solution.
3. Insert the tip of the needle (21-gauge) about 1 cm distal to the point of maximal tenderness and about 1 cm proximal to the radial styloid (Fig. 2.31).
4. Advance the needle almost parallel to the skin along the line of the tendon.
5. Inject about 0.5 mL of the corticosteroid suspension into the tendon sheath. If the needle is in the sheath, very little resistance to the plunger should be felt and the injection will cause the tendon sheath to billow out. Complete the injection of 2 mL.

Alternative method

1. Advance the needle into the tendon, where there will be resistance to the attempted injection in addition to a firm, gritty feel to the needle.
2. Slowly withdraw the needle until the resistance to depressing the plunger disappears.
3. Inject the corticosteroid.

The ideal site for this injection is into the sheath of the abductor tendons to the thumb just above the radial styloid. It is important, therefore, to avoid injecting into the radial artery, which should always be identified beforehand.

Note: It should be emphasised that the common problem of de Quervain disease (also known as 'washerwoman's sprain') is best treated by resting and avoiding the causative stresses and strains on the thumb abductors.

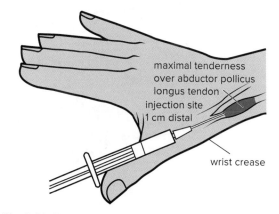

maximal tenderness over abductor pollicus longus tendon

injection site

1 cm distal

wrist crease

Fig. 2.31 Tendon sheath injection

INJECTION FOR PLANTAR FASCIITIS

Plantar fasciitis can be treated by injecting local anaesthetic and long-acting corticosteroid into the site of maximal tenderness in the heel. An alternative is to inject the corticosteroid into the anaesthetised heel. On the other hand, to minimise the pain of injecting through the heel, apply liquid nitrogen beforehand and immediately inject through that spot.

Method

1. Perform a tibial nerve block. (The area of maximal tenderness should be marked prior to the nerve block.) Refer to Figure 2.14.
2. When anaesthesia of the heel is present (about 10 minutes after the tibial nerve block), insert a 23-gauge needle with 1 mL of long-acting corticosteroid perpendicular to the sole of the foot at the premarked site (Fig. 2.32). Insert the needle until a 'give' is felt as the plantar fascia is pierced.
3. Inject half the steroid against the periosteum in the space between the fascia and the calcaneus.
4. Reposition the needle to infiltrate into the fascial attachments over a wider area.

Alternative approach

For the non-anaesthetised heel, introduce the needle containing 3–4 mL of LA with steroid into the softer part of the heel medially and guide it to the most tender site.

Tip for plantar fasciitis: Massage the sole of the foot over a wooden foot massager, golf ball, bottle filled with water or frozen water bottle for 5 minutes daily to help prevent recurrence (refer to Chapter 7).

INJECTION FOR TROCHANTERIC BURSALGIA

Pain around the greater trochanter

Pain around the lateral aspect of the hip is a common disorder, and is usually seen as lateral hip pain radiating down the lateral aspect of the thigh in older people engaged in walking exercises, tennis and similar activities. It is analogous in a way to the shoulder girdle, where supraspinatus tendinopathy and subacromial bursitis are common wear-and-tear injuries.

The two presumed common causes are tendinopathy of the gluteus medius tendon, where it inserts into the lateral surface of the greater trochanter of the femur, and bursitis of one or both of the trochanteric bursae. Distinction between these two conditions is difficult, and it is possible that, as with the shoulder, both are related. The pain of bursitis tends to occur at night when lying on the affected side; that of tendinopathy occurs with such activity as long walks and gardening.

Method

Treatment for both is similar.
1. Determine the points of maximal tenderness over the trochanteric region and mark them. (For tendinopathy, this point is immediately over or above the superior aspect of the greater trochanter; see Fig. 2.33.)
2. Keeping the needle perpendicular to the skin, direct it down to the point of maximal tenderness until the underlying bone is touched; withdraw about 2 mm before injecting.
3. Inject aliquots of a mixture of 1 mL of long-acting corticosteroid with 5–8 mL of LA into the tender area, which usually occupies an area similar to that of a standard marble.

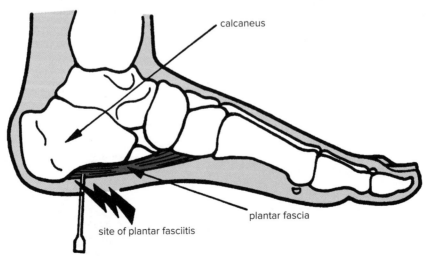

Fig. 2.32 Injection approach in plantar fasciitis

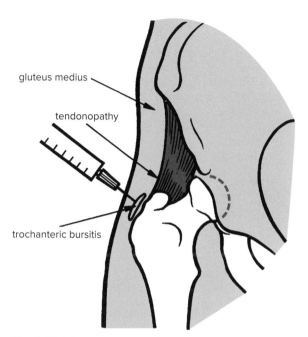

Fig. 2.33 Injection technique for gluteus medius tendinopathy (into area of maximal tenderness)

The injection is invariably very effective. Follow-up management includes sleeping with a small pillow under the involved buttock, and stretching the gluteal muscles with knee–chest exercises. One, two or three repeat injections over 12 months may be required. Surgical intervention may be necessary for a severe persistent problem but is best avoided. A more precise injection can be given under ultrasound guidance.

Extra tips to alleviate pain

- Local application of cold pack if acute.
- Perform straight-leg stretching in dependent adduction (see Fig. 11.63).
- Develop a 'Charlie Chaplin' gait—legs in external rotation for walking.
- Massage lateral thigh for 2 to 5 minutes daily using a glass or plastic (preferably grooved) bottle, full of water, as a rolling pin.

INJECTION OF THE CARPAL TUNNEL

An injection of long-acting corticosteroid into the carpal tunnel may relieve symptoms permanently or, more commonly, temporarily. It may therefore be useful as a diagnostic test and also to provide symptomatic relief while awaiting surgery.

Note: The injections may be repeated. Do not use local anaesthetic in the injection.

Method

1. The patient sits by the side of the doctor with the hand palm upward, the wrist slightly extended (a crepe bandage under the wrist helps this extension).
2. Identify the palmaris longus tendon, which lies above the median nerve (best done by flexing the wrist against resistance or opposing the thumb with the little finger) and the ulnar artery.
3. Insert the needle (23-gauge) at a point about 2 cm proximal to the main transverse crease of the wrist and midway between the palmaris longus tendon and the flexor carpi ulnaris or the ulnar artery (Fig. 2.34). Take care to avoid the superficial veins.
4. Advance the needle distally, parallel to the tendons and nerve at about 25° to the horizontal. It should pass under the transverse carpal ligament (flexor retinaculum) and come to lie in the carpal tunnel.
   Note: The needle can be slightly bent to facilitate entry.

(a)

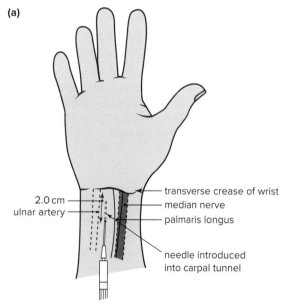

(b)

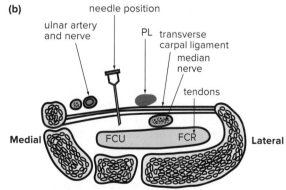

Fig. 2.34 Needle introduced into carpal tunnel:
(a) anterior view; **(b)** section

5. Inject 1 mL of corticosteroid. This is usually painless and runs freely. Place the free thumb proximal to the needle and apply pressure to facilitate flow of fluid distally. Ensure that the patient feels no severe pain or paraesthesia during the injection. If so, immediately withdraw the needle. The medial nerve lies below and between the palmaris longus and the flexor carpi radialis tendons.

6. Withdraw the needle and ask the patient to flex and extend the fingers for 2 minutes. Remind the patient that there may be pain for up to 48 hours and to rest the arm for 24 hours.

INJECTION NEAR THE CARPAL TUNNEL

A study[6] recommended giving a single injection of corticosteroid, e.g. 40 mg methylprednisolone with lidocaine 1%, close to but not into the tunnel (to avoid potential damage to the median nerve). The results were considered to be as good as giving it into the tunnel.

INJECTION OF THE TARSAL TUNNEL

Tarsal tunnel syndrome is caused by an entrapment neuropathy of the posterior tibial nerve in the tarsal tunnel beneath the flexor retinaculum on the medial side of the ankle (Fig. 2.35). The condition, which is uncommon, is due to dislocation or fracture around the ankle or tenosynovitis of tendons in the tunnel from injury, rheumatoid arthritis and other inflammations.

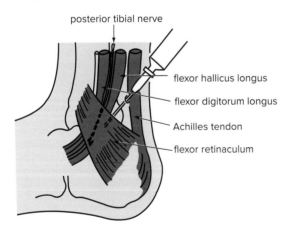

posterior tibial nerve
flexor hallicus longus
flexor digitorum longus
Achilles tendon
flexor retinaculum

Fig. 2.35 Sites of injection for tarsal tunnel syndrome (above or below the flexor retinaculum that roofs the 'tunnel'). This medial view of the right foot shows the relationship of the posterior tibial nerve to the tendons.

Symptoms and signs

- A burning or tingling pain in the toes and sole of the foot, occasionally the heel.
- Retrograde radiation to the calf.
- Discomfort often in bed at night and worse after standing.
- Removal of the shoe may give relief.
- Sensory nerve loss is variable (may be no loss).
- The Tinel test (finger or reflex hammer tap over the nerve below and behind the medial malleolus) may be positive.
- A tourniquet applied above the ankle may reproduce symptoms.
   The diagnosis is confirmed by electrodiagnosis.

Treatment

- Relief of abnormal foot posture with orthotics.
- Corticosteroid injection.
- Decompression surgery if other measures fail.

Injection method

Using a 23-gauge 32 mm needle, inject a mixture of corticosteroid in 1% xylocaine or procaine into the tunnel either from above or below the flexor retinaculum. The sites of injection are shown in Figure 2.35. Be careful not to inject the nerve.

INJECTION FOR ACHILLES PARATENDINOPATHY

Management

Inflammation of and around the tendon can be a resistant problem, and conservative measures such as rest, a heel raise and NSAIDs should be adopted. As a rule, injections around the Achilles tendon should be avoided but for resistant painful problems an injection of corticosteroid can be helpful. The inflammation must be localised, such as a tender 2 cm area.

   Avoid giving the corticosteroid injection in the acute stages and never lodge it in the tendon.

Method

1. Mark the area of paratendinopathy, which usually lies immediately anterior and deep to the tendon just above the calcaneus.
2. Infiltrate this tender area adjacent to the tendon with 1 mL of plain local anaesthetic (e.g. 1% lidocaine) and 1 mL of long-acting corticosteroid (Fig. 2.36). The solution should run freely, and care should be taken to avoid the tendon.

INJECTION FOR TIBIALIS POSTERIOR TENDINOPATHY

This is a common and under-diagnosed condition in people presenting with foot and ankle pain, especially on the medial side.

   It is usually found in middle-aged females, in ballet dancers and in those with flat feet with a valgus deformity.

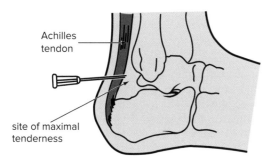

Fig. 2.36 Usual approach for the injection of Achilles paratendinopathy

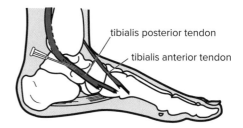

Fig. 2.37 Method of injecting the tendon sheath of tibialis posterior

Pain is reproduced on:
- palpation anterior and inferior to the medial malleolus
- stretching by passive inversion of the foot
- resisted inversion of the foot.

Tibialis posterior tendinopathy can cause the tarsal tunnel syndrome. The diagnosis can be confirmed by ultrasound imaging.

Preferred treatment
- Conservative with inversion/eversion exercises
- Orthotics

Method of injection

Reserved for painful recalcitrant cases.
1. Mark the tender area of the tendon.
2. Use a lower-gauge needle with a syringe containing 0.5–1 mL LA corticosteroid with 0.5–1 mL local anaesthetic.
3. Approach the tendon at a very shallow angle, either proximally or distally, and inject into the sheath, taking care to avoid injecting the tendon (Fig. 2.37).
   Note: The tibialis posterior tendon is prone to rupture.

INJECTION OR ASPIRATION OF JOINTS

Intra-articular injections of corticosteroids can be very therapeutic for some acute inflammatory conditions, particularly severe synovitis caused by rheumatoid arthritis (especially monarticular rheumatoid arthritis). The common indication for the glenohumeral joint of the shoulder is adhesive capsulitis, although hydrodilatation under imaging is the preferred method. This use is limited in osteoarthritis but can be very effective for a particularly severe flare-up of osteoarthritis such as in the knee or the acromioclavicular joint. Corticosteroids can cause degeneration of articular cartilage and hence restricted usage is important. Strict asepsis is essential, using disposable equipment.

Acromioclavicular joint
Method

1. The patient sits with the arm hanging loosely by the side and externally rotated. The joint space is palpable just distal (lateral) to the bony enlargement of the clavicle. It is about 2 cm medial to the lateral edge of the acromion.
2. Palpate the 'gap' for maximal tenderness.
3. Insert a 25-gauge needle, which should be angled according to the different surfaces encountered (Fig. 2.38). It may be helpful to 'walk' the needle along the acromion to get the feel of the joint. It should reach a depth of about 0.5–1 cm when it is certainly intra-articular.
4. Inject a mixture of 0.25–0.5 mL of corticosteroid with 0.25–0.5 mL of 1% lidocaine.

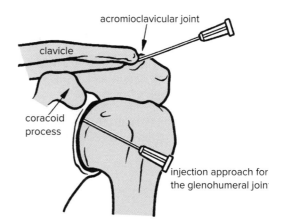

Fig. 2.38 Approaches for injections into the acromioclavicular joint and the glenohumeral joint of the shoulder

Shoulder (glenohumeral) joint
Method 1: Anterior approach

1. The patient sits in the same position as for the acromioclavicular joint injection.

2. Use an anterior approach and insert a 21- to 23-gauge needle just medial to the head of the humerus. Feel for the space between the head of the humerus and the glenoid cap. (If in doubt, feel for it by rotating the humerus externally or alternating external and internal rotation.)
3. This insertion should also be 1 cm below and just lateral to the coracoid process (Fig. 2.38). Then aim the needle posteriorly towards the glenoid fossa.
4. Inject a mixture of 1 mL of corticosteroid and 1 mL of 1% lidocaine.

Method 2: Posterior approach

This uses the same approach as for the posterior injection into the subacromial space, that is, into the 'soft spot' 2 cm inferior to and 1 cm medial to the edge of the acromion.

Aim the needle to the tip of the coronoid process and inject when the joint space is reached.

Elbow joint

Intra-articular injections may alleviate synovitis, either arthritic or post-traumatic.

The objective is to inject the solution into the middle of the joint by identifying the soft entry point near the middle of the isosceles triangle formed by the lateral epicondyle, the radial head and the tip of the olecranon (Fig. 2.39).

Method

1. The patient sits with the elbow flexed to 70–90° and the wrist pronated.
2. Mark the three key points of the triangle and palpate the soft entry point.
3. Using a posterolateral approach, insert a 23-gauge needle with 1 mL of steroid and 2 mL of local anaesthetic into the space.
4. The needle should easily enter the joint. Aim for the middle of the joint and to a depth of about 2 cm. A slight readjustment of the needle may be necessary.

Wrist joint

Method

Inject on the dorsal surface in the space just distal to the ulnar head at its midpoint.
1. Palpate the space between the ulnar head and the lunate.
2. Insert the needle at right angles to the skin between the extensor tendons of the fourth and fifth fingers.
3. Insert to a depth of about 1 cm.
4. Inject 0.5 mL of corticosteroid and 0.5 mL of 1% lidocaine.

First carpometacarpal joint of thumb

Method

1. Palpate the proximal margin of the first metacarpal in the anatomical snuffbox.
2. Insert the needle to a depth of about 1 cm between the long extensor and long abductor tendons into the joint space.
3. Inject 0.5 mL of corticosteroid.

Finger joint

The technique for injections of the metacarpophalangeal and interphalangeal joints is similar.

Method

It is important to have an assistant for this injection.
1. The joint is flexed to an angle of 30°, and this position is maintained by the assistant who simultaneously applies longitudinal traction to 'gap' the dorsal aspect of the joint.
2. Insert the needle, which is kept at right angles to the base of the more distal phalanx, from the dorsal aspect in the midline.
3. Direct the needle through the tendon of extensor digitorum just distal to the head of the more proximal bone (phalanx or metacarpal) to a depth of 3–5 mm (Fig. 2.40).

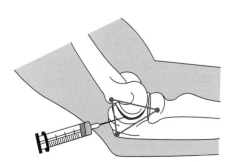

Fig. 2.39 Injection into the centre of triangular space of the elbow joint

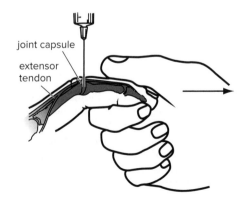

joint capsule

extensor tendon

Fig. 2.40 Injection of the proximal interphalangeal joint

Hip joint

Method

1. The patient lies supine with the hip in extension and internal rotation.
2. Use an anterior approach, with the insertion point being 2.5 cm below the inguinal ligament and 2 cm lateral to the femoral artery.
3. Use a 20-gauge 6–7 cm needle and insert it at about 60° to the skin.
4. Introduce the needle downwards and medially until bone is reached (Fig. 2.41).
5. Withdraw it slightly and inject the mixture of 1 mL of corticosteroid and 2 mL of 1% lidocaine.

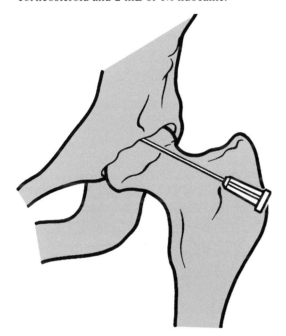

Fig. 2.41 Injection approach for the hip joint

Knee joint

Injections can be given into one of four 'safe' zones at the four corners of the patella.

Method for infrapatellar route (inferior safe zone)

1. The patient flexes the knee to a right angle. (The patient can sit on the couch with the leg over the side.) Alternatively, the knee can be extended with the quadriceps relaxed.
2. A 21-gauge needle can be inserted either medially (preferably) or laterally.
3. Insert the needle in the triangular space bounded by the femoral condyle, the tibial condyle and the patellar ligament (Fig. 2.42).
4. Direct the needle inwards and slightly posteriorly in a plane pointing slightly upwards to the horizontal (to avoid the infrapatellar fat pad).

5. Inject 1 mL of LA corticosteroid (an anaesthetic agent isn't necessary).

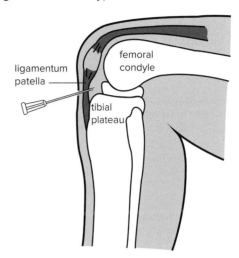

Fig. 2.42 Injection of the knee joint (note the needle angled into the triangular space)

Temporomandibular joint

This injection is useful in the treatment of painful rheumatoid arthritis, osteoarthritis or temporomandibular joint dysfunction that is not responding to conservative measures.

Method

1. The patient sits on a chair, facing away from the doctor. The mouth is opened to at least 4 cm.
2. Palpate the joint line anterior to the tragus of the ear. This is confirmed by opening and closing the jaw.
3. Insert a 25-gauge needle into the depression above the condyle of the mandible, below the zygomatic arch and one finger breadth (2 cm) anterior to the tragus.
4. Direct the needle inwards and slightly upwards so that it is free within the joint cavity (Fig. 2.43).
5. Inject the 1 mL solution containing 0.5 mL of local anaesthetic and 0.5 mL of corticosteroid, which should flow freely.

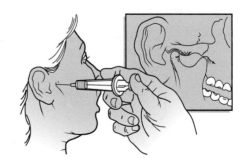

Fig. 2.43 Injection of the temporomandibular joint

ACUTE GOUT IN THE GREAT TOE

Injection technique

Acute gouty arthritis invariably presents with exquisite pain in the great toe and the diagnosis and relief of pain is a special challenge to the general practitioner.

An effective and caring, albeit invasive, treatment is as follows:

- Perform a modified digital block using 1% plain local anaesthetic to the affected toe.
- When anaesthesia has been obtained, use a 19-gauge needle to aspirate fluid from the joint or the periarticular region.
- Examine the fluid under polarised light microscopy. The presence of long, needle-shaped urate crystals is diagnostic.
- If sepsis is eliminated, inject corticosteroids, e.g. 0.5–1.0 mL of triamcinolone, into the joint (Fig. 2.44).

Drug treatment

Two NSAIDs options are usually employed, one a heavier dosage than the other. Indomethacin is the preferred one but others can be used.

Conventional method

Indomethacin 50 mg (o) 8 hourly for 24 hours, then 25 mg (o) 6 hourly until resolution.

'Shock' method

Indomethacin 100 mg (o) statim, 75 mg 2 hours later, then 50 mg (o) 8 hourly (relief is usual within 48 hours)
plus
Metoclopramide (Maxolon) 10 mg (o) 8 hourly (or other anti-emetic).

Other corticosteroids

- Prednisolone 50 mg/day for 3 to 5 days
  or
- Corticotrophin (ACTH) IM
- Colchicine
  Consider if NSAIDs are not tolerated.
  0.5–1.0 mg statim, then 0.5 mg every 2 hours until pain disappears or GIT side effects develop.

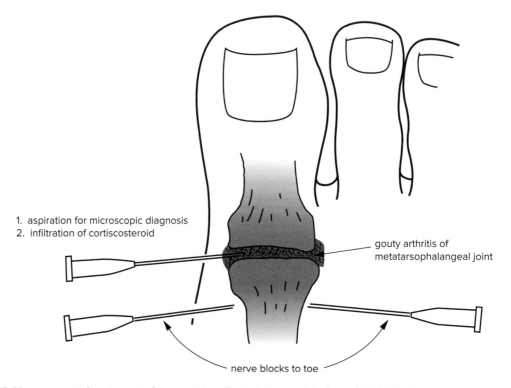

1. aspiration for microscopic diagnosis
2. infiltration of cortiscosteroid

gouty arthritis of metatarsophalangeal joint

nerve blocks to toe

Fig. 2.44 Management of acute gout of the great toe, illustrating nerve blocks and joint injection

References

1. Penfield W, Boldrey E. Somatic motor and sensory representation in the cerebral cortex of man as studied by electrical stimulation. Brain, 1937; 60: 389–443.
2. Claesson M, Short R. Lancet with less pain. Lancet, 1990; December 22–9: 1566–7.
3. Mohan PP. Epinephrine in digital nerve block. Emergency Medicine Journal, 2007; November 24–11: 789–90.
4. Chowdhry S, Seidensticker L, Cooney DS, Hazani R, Wilhelmi BJ. Do not use epinephrine in digital blocks: myth or truth? Part II. A retrospective review of 1111 cases. PubMed. 2010, December 126(6): 2031–4.
5. Kenna C and Murtagh J. *Back pain and spinal manipulation*. Sydney: Butterworths, 1989.
6. Dammers JW, Veering MM, Vermeulen M. Injection of methylprednisolone proximal to the carpal tunnel: Randomised double-blind trial. BMJ, 1999; 319: 884–886.

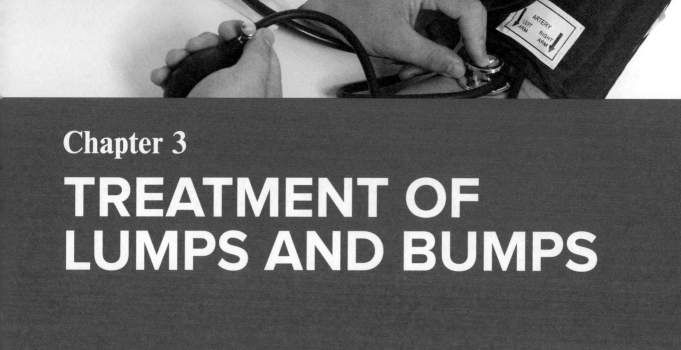

Chapter 3
TREATMENT OF LUMPS AND BUMPS

REMOVAL OF SKIN TAGS

Skin tags (fibroepithelial polyps) are very benign tumours, and can safely be left. However, patients often request their removal for cosmetic reasons. There are several ways to remove skin tags. These include:

- simple excision (see also *Perianal skin tags* for elliptical excision)
- cutting with scissors
- electrocautery (to base); a very effective method
- tying a fine thread around the base
- crushing with bone forceps
- liquid nitrogen therapy.

Liquid nitrogen therapy

1. Use a pair of forceps (dissecting or artery) to grasp the skin tag, preferably on the base or stalk.
2. Holding the skin tag upright and taut, apply liquid nitrogen (spray or soaked cotton bud) to the forceps close to the tumour (Fig. 3.1).
3. Apply for several seconds to freeze the tumour. It can be left or cut off with scissors.

A variation

The tips of the forceps can be dipped directly into a polystyrene cup of liquid nitrogen and then clamped onto the base of the skin tag. Multiple tags can be frozen rapidly in this way.

Bone forceps method

A simple procedure is to crush the base of the skin tag flush with the skin using bone forceps (Fig. 3.2a). The advantages are that:

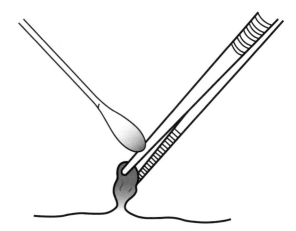

Fig. 3.1 Removal of skin tag by liquid nitrogen

- no local anaesthetic is required
- the procedure is relatively painless
- the procedure is very quick
- immediate haemostasis is achieved (Fig. 3.2b).

REMOVAL OF EPIDERMOID (SEBACEOUS) CYSTS

There are several methods for removal of epidermoid cysts after infiltration of local anaesthetic over and around the cyst. They are the most common cutaneous cysts, which contain a cheesy keratin material (not sebum). They can occur anywhere but most commonly on the face, scalp and trunk. These include the following methods.[1]

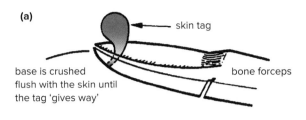

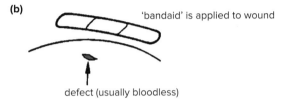

Fig. 3.2 Removal of skin tag using bone forceps method

Incision into cyst

Make an incision into the cyst to bisect it, squeeze the contents out with a gauze swab and then avulse the lining of the cyst with a pair of artery forceps or remove with a small curette.

Punch biopsy method

Use a 2, 3, 4 or 5 mm punch biopsy to punch a hole into the apex of the cyst. Squeeze vigorously to express the contents. Look for the cyst wall, grasp it with forceps or a skin hook and *carefully* enucleate it. A suture is not necessary.

Incision over cyst and blunt dissection

Make a careful skin incision over the cyst, taking care not to puncture its wall. Free the skin carefully from the cyst by blunt dissection. When it is free from adherent subcutaneous tissue, digital pressure will cause the cyst to 'pop out'.

Standard dissection

Incise a small ellipse of skin to include the central punctum over the cyst (Fig. 3.3a). Apply forceps to this skin to provide traction for dissection of the cyst from the adherent dermis and subcutaneous tissue. Ideally, forceps should be applied at either end. The objective is to avoid rupture of the cyst. Insert curved scissors (e.g. McIndoe scissors) and free the cyst by gently opening and closing the blades (Fig. 3.3b). Bleeding is not usually a problem. When the cyst is removed, obliterate the space with subcutaneous absorbable sutures. The skin is sutured with a vertical mattress suture to avoid a tendency to inversion of the skin edges into the slack wound. Send the cyst for histopathology.

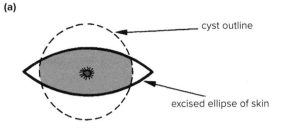

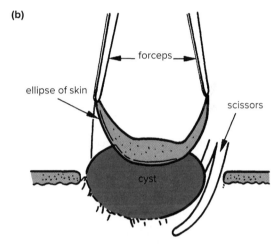

Fig. 3.3 Standard dissection of sebaceous cyst

Electrocautery method

On the *first visit,* inject LA into the overlying skin. Insert a heated electrocautery needle in the cyst and cauterise the contents for several seconds (Fig. 3.4).

On the *second visit,* 7 to 10 days later, inject LA, then make a small incision in the cyst and express the contents. Ideally, the cautery will prevent recurrence even though the cyst wall is not removed.

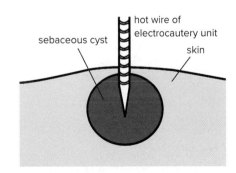

Fig. 3.4 Electrocautery to sebaceous cyst

Simple deroofing method

This method simply unroofs the cyst and allows healing by dressings over an open area. It should be avoided on the face or other areas where a puckered scar is unacceptable. It is very useful for an infected cyst.

Method

1. Infiltrate the skin over the cyst with local anaesthetic.
2. Unroof the cyst by removing a disc of skin with scalpel or scissors. This disc should be slightly smaller than the diameter of the cyst (Fig. 3.5).
3. Evacuate the contents of the cyst and pack with paraffin gauze.
4. Apply pressure if bleeding is a problem.
5. Apply non-adherent dressings daily.

THE INFECTED EPIDERMOID CYST

When an infected cyst is encountered, it is appropriate to open it and drain the pus through a cruciate incision or a 4–6 mm punch biopsy (under local anaesthetic). Evacuate the contents with sterile gauze and determine if it is possible to avulse the cyst wall. Usually it heals, often definitively, through open healing. If not, the cyst can be later excised as outlined above.

SEBACEOUS HYPERPLASIA

Sebaceous hyperplasia presents as a single or multiple nodules on the face, especially in older persons. The nodules are small, yellow-pink, slightly umbilicated and are found in a similar distribution to basal cell carcinoma, for which they may be mistaken. There is no need for surgical excision.

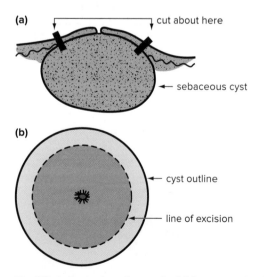

Fig. 3.5 A simple deroofing method: **(a)** cross-sectional view; **(b)** surface view

DERMOID CYSTS

Subcutaneous dermoid cysts arise from a nest of epidermal cells in the subcutaneous tissues. There are two forms.

Developmental (inclusion) dermoid cyst

The most common is the external angular dermoid, which lies at the junction of the outer and upper margins of the orbit, in the line of fusion of the maxilla and frontal bones (Fig. 3.6). It is usually fluctuant and transilluminable. It should not be treated in the office as an excision of a simple cyst, but referred for expert dissection under general anaesthetic, as it can extend into the cranium. Imaging (CT or MRI) is advisable.

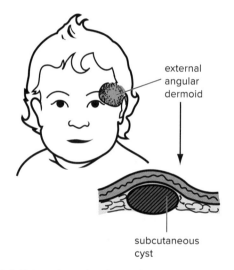

Fig. 3.6 External angular dermoid

Traumatic (implantation) dermoid cyst

This is a common lesion of the fingers and palms in adults. It is lined by squamous epithelium and contains sebum, degenerate cells, mucus and occasionally hair. It is caused by implantation of epithelial cells from repeated occupational trauma (puncture wounds) and may be seen in tailors, wire workers and hairdressers. It initially presents as a small (< 1 cm) cystic nodular swelling beneath the skin surface and attached to it, commonly on the finger pulp (Fig. 3.7). There may be an overlying puncture wound or scar. It is often painful and tender, and should be removed by a simple incision removal under local anaesthetic (deroof the cyst and enucleate its contents by curette or scraping). If asymptomatic, it can be left.

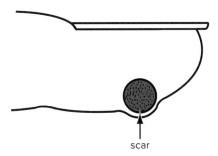

Fig. 3.7 Implantation cyst of finger

ACNE CYSTS

Acne cysts can be treated by an injection of a long-acting corticosteroid preparation in such a way as to flush out the follicular contents and subdue the sterile inflammation. The treatment is suitable for small numbers of cysts.

Equipment

You will need:
- 25-gauge needles
- small syringe
- 1 mL long-acting corticosteroid (e.g. triamcinalone acetonide, methylprednisolone acetate).

Method

1. Introduce a 25-gauge needle into one side of the cyst and inject a small quantity of steroid. Remove the needle (Fig. 3.8a).
2. Introduce a needle into the opposite side of the cyst. Inject steroid so that material is flushed out through the initial entry point (Fig. 3.8b). This removes the follicular material and leaves residual amounts of steroids in a depot form.

BIOPSIES

There are various methods for taking biopsies from skin lesions. These include scraping, shaving and punch biopsies, which are useful but not as effective or safe as excisional biopsies.

Shave biopsies

This simple technique is generally used for the tissue diagnosis of premalignant lesions and some malignant tumours, but not melanoma.

Method

1. Infiltrate with LA.
2. Holding a no. 10 or 15 scalpel blade horizontally, shave off the tumour just into the dermis (Fig. 3.9).
3. Diathermy may be required for haemostasis.

The biopsy site usually heals with minimal scarring.

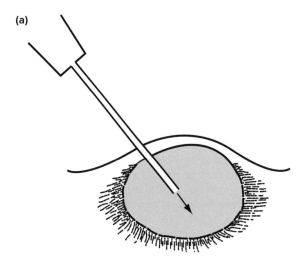

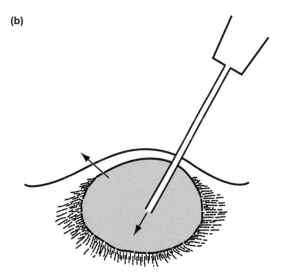

Fig. 3.8 Treatment of acne cyst

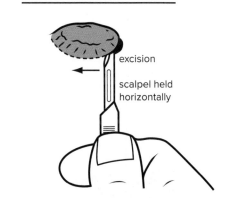

Fig. 3.9 Shave biopsy

Punch biopsy

This biopsy has considerable use in general practice, where full-thickness skin specimens are required for histological diagnosis. Take care not to crush the specimen with forceps; an alternative is to 'stab' horizontally through the specimen with the anaesthetic needle to lift it out. Although a single suture is always optional, the procedure is simpler using tape (e.g. Steri-Strips), particularly for the most common 3–4 mm punch sizes. For larger sizes requiring a suture (e.g. 8–10mm), stretch the skin along one axis before the punch; the circle will contract back into more of an ovoid shape, less prone to 'dog ears' after suturing across the narrow diameter.

Method

1. Clean the skin.
2. Infiltrate with LA.
3. Gently stretch the skin between the finger and thumb to limit rotational movement.
4. Select the punch size and hold it vertically to the skin.
5. Rotate (in a clockwise, screwing motion) with firm pressure to cut a plug through the dermis into the subcutaneous fat layer, about 3 mm in depth (Fig. 3.10). Remove the punch.
6. Use fine-toothed forceps, tissue hook or needle to grip the outer rim of the plug.
7. Exert gentle traction and undercut the base of the plug parallel to the skin surface using fine-pointed scissors or a scalpel.
8. Place the specimen in fixative.

9. Secure haemostasis by firm pressure or by diathermy.
10. Apply a dry dressing or a single suture to the defect.

TREATMENT OF GANGLIONS

Ganglions have a high recurrence rate after treatment, with a relapse of 30% after surgery. Most ganglions are around the dorsal area of the wrist and associated with the scapulolunate joint, while about 25% are volar (palmar).

A simple, relatively painless and more effective method is to use intralesional injections of long-acting corticosteroid, such as methylprednisolone acetate.[2]

Method 1

1. Insert a 19- or 21-gauge needle attached to a 2 mL or 5 mL syringe into the cavity of the ganglion.
2. Aspirate some (not all) of its jelly-like contents, mainly to ensure that the needle is in situ.
3. Keeping the needle exactly in place, swap the syringe for an insulin syringe containing up to 0.5 mL of steroid.
4. Inject 0.25–0.5 mL (Fig. 3.11).
5. Rapidly withdraw the needle, pinch the overlying skin for 1 to 2 minutes and then apply a firm dressing.
6. Review in 7 days and, if still present, repeat the injection using 0.25 mL of steroid.

Up to six injections can be given over a period of time, but 70% of ganglions will disperse with only one or two injections.

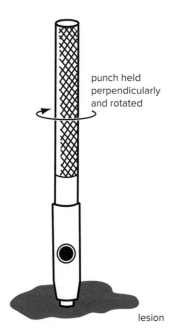

Fig. 3.10 Punch biopsy

punch held perpendicularly and rotated

lesion

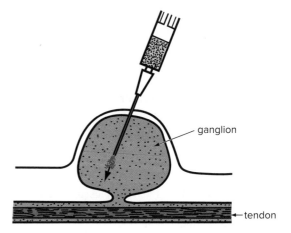

ganglion

tendon

Fig. 3.11 Injection treatment of ganglion

Method 2

Insert a larger gauge catgut suture through the middle of the ganglion and firmly tie it over the ganglion. Side pressure may express the contents through the needle holes. Remove the knot 12 days later.

OLECRANON AND PRE-PATELLAR BURSITIS

Simple aspiration–injection technique

Chronic recurrent traumatic olecranon or pre-patellar bursitis with a synovial effusion may require surgery, but most cases can resolve with partial aspiration of the fluid and then injection of long-acting corticosteroid through the same needle.

EXCISION OF LIPOMAS

Lipomas are benign fatty tumours situated in subcutaneous tissue. They are common on the back, but can occur anywhere. Ultrasound imaging can be useful for gauging the depth of a lipoma.

Lipomas rarely require removal, but removal may be desired for cosmetic reasons or to relieve discomfort from pressure. Many lipomas can be simply enucleated using a gloved finger, but there are a few traps: some are deeper than anticipated, and some are adjacent to important structures such as large nerves and blood vessels. Others are tethered by fibrous bands, and recurrence can occur if excision is incomplete. Beware of lipomas on the back that can be difficult to remove and in the axilla and supraclavicular areas where they can be misleadingly extensive.

Larger lipomas (> 5 cm) may require referral.

Method

The principle is CUT, SQUEEZE, POP.
1. Outline the extent of the lipoma and mark it with a ballpoint pen. Note its anatomical relationships.
2. Infiltrate the area with 1% lidocaine with adrenaline. (Include the deepest part of the lipoma.)
3. Make a linear incision (Fig. 3.12a) in the overlying skin, preferably in a natural crease line, for about three-quarters of its length. The lipoma should bulge through the wound. For large lipomas, incise an ellipse of skin (Fig. 3.12b).
4. Deepen the incision until the lipoma can be seen.
5. Insert a gloved finger between the skin and fatty tumour to find a plane of dissection and to determine whether it will shell out.
6. It is important to seek the outer edge of each lobule, dissect it and bring it to the wound surface (Fig. 3.12c). If necessary, insert curved scissors and use a blunt opening action to free any fibrous bands tethering the lipoma (Fig. 3.12d).
   Note: The best way to prevent bleeding is not to dissect around the fatty tissue but to incise it, invert the tumour through the wound and then remove it.
7. Ensure that all the fatty tissue is removed. Send it for histological examination. Clipping and ligation of persistent bleeding vessels may be required. Haemostasis should be meticulous.

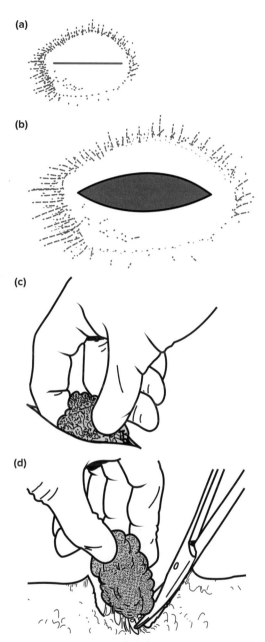

Fig. 3.12 (a) Linear incision for small lipomas; **(b)** elliptical incision for large lipomas; **(c)** gloved finger dissection to bring lipoma to the surface; **(d)** blunt scissors dissection to free lipoma from tethering fibrous bands**(d)**

8. Use a gauze swab to control bleeding and remove debris from the dead space.
9. Close the dead space with interrupted catgut sutures. Consider a small suction drain tube if oozing persists in an extensive dissection area.
10. Close the skin with interrupted or subcuticular sutures.
    Note: A punch biopsy method can be used to remove a lipoma.

KERATOACANTHOMA

Most keratoacanthomas (KAs) occur singly on light-exposed areas. They are regarded as a variant of squamous cell carcinoma and should be treated as such.

Although KAs can be treated by curettage and cautery, the recommended treatment is surgical excision and histological examination. Ensure a 2–3 mm margin for excision. Most patients will not tolerate a tumour on an exposed area such as the face for 6 months while waiting for a spontaneous remission to confirm the clinical diagnosis.

Note: SCCs on the ear metastasise 15 times more rapidly than elsewhere. The relative growth rates of SCC, KAs and basal cell carcinomas (BCCs) are shown in Figure 3.13.

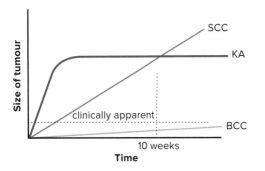

Fig. 3.13 Relative growth rates of three types of skin tumours

BASAL CELL CARCINOMA (BCC)

BCCs are the most common type of skin cancer. They can occur on any part of the body, but the most common site is on the face, especially next to the eyes or nose. It is useful to think of it as the area covered by an eye mask (Fig. 3.14). Another common area is the neck, and the upper back and chest are becoming more common sites.

Increased risk occurs with:

- age over 50 years
- exposure to excessive sunlight
- fair complexion
- lack of sun protection.

Treatment guidelines

- Surgery is the primary treatment: use a simple ellipse (where possible) under local anaesthetic with a 3 mm margin (in most cases).
- Cryotherapy is suitable for primary, well-defined, histologically confirmed superficial tumours, at sites away from the head and neck. Contraindicated for morphoeic or ill-defined tumours. Good results are obtained for small BCCs (< 1 cm) with sharply demarcated borders.
- Superficial X-ray therapy is an option in larger tumours in older people. Use with discretion and infrequently.
- Imiquimod: Suitable for biopsy-proven superficial BCC, but not on nose or around eyes. Treatment Monday to Friday, 5 times weekly for 6 weeks.
- Curettage and electrodesiccation: A curette is first used to remove friable tumour tissue, leaving firm normal tissue. Electrodesiccation of the margins of the defect is then performed. Careful follow-up is essential.

SQUAMOUS CELL CARCINOMA (SCC)

SCCs usually develop in skin exposed to the sun, in particular the face (especially the lower lip), ears, neck, forearm, back of the hands and lower legs (Fig. 3.15). A special trap is on the scalps of men who are bald or have thin scalp hair.

Increased risk occurs with:

- age over 60 years
- fair complexion
- outdoor occupations
- development of sunspots (solar keratoses).

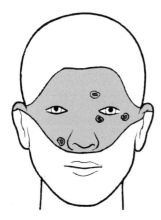

Fig. 3.14 Typical sites of basal cell carcinoma: the 'mask' area of the face

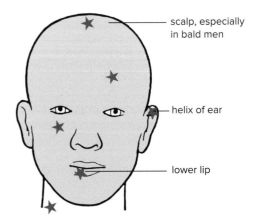

Fig. 3.15 Important common sites of squamous cell carcinoma on the head and face

Treatment guidelines

- Surgery is the treatment of choice—use a simple ellipse under LA with a 4 mm margin (in most cases).
- Superficial X-ray therapy is an option in a primary untreated tumour when surgery is not feasible. Cryotherapy and curettage are not treatments of choice.

PYOGENIC GRANULOMA

These solitary, raised, bright red tumours (granuloma telangiectaticum) tend to bleed profusely. The most effective treatment is curettage and electrocautery under local anaesthesia.

However, it must be stressed that histological confirmation of the diagnosis is essential to exclude anaplastic squamous cell carcinoma or amelanotic melanoma. Thus, after the tumour has been shaved off or curetted, it should be sent for examination.

SEBORRHOEIC KERATOSES

Regular applications of liquid nitrogen may remove these benign skin tumours, or at least decolourise them.

Immediately after freezing you can use a scalpel (e.g. size 15 blade) to scrape off the lesion at skin level.

Another method is to carefully apply concentrated phenol solution. Repeat in 3 weeks if necessary.

Yet another method is to apply trichloroacetic acid to the surface and instil it gently by multiple pricks with a fine gauge needle. Perform twice weekly for 2 weeks.

Stucco keratoses

This subtype of seborrhoeic keratoses are multiple non-pigmented small friable keratoses over the lower legs. They can be treated with a topical keratolytic such as 3–5% salicyclic acid in sorbolene.

CHERRY ANGIOMA

A cherry angioma, also referred to as a red mole or Campbell de Morgan spot, is best left but if removed for cosmetic or other reasons, the options are:
- electro cauterisation
- cryosurgery
- laser surgery, e.g. pulsed dye laser
- radiofrequency ablation (specialist device)
- shave biopsy.

CHONDRODERMATITIS NODULARIS HELICUS

This lump, which is not an SCC or other neoplasm, presents as a painful nodule on the most prominent part of the helix or antihelix of the ear (Fig. 3.16). It is seen more often on the helix in men, while it is found

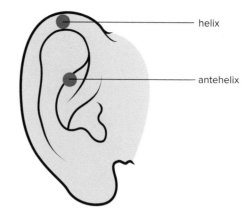

Fig. 3.16 Typical sites of chondrodermatitis nodularis helicus

more often on the antihelix in women. It is caused by sun damage and pressure degeneration from excessive sleeping on the affected side. It causes pain at night.

Histologically, a thickened epidermis overlies inflamed cartilage. It looks like a small corn, is tender and affects sleep if that side of the head lies on the pillow. The first line treatment is cryotherapy. Adding a layer of 'bubble wrap' to the dressing helps protect the lesion for the first night or two. If that fails, wedge resection (see 'Wedge resection of ear') with a minimal border or a simple superficial elliptical excision (Fig. 3.17) under local anaesthesia is an effective treatment. Send the specimen for histological examination.

ORF

Rapid healing of the skin lesion orf can be achieved by injecting corticosteroids into the pustular nodule.

Precautions

- Ensure that the diagnosis of orf is correct.
- Warn the patient of likely increased discomfort for 24 hours.

Method

- Mix 0.5 mL of 1% plain lidocaine with 0.5 mL of long-acting corticosteroid, e.g. triamcinolone. Use more solution for a larger lesion.
- Infiltrate the solution into the lesion, around its margins and into its base.
- The lesion is left to heal without dressings.

Rapid healing occurs within 5 to 10 days. Otherwise it takes 3 to 4 weeks.

MILKER'S NODULES

These nodules can heal more rapidly if the same intralesional corticosteroid injection is given as for orf.

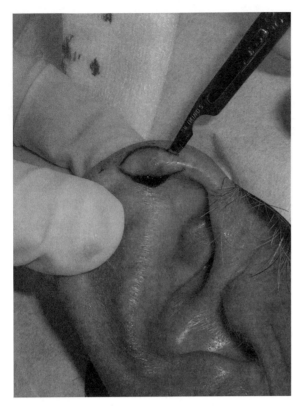

Fig. 3.17 Elliptical excision of chondrodermatitis nodularis helicis

Courtesy of Richard P. Usatine, MD.

HAEMANGIOMA OF THE LIP

Attempted excision of these common lesions should be avoided because of bleeding. Perform a mental nerve block (preferable to local infiltration) and insert the needle of the electrocautery into the centre of the haemangioma. More than one treatment may be necessary.

ASPIRATION OF BAKER CYST

A distended tender popliteal cyst (Baker cyst) of the knee is really a bursa that communicates with the knee joint. It may be associated with rheumatoid arthritis, osteoarthritis, traumatic knee disruption or a normal joint.

Aspiration and injection may alleviate the symptoms of swelling and tenderness.

Method

1. The patient should be prone, with a small pillow under the knee to produce slight hyperextension of the joint and obvious distension of the bursa.
2. Using a sterile, no-touch technique, insert a 21-gauge 38 mm needle attached to a 20 mL syringe into the bursa.

3. Completely aspirate the fluid, which is usually a clear yellow.
4. Leave the needle in situ and exchange the 20 mL syringe for a 2 mL syringe containing 1 mL of long-acting corticosteroid, which is then injected (Fig. 3.18).
5. Recurrence is common. An alternative treatment is to inject 5 mL of 2.5–3% aqueous phenol or 3% sodium tetradecyl sulfate (STD) solution instead of corticosteroid.

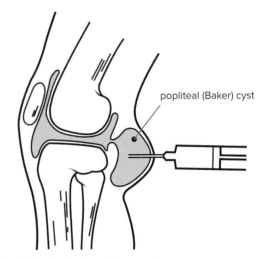

Fig. 3.18 Aspiration of Baker cyst

ASPIRATION AND INJECTION OF HYDROCELE

Aspiration, followed by an injection of dilute aqueous phenol or STD, can be a very useful treatment technique for primary hydroceles—especially where definitive surgery is inappropriate. Aspiration alone rarely corrects a hydrocele, but the aspiration/injection combination performed 2 or 3 times can often cure the problem.

Method

1. Inject LA into the scrotal skin down to the sac.
2. Insert an 18- or 19-gauge intravenous cannula through this site into the sac and remove the stilette, leaving the soft cannula in the sac (Fig. 3.19).
3. Remove the serous fluid initially by free drainage, possibly aided by manual compression on the sac and then by aspiration with a 20 mL syringe.
4. Record the volume.
5. Inject 2.5–3% sterile aqueous phenol into the empty sac (10 mL for 200 mL of fluid removed, 15 mL for 200–400 mL and 20 mL for over 400 mL). An alternative and simpler solution is to use 3% STD. Use 2–5 mL.

The procedure can be repeated after 6 weeks.

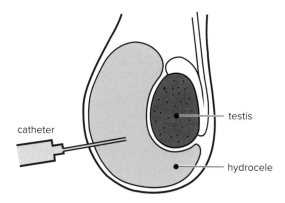

Fig. 3.19 Aspiration of hydrocele

EPIDIDYMAL CYSTS

The same method as for hydroceles can be used. Aspirate and then inject sclerosant.

TESTICULAR TUMOURS

It has been shown that scrotal needling such as for needle biopsy of testicular tumours has the potential risk of implanting malignant cells in the scrotal wall. The same applies to a scrotal incision to remove testicular cancer. For this reason, incisions to remove testicular cancer are made in the inguinal area. Testicular cancer is spread by the lymphatics to the para-aortic nodes, and not to the inguinal nodes.

TORSION OF THE TESTICLE

- Follow the 4 to 6 hour intervention rule.
- Don't waste time with investigations, such as ultrasound.
- Consider manipulation from the horizontal position, although it is painful.

STEROID INJECTIONS INTO SKIN LESIONS

Indications

Suitable lesions for steroid injections are:
- granuloma annulare
- hypertrophic scars (early development)
- keloid scars (early development)
- alopecia areata
- lichen simplex chronicus
- necrobiosis lipoidica
- hypertrophic lichen planus
- plaque psoriasis.
 Triamcinolone is the appropriate long-acting corticosteroid (10 mg/mL). It may be diluted in equal quantities of saline.

Method

1. The steroid should be injected into the lesion (not below it).
2. Insert a 25- or (preferably) 27-gauge needle, firmly locked to a small insulin-type 1 mL syringe, into the lesion at the level of the middle of the dermis (Fig. 3.20).
3. High pressure is required with some lesions. Keloids may be softened by thawing after a burst of liquid nitrogen spray.
4. Inject sufficient steroid to make the lesion blanch.
5. Several sites will be needed for larger lesions, so preceding LA may be required in some instances. Avoid infiltration of steroid in larger lesions: use multiple injections.

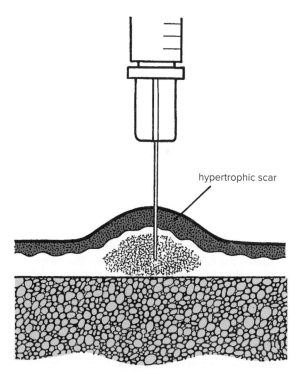

Fig. 3.20 Injection of corticosteroid into mid-dermis

STEROID INJECTIONS FOR PLAQUES OF PSORIASIS

An excellent, effective treatment of small to moderately sized plaques of psoriasis is by intralesional infiltration using a long-acting corticosteroid.

Requirements

- Triamcinolone 10 mg/mL solution (or other corticosteroid)
- 1% (plain) lidocaine (or similar local anaesthetic)
- 25-gauge needle (or 23-gauge if larger plaque)

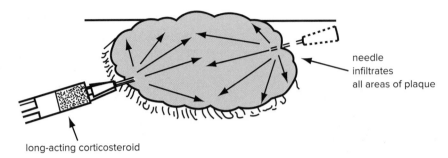

long-acting corticosteroid

needle
infiltrates
all areas of plaque

Fig. 3.21 Intralesional corticosteroid injection technique for psoriatic plaque (requiring double injection; small plaques cope with one infiltration)

Method

1. Mix equal parts of corticosteroid and local anaesthetic.
2. Swab the lesion.
3. Insert the needle at the margin of the plaque and infiltrate the lesion at an intradermal level, avoiding going deep into the subcutaneous tissue.
4. Infiltrate the whole plaque.
5. A larger plaque may require needle insertion at two sites (Fig. 3.21).

This treatment, which is ideal for a persistent elbow or knee plaque, is rapidly effective and tends to induce a long remission.

HYPERTROPHIC SCARS: MULTIPLE PUNCTURE METHOD

Hypertrophic scars are usually treated by multiple intradermal injections of long-acting corticosteroids. The injections are not normally painful, but the procedure can be distressing, particularly to children.

It is possible to achieve the same results without 'an injection', delivering the steroid by the multiple-pressure technique used for smallpox vaccinations.

Method

1. The patient is positioned so that the scar to be treated is in the horizontal plane.
2. Cleanse the skin thoroughly with an alcohol swab and allow it to dry.
3. Draw injectable corticosteroid up into a syringe, preferably before the patient enters the treatment room.
4. Spread a film or layer of the steroid aseptically over the scar.
5. Make multiple pressures through the solution into the scar, using a 21-gauge needle held tangentially to the skin. The point of the needle should just penetrate the epidermis and not be deep enough to cause bleeding.
6. There should be approximately 20 pressures per cm^2.
7. Allow the steroid to dry and cover the area with a dressing if desired.

Treatment can be repeated every 6 weeks if necessary; most simple hypertrophic scars, however, settle after one treatment.

Silicon adhesive gel/dressings

Silicon sheet dressings (e.g. Cica-Care) worn continuously over a wound may prevent hypertrophy of the wound. An adhesive gel sheet can be purchased and a piece cut out to fit the wound. The gel sheet should be re-applied daily for 12 weeks.

Alternatively, silicon gels massaged firmly into the wound each day after the wound has re-epithelialised may help.

Elastoplast Scar Reduction Patch

These patches can be used to treat or prevent hypertrophic scars. The patch is applied over the scar and changed every 24 hours. It should not be applied to open wounds or burns.

KELOIDS

Methods

- Multiple puncture method.
- Inject long-acting corticosteroid, e.g. triamcinolone 10 mg/mL (usually three treatments, 6 weeks apart).
- Apply liquid nitrogen, then inject with corticosteroid about 5 to 15 minutes later—the softer oedematous tissue is easier to inject.
- Radiotherapy.

Prevention of keloids (in susceptible patients)

- Apply high-potency topical corticosteroid with occlusive dressing for 2 to 3 days.
- Inject long-acting corticosteroid into the recess of the wound immediately following suture of the wound (Fig. 3.22).
- Inject long-acting corticosteroid immediately following suture removal.

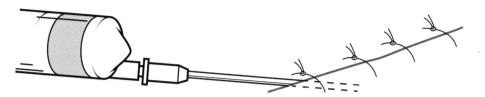

Fig. 3.22 Injecting corticosteroid into wound

DUPUYTREN CONTRACTURE

If the palmar nodule is growing rapidly, an injection of long-acting corticosteroid or collagenase (e.g. Xiaflex) into the cord or nodule may be very effective. It can be repeated in 6 weeks, but surgical intervention is indicated for a significant flexion deformity.

DRAINAGE OF BREAST ABSCESS

Acute bacterial mastitis

Resolution without progression to an abscess will usually be prevented by antibiotics (e.g. flucloxacillin 500 mg 4 times a day orally or cephalexin 500 mg 4 times a day orally). In addition, therapeutic ultrasound (2 W/cm^2 for 6 minutes) daily for 2 to 3 days will assist resolution.

The breast abscess

If an abscess develops, repeated aspiration or occasionally incision and drainage will be required.

Aspiration drainage

This is the preferred treatment and best performed under ultrasound guidance. However, if US is unavailable it can be drained with an 18- to 21-gauge needle under local anaesthetic every second day until resolution.

Surgical drainage under general anaesthesia

The surgical incision should be placed as far away from the areola and nipple as possible and the dressings kept clear of the areola to allow breastfeeding to continue. The incision is best placed in a radial orientation (like the spoke of a wheel) to minimise the risk of severing breast ducts or sensory nerves to the nipple.

Method

1. Make an incision over the point of maximal tenderness, preferably in a dependent area of the breast (Fig. 3.23a).
2. Use artery forceps to separate breast tissue to reach the pus.
3. Take a swab for culture.
4. Introduce a gloved finger to break down the septa that separate the cavity into loculations (Fig. 3.23b). Flush the cavity with sterile saline solution.
5. Insert a corrugated drainage tube into the cavity. Fix it to the skin edge with a single suture (Fig. 3.23c).

(a)

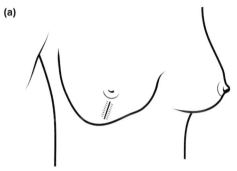

(b)

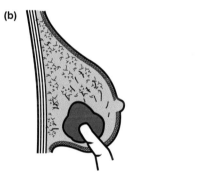

(c)

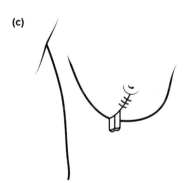

Fig. 3.23 Drainage of breast abscess: **(a)** linear incision; **(b)** exploring abscess cavity; **(c)** drainage tube in situ

Remove the tube 2 days after the operation. Change the dressings daily until the wound has healed. Continue antibiotics until resolution of the inflammation. Continue breastfeeding from both breasts, but if breastfeeding is not possible because of the location of the incisions and drains, milk should be expressed from that breast.

ASPIRATION OF BREAST LUMP

This simple technique is very helpful, especially if the lump is a cyst, and will have no adverse effects if the lump is malignant. If so, the needle biopsy will help with the pre-operative cytological diagnosis.

Clues to diagnosis of breast cysts

- Sudden onset; past history of surgery
- Discrete breast mass, firm, rarely fluctuant, relatively mobile

Method of aspiration and needle biopsy

1. Avoid LA; use an aqueous skin preparation.
2. Use a 21-gauge needle and a 5 mL sterile syringe.
3. Identify the mass accurately and fix it by placing three fingers of the dominant hand firmly on three sides of the mass (Fig. 3.24a).
4. Introduce the needle directly into the area of the swelling, and once in subcutaneous tissue apply gentle suction as the needle is being advanced (Fig. 3.24b).
5. If fluid is obtained (usually yellowish green), aspirate as much as possible.
6. If no fluid is obtained, try and get a core of cells from several areas of the lump in the bore of the needle.
7. Make several passes through the lump at different angles, without exit from the skin and maintaining suction.

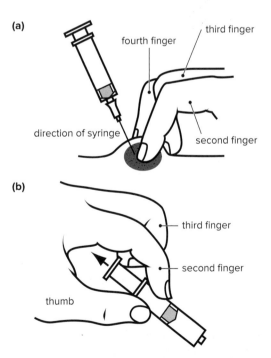

(a)

fourth finger

third finger

direction of syringe

second finger

(b)

third finger

second finger

thumb

Fig. 3.24 Fixation of the cyst: **(a)** lateral view; **(b)** position of other hand: second (index) finger and thumb steady the syringe while the third (middle) finger slides out the plunger to create suction

8. Release suction before exit from the skin so as to keep the cells in the needle (not in the syringe).
9. After withdrawal, remove the syringe from the needle, fill with 2 mL of air, reattach the needle and produce a fine spray on two prepared slides.
10. Fix one slide (in Cytofix) and allow one to air dry, and forward to a reputable pathology laboratory.

Indications for biopsy of lump

- The cyst fluid is bloodstained.
- The lump does not disappear completely with aspiration.
- The swelling recurs within 1 month.

Recurrent cysts

After aspiration, leave the needle in situ and inject 2–5 mL of air. This method reduces the recurrence rate.

MARSUPIALISATION TECHNIQUE FOR BARTHOLIN CYST

A Bartholin cyst presents as a swelling at the posterior end of the labium majus, close to the fourchette. The correct treatment of both cyst and abscess is marsupialisation, not excision (which is difficult, bloody and leads to scarring) or incision (which is usually followed by recurrence).

The procedure can be carried out on an outpatient using local anaesthesia.

Method

1. With the patient in the lithotomy position, swab and drape the vulva.
2. Infiltrate the skin over the medial part of the cyst with 1% lidocaine with adrenaline, using a fine needle and a slow injection.
3. Make a narrow elliptical incision over the medial part of the cyst, at least 3 cm in length (Fig. 3.25a). (As this ostium later contracts, it is a fault to make it too small.)
4. Excise the ellipse of skin, then open the wall of the cyst in the same line and carefully grasp its edges with mosquito forceps.
5. After the contents of the cyst escape, wash out the cavity with saline and inspect it, then dry it carefully. Any deep loculi must be opened widely. On the postero-inferior cyst wall it is usual to find a punctum leading into the proximal remnant of the duct.
6. Suture the cyst wall to the skin edge at four points using fine catgut, thus creating a pouch (Fig. 3.25b). No dressing is applied and the patient is instructed to take a sitting bath twice a day for a week. Healing is rapid, without pain, and the result is a permanent ostium close to the hymen which delivers free-draining secretion close to the normal site (Fig. 3.25c). If this ostium is too lateral, the woman may complain of discharge and wetness of the skin.

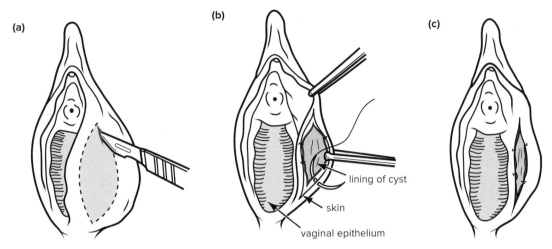

Fig. 3.25 Marsupialisation technique: **(a)** start of operation; **(b)** final suture; **(c)** post-operative appearance

With this technique, even the inexperienced operator will have no difficulty achieving good results with Bartholin cysts. Abscesses can be more difficult if the lining is friable or necrotic. For this reason, early operation should be advised in the presence of inflammation.

CERVICAL POLYPS

Women presenting with small cervical polyps can be readily and simply treated in the office with sponge-holding forceps and a silver nitrate stick. Patients with large polyps require a different approach and referral may be appropriate.

Method

1. Grasp the polyp with sponge-holding forceps and gently twist the polyp until it separates (Fig. 3.26a).
2. Place the polyp in a specimen bottle and send it for histological examination.
3. Cauterise the base of the polyp at the cervical os (Fig. 3.26b) with silver nitrate or by electrocautery.

LIQUID NITROGEN THERAPY

Ideally, liquid nitrogen is stored in a special, large container and decanted when required into a small thermos flask, a spray device or a small polystyrene cup (for each individual patient). The temperature is −193°C.

The application to superficial skin tumours (see Table 3.1) is via a carefully targeted spray or a ball of cotton wool rolled rather loosely on the tip of a wooden applicator stick. The ball should be slightly smaller than the lesion, to prevent freezing of the surrounding skin.

Beware of application to the following:

- dark skin
- upper lips
- nerves
- eyelids

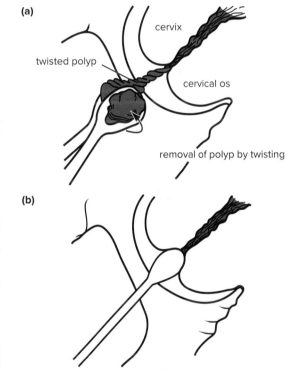

Fig. 3.26 Cervical polyp excision: **(a)** removal by twisting; **(b)** cauterising base with silver nitrate

Table 3.1 Superficial skin tumours suitable for cryotherapy

Warts (plane, periungual, plantar, anogenital)
Skin tags
Seborrhoeic keratoses
Molluscum contagiosum
Solar keratoses

- beard (alopecia risk)
- nails (do not freeze over nail matrix).

Cryotherapy spray method

Spraying liquid nitrogen under high pressure (the timed spot freeze open-spray technique) is the most efficient method of cryotherapy. It produces sufficient intense cold to treat deeper lesions, with the deepest freeze being at the centre of the white circle that forms on the skin. This 'halo' is not nitrogen, but ice particles formed from water in the air. Direct the spray at a 90° angle at a distance of 1 cm from the skin surface (Fig. 3.27).

For the nervous patient, use an initial brief burst to 'reset the pain receptors' before fully spraying. Children may benefit from topical anaesthetic cream (e.g. EMLA) an hour prior. The targeted tissue necrosis is more effective at a lower spray rate for a longer time period, rather than a brief full blast.

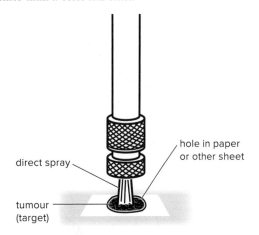

Fig. 3.27 Cryotherapy—spray gun method

direct spray

hole in paper or other sheet

tumour (target)

Small lesions may require pulsing the trigger on and off every couple of seconds, because the minimum flow rate is too high. If the spray is too diffuse for the lesion, protect the surrounding skin from collateral damage:

- Place the small opening of an otoscope earpiece over the lesion and spray into the large opening. Disadvantages are the cold earpiece (wear thick gloves), and the difficulty judging how much spray is hitting the hidden lesion.
- Punch or cut a hole the size of the target lesion into a piece of paper or cardboard and place it over the lesion.
- Hold a tissue over the eye for lesions on the cheek or forehead.
- Apply a thick film of petroleum jelly or spray 'plastic skin' such as OpSite on surrounding skin.

Ice particles can block the nozzle—unclog it with a 25-gauge needle or run water over the outside of the nozzle (not through it).

Cotton wool application method (basic steps)

1. Tell the patient what to expect.
2. Pare excess keratin with a scalpel.
3. Use a cotton wool applicator slightly smaller (not larger—see Fig. 3.28a) than the lesion.
4. Immerse it in nitrogen until bubbling ceases.
5. Gently tap it on the side of the container to remove excess liquid.
6. Hold the lesion firmly between thumb and forefinger.
7. Place the applicator vertically (Fig. 3.28b) on the tumour surface.
8. Apply with firm pressure: *do not dab.*
9. Redip the applicator every 5 to 10 seconds.
10. Freeze until a 2–5 mm white halo appears around the lesion.

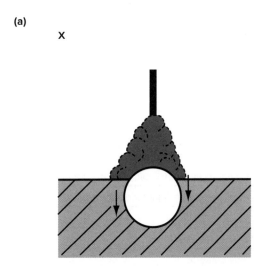

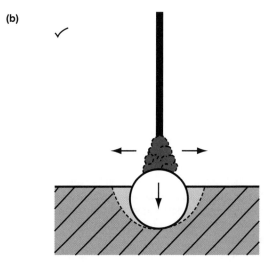

(a) X

(b) ✓

Fig. 3.28 Shows **(a)** applicator too large; **(b)** correct size and approach of applicator

Table 3.2 Recommended treatment times for cryotherapy

Solar keratoses, solar lentigos	5 seconds
Seborrhoeic keratoses	single cycle 5–10 seconds
Skin tags	5–10 seconds
Warts—hands	single cycle 30 seconds
Warts—feet	two cycles 30 seconds with complete thaw in between
Molluscum contagiosum	5 seconds

The appropriate length of application varies (see Table 3.2).

Explain likely reactions to the patient, such as the appearance of blisters (possibly blood blisters). The optimal time for retreatment of warts is at 2–3 weeks.

Post-cryotherapy

The application of an alcohol swab to the site immediately after cryotherapy provides some immediate pain relief because of the evaporative effect. Patients can usually return to work and exercise on the same day of treatment. Expect a scab to appear, and fall off within 10 days.

TRICHLOROACETIC ACID

Trichloroacetic acid, which should be readily available from pharmacies, has good use as a chemical ablative agent, but it requires careful application on skin lesions. It is usually applied twice weekly, and can be introduced into the lesions, e.g. seborrhoeic keratoses, with fine needle pricks.

Suggested uses

- Seborrhoeic keratoses
- Xanthelasma
- Other flat hyperpigmented lesions

SIMPLE REMOVAL OF XANTHOMA/ XANTHELASMAS

General practitioners receive many requests to remove cosmetically unacceptable xanthomas (xanthelasmas) of the eyelid. A simple method of removal is described. It is suitable for most sizes, but works best for smaller nodular xanthomas that are bulging and 'ripe' for removal.

Equipment

- A 21-gauge sterile disposable needle
- Manicure tweezers (flat or slanted, not pointed)

Method

1. Explain the method to the patient, indicating that there is slight discomfort only.

2. Although it is not necessary for all patients, apply some ice or other surface 'anaesthetic' to the xanthoma to lessen the discomfort.
3. Stretch the overlying skin and make a small incision in the skin with the tip of the needle (or a fine scalpel) (Fig. 3.29a).
4. Compress the xanthoma along its axis with the tweezers. It is invariably easily expelled (Fig. 3.29b).

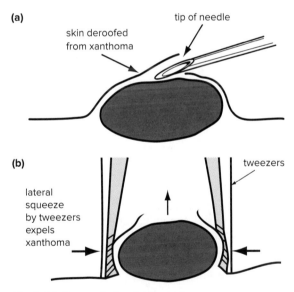

Fig. 3.29 Removal of nodular xanthoma

Infiltrative xanthelasmas

The flat yellowish xanthelasma around the eyes is difficult to treat surgically. The simplest method is to use ablative therapy, such as laser or very careful application of trichloracetic acid.

WARTS AND PAPILLOMAS

Warts are skin tumours caused by the human papilloma virus that are transmitted by direct or fomite contact and may be autoinnoculated from one area to another.

The various types include common warts, filiform warts (fine elongated growths usually on the face and neck), digitate warts (finger-like projections, usually on scalp), genital and plantar warts. We should keep in mind the fact that about 25% of warts resolve spontaneously in 6 months and 70% in 2 years. They can be tricky to reliably cure—particularly longstanding plantar warts—which is perhaps why such a variety of methods exist.

Treatment options

Topical applications

- Salicylic acid, e.g. salicylic acid 5–20% in flexible collodion (apply daily or bd), salicylic acid 17% + 17% lactic acid (apply once daily)
- Formaldehyde 2–4% alone or in combination
- Podophyllotoxin 0–5%, for warts on mucosal surfaces, e.g. anogenital warts
- Cytotoxic agents, e.g. 5-fluorouracil, very good for resistant warts such as plantar warts and periungual warts
- The immunomodulator, imiquimod

Cryotherapy

- Carbon dioxide (−56.5°C) or liquid nitrogen (−195.8°C)
- Excessive keratin must be pared before freezing

Curettage

A most common treatment, some plantar warts can be removed under LA with a sharp spoon curette. The problem is a tendency to scar.

Electrodessication

A high-frequency spark under LA is useful for small or digitate warts. A combination of curettage and electrodessication is suitable for large and persistent warts.

Vitamin A and the retinoids

- Topical retinoic acid (e.g. tretinoin 0.1% cream-Retin-A) for plane warts
- Systemic oral retinoid, acitretin (Neotigason) for recalcitrant warts (with care)

Medication

Oral cimetidine has been postulated as treatment for a large crop of warts, but no evidence beyond anecdote supports its use.[3]

Specialised treatments

Bleomycin, cantharidin, immunotherapy (e.g. topical diphenyl-cyclo-propenone [DCP]). Consider DCP treatment for recalcitrant warts.[4]

Specific wart treatment

The method chosen depends on the type of wart, its site and the patient's age.

- Plane warts: liquid nitrogen (after paring) to each wart every 2 to 4 weeks; consider tretinoin 0.05% cream (once daily for face) or 5-fluorouracil cream
- Filiform or digitate warts: liquid nitrogen or electrodessication
- Plantar warts: refer to 'Treatment of plantar warts' in Chapter 7
- Periungual warts (fingernails): consider 5-fluorouracil or liquid nitrogen with care. Always use a paint rather than ointment or paste on fingers
- Common warts (see below)

Topical options for common warts: helpful hints

1. Soak the wart/s in warm soapy water.
2. Rub back the wart surface with a pumice stone.
3. Apply the anti-wart agent—options:
   - Adults: 17% salicylic acid, 17% lactic acid in collodion paint (Dermatech, Duofilm), apply daily.
   - Children: 8% salicylic acid, 8% lactic acid in collodion.
   - Formulated paint: formalin 5%, salicylic acid 12%, acetone 25%, collodion to 100%; apply daily or every second day.
4. Consider protecting the surrounding skin with nail polish or Vaseline.
5. Remove dead skin between applications.
6. Salicylic 70% paste in linseed oil: available as extemporaneous prescription on the PBS. Store the jar in a safe place in the surgery—do not give it to the patient. Cut a hole in thick sports tape by folding it in half (sticky side out) and cutting out a double-layered semicircle which unfolds into a circular hole that fits over the wart. Apply the paste with a tongue depressor, then cover with more sports tape. Leave 1 week (the dead skin will look messy), then pare and freeze base with liquid nitrogen.

Maverick tip (from personal communications): Apply superglue weekly to stubborn common warts.

MOLLUSCUM CONTAGIOSUM

Individual lesions usually involute spontaneously over several months. There are several simple treatments available for this viral tumour of the skin, the choice being influenced by the person's age. The great range of possible treatments reflects the difficulty of achieving rapid resolution.

Treatment choices are:
- liquid nitrogen (a few seconds)
- pricking the lesion with a pointed stick soaked in 1% or 3% phenol

- application of 15% podophyllin in Friar's Balsam (compound benzoin tincture)
- application of 30% trichloroacetic acid
- application of 5% benzoyl peroxide
- application of 17% salicylic acid + 17% lactic acid in collodion (Dermatech or Duofilm)
- application of wheatgrass topical cream or spray (a wheatgrain extract—see www.drwheatgrass.com.au)
- destruction by electrocautery or diathermy
- ether soap and friction method
- lifting open the tip with a sterile needle inserted from the side (parallel to the skin) and applying 10% povidone-iodine (Betadine) solution or 2.5% benzoyl peroxide (parents can be shown this method and continue it at home for multiple tumours)
- paint with clear nail polish
- cover with a piece of duct tape or Micropore (or similar paper-based tape) and change every day (may take a few months)
- inject a larger single lesion with corticosteroid, e.g. triamcinolone 10 mg/mL solution.

Most effective method

Extract the core with a curette or large needle, then apply 10% povidone-iodine solution. Given how long this takes for many dozens of lesions, it may be more practical for a parent to do at home, following a demonstration in the surgery.

For large areas of multiple molluscum contagiosum

Apply aluminum acetate (Burow's solution 1:30) twice a day.

New alternative treatments

- Extract of the Cantharis beetle (prepared as Cantharone) is reportedly very effective (if available)
- Imiquimod (Aldara) cream, thrice weekly for 3 weeks
- Diphenyl-cyclo-propenone (DCP) ointment

References

1. Marwood J. Sebaceous cyst excision. General Practitioner, 1994; 2: 4–5.
2. LaVilla G. The action of methylprednisolone acetate in local therapy of ganglions. Clinical Therapeutics, 1968; 47: 455–75.
3. Tam M. Oral cimetidine as the treatment of common warts. Morsels of Evidence, 2019, https://evidencebasedmedicine.com.au/?p=1756.
4. Buckley DA, Keane FM, Munn SE, Fuller LC, Higgins EM, Du Vivier AW. Recalcitrant viral warts treated by diphencyprone immunotherapy. Br J Dermatology, 1999; 141(2): 292–6.

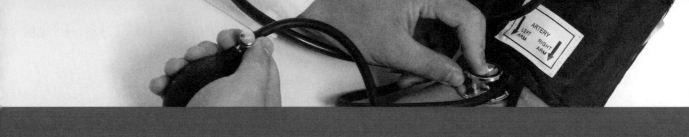

Chapter 4
BASIC PRACTICAL MEDICAL PROCEDURES

VENEPUNCTURE AND INTRAVENOUS CANNULATION

Basic venepuncture

Purpose

Collection of blood, including large volume collection for transfusion. The ideal site is the basilic vein or median cubital vein, otherwise the dorsum of the hand or others according to availability (Fig. 4.1). Use local anaesthetic for large volume blood collection.

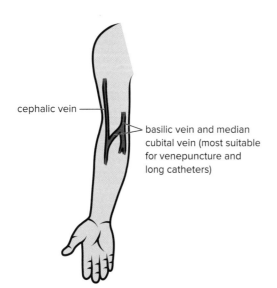

cephalic vein

basilic vein and median cubital vein (most suitable for venepuncture and long catheters)

Fig. 4.1 Main veins of arm for venepuncture

Method

1. Explain the method to the patient. Ensure the patient is warm and comfortable.
2. Wear gloves.
3. Dilate the vein by means of a tourniquet applied to occlude venous return.
4. Place a padded block under the arm to keep it straight.
5. After using a sterile swab to prepare the site, place the needle with attached syringe on the skin. Using downwards oblique pressure, puncture the vein firmly, ensuring the needle lies well within the vein. Remove the tourniquet.

Venepuncture in children

The same process for adults applies to adolescents and older children, but in infants and small children a 23-gauge butterfly needle provides more stability. A palpable vein is more likely to be successful than a visible but non-palpable vein. An assistant is necessary to support the limb and provide a tourniquet in small children.

For analgesia consider topical anaesthesia (amethocaine or EMLA), sucrose in infants < 3 months or consider sedation with midazolam (oral, intranasal or buccal) or nitrous oxide in children > 2 years.

Tips to aid dilation of veins

There are several ways in which peripheral veins can be dilated to facilitate venepuncture. The following are some of the methods used.

Vasodilation methods

- Apply a warm flannel for 60 seconds
- Rub glyceryl trinitrate ointment over the vein
- Give the patient half a glyceryl trinitrate tablet (if no contraindications).[1]

Sphygmomanometer methods[2]

- Dilate the vein by means of the sphygmomanometer to a pressure of about 80–90 mmHg (veins will stand out).
  or
- Using the sphygmomanometer, inflate it to a pressure around 30 mmHg above systolic arterial pressure for 1 to 2 minutes while the patient opens and closes their hand. Thereafter it is deflated to around 80 mmHg and the resulting reactive hyperaemia is effective in filling even the shyest of veins. According to Wishaw, this is the method par excellence.[3]

Venesection tourniquet method[3]

Apply the tourniquet tightly and then release. After a reactive hyperaemia occurs reapply it and the veins should stand out well.

Intravenous cannulation

Use sterile gloves for this procedure.

Best site

- Choose a suitable prominent vein in the non-dominant forearm (not over a joint), e.g. dorsum of hand, cephalic vein just above wrist (dorsolateral position).
- Use cubital fossa veins as last resort.
- Choose a relatively fixed vein, e.g. where it penetrates the fascia.
- Choose a vein running parallel to the long axis of the arm.

Method

1. Apply a small bleb, e.g. 0.2–0.5 mL of local anaesthetic, over or adjacent to the vein (keep very superficial) and wait 5 minutes, or apply EMLA cream at least 60 to 90 minutes beforehand (note that all cannulae hurt).
2. Insert the needle and catheter unit (6-gauge is suitable) through the skin beyond the shoulder of the plastic part.
3. Pierce the vein and ensure that the unit lies flat as it is guided along the vein lumen for a short distance, at an angle of 10–15°.
4. When blood enters the chamber, put a finger over the vein to stop backflow. Remove the tourniquet and guide the plastic catheter into the vein.
5. Fix the cannula in position, e.g. use transparent 'Tegaderm'.

Cannulation in children

The preferred site is the dorsum of the non-dominant hand and consider the need for subsequent splinting. The same rules of local anaesthesia apply with an injection of LA considered for older children (see p. 212).

Note the advisory grasp if using the dorsum of the hand for infants (Fig. 4.2). Grasp the wrist between the index and middle finger, with the thumb over the child's fingers, flexing the wrist.[4]

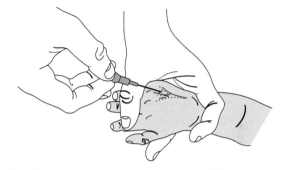

Fig. 4.2 Intravenous cannula insertion in children
Reproduced from Thomson, K., Tey, D. and Marks, M. (eds), *Paediatric Handbook* (8th Edn), 2009, Wiley-Blackwell, Sydney, p. 32.[4]

RAPID INTRAVENOUS INFUSION CATHETER (RIC)

This is a very useful device for the rapid infusion of fluids in emergencies, particularly where there has been severe blood loss. It allows rapid upsizing of a cannula to a larger bore in a peripheral vein. It is based on the principle that for every doubling of the radius, the flow increases by the 4th power (or 16 times). The method does require practice since skilful technique is required. After the normal IV catheter is inserted, a guide wire is introduced. This permits the insertion of the RIC with a 7 FG or larger diameter.

See product instructions for further instructions on use.

NASOGASTRIC TUBE INSERTION

Indications

- Intestinal obstruction—to drain stomach
- Diagnostic—aspiration of stomach contents
- Administer enteral nutrition

Equipment

- Radio-opaque nasogastric tube e.g. 16 FG for aspiration, fine bore for feeding (more comfortable).
- Assess correct length of tube—measure from the end of the nose to the earlobe and then 5 cm below the end of the xiphisternum.
- Lidocaine spray and lubricating jelly (consider lidocaine).
- 50–60 mL syringe for aspiration.

Method

1. Explain the procedure to the patient including anticipated times of discomfort.

2. Sit the patient upright. Inspect the nose for any deformity and the best possible passage. As a rule, the right nostril is easier to negotiate than the left.
3. Use a local anaesthetic spray to anaesthetise the nasal passage. Consider also lubrication with lidocaine jelly. Wait 5 minutes.
4. Lubricate the tube and pass it backwards along the floor of the nasal passage (Fig. 4.3). Advance it directly backwards (avoid going upwards). Resistance will be felt when the tube passes from the nasopharynx to the oropharynx. Warn the patient that a retching sensation may be experienced.
5. Now ask the patient to swallow (with the assistance of a 'feeder' of water if not contraindicated) as the tube continues to advance with each swallow.
6. The tube should pass down the oesophagus without resistance (never force it down. If retching, take it slowly and only advance with each act of swallowing). The distance from the nostril to the stomach in adults is approximately 35–40 cm.
7. Ideally 10–15 cm of tube should be placed in the stomach. Confirmation of its presence in the stomach is confirmed by free aspiration of gastric contents and testing for acidity with litmus paper. If pH > 5.5 or in doubt, check the position radiologically.
8. Once in place, the tube is fixed to the nose with adhesive tape.

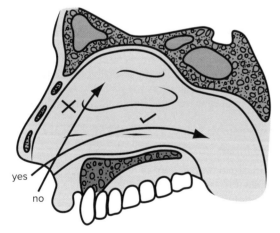

Fig. 4.3 Nasogatric intubation: note the correct direction for inserting the tube

NASOGASTRIC TUBE INSERTION IN CHILDREN

See Fig. 4.4.

Indications

- Decompression of stomach, e.g. intestinal obstruction
- Administration of medication, e.g. charcoal
- Oral rehydration/enteral nutrition

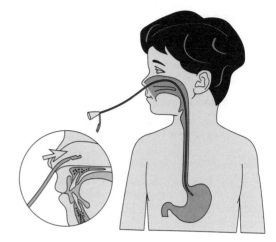

Fig. 4.4 Nasogastric tube insertion in children

Reproduced from Thomson, K., Tey, D. and Marks, M. (eds), *Paediatric Handbook* (8th Edn), 2009, Wiley-Blackwell, Sydney, p. 32.[4]

Method

- Same principles as for adults, including topical anaesthetic spray.
- Tube size: 8 FG neonates, 10–12 FG 1–2 years, 14–16 FG adolescents.
- Correct length: Place distal end of tube at end of nose, run it to the ear and 3.5 cm beyond the xiphisternum.
- If the child coughs and gasps, or gets a hoarse voice or the tube appears in the mouth, pull the tube back into the nasopharynx and retry.

URETHRAL CATHETERISATION OF MALES

'To start catheterising before the anaesthetic works is barbarous'—C.G. Fowler, *British Medical Journal*.
    The adult male urethra is 18–20 cm long.

Preliminary questions

1. What is the aim of this procedure and can it be achieved without urethral catheterisation?
2. How long must the catheter remain in situ?
3. Can I avoid introducing urinary infection?
4. Do I have the skill to perform the procedure safely?

Equipment

You will need:
- prepackaged set including swabs
- aqueous (not alcoholic) skin antiseptic
- one or two pairs of forceps
- sterile kidney dish to collect urine
- suitable catheter—usually medium size
- sterile lubricant, e.g. lidocaine jelly in syringe
- sterile syringe

- suitable catheter drainage bag
- catheter dressing
- sterile gown and mask.

Technique essentials

1. Explain the procedure to the patient, who is best placed in the heel-to-heel position.
2. Sterile preparation/clean suprapubic area and glans penis. A sterile drape is placed over the scrotum and thighs and the penis is lowered onto this.
3. A small amount of lidocaine jelly (2%) is put aside onto a sterile bowl to lubricate the tip of the catheter. Fit nozzle to the syringe of lidocaine jelly and insert gently into the penile meatus (warn the patient that this brief introduction is very uncomfortable)—instil the 10–20 mL jelly slowly: massage the gel carefully down the urethra to the sphincter; compress the glans and leave for a minimum of 5 minutes.
4. Grasp the catheter a few centimetres from its tip with forceps (the funnel end rests in the kidney dish). Apply lidocaine jelly to the tip of the catheter.
5. Hold the penis upwards and straight with one hand and gently insert and slowly advance the catheter. Ask the patient to slowly take deep breaths in and out. Do not rush or use force (Fig. 4.5).
6. When the catheter reaches the penoscrotal junction (it now rests against the external sphincter), pull the penis downwards between the patient's thighs.
7. Continue insertion through the sphincter or prostatic urethra until the entire length is inserted, even if urine emerges before then.
8. Non-retaining catheter: Ensure urine is flowing, then withdraw a few centimetres. Eventually press on the abdomen to ensure the bladder is empty.
   Retaining catheter: Inflate balloon (usually 5 mL of water) and gently withdraw until the balloon impinges on the bladder neck.

Note: Ensure the catheter is in the bladder with urine coming out (get the patient to cough to confirm this) before inflating the balloon.

9. Replace the retracted prepuce over the glans (to prevent paraphimosis).

Method of overcoming prostatic obstruction

If difficulty is experienced from prostatic urethral obstruction, it is worth attempting the catheter balloon stretching method. For example, if a size 16 catheter (often used but quite large) is obstructed, rather than changing to a smaller size, try the following method. While gently pushing on the catheter, get an assistant to inflate the balloon with a few mL of water, remove the water and repeat a few times. The stretched prostatic urethra allows free passage of the catheter.

URETHRAL CATHETERISATION OF FEMALES

Anatomical considerations

The female urethra is comparatively short and straight: 3–4 cm long and 6 mm in diameter. The urethral orifice lies approximately halfway between the clitoris and the vaginal opening and may be partly obscured by a fringe of soft tissue (Fig. 4.6).

Explanation

Despite the shorter length of the urethra the procedure is most uncomfortable and local anaesthesia is important. Explain the procedure to the patient with appropriate reassurance. Indicate that the introduction of the nozzle and anaesthetic jelly is uncomfortable and advise about slow deep breathing during introduction of the jelly and subsequently the catheter.

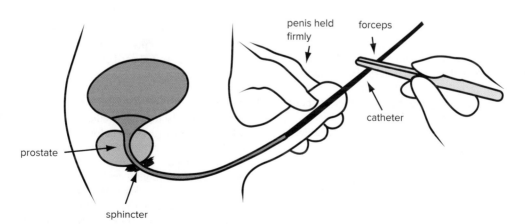

Fig. 4.5 Urethral catheterisation: initial phase of the procedure where the catheter is gently guided with forceps

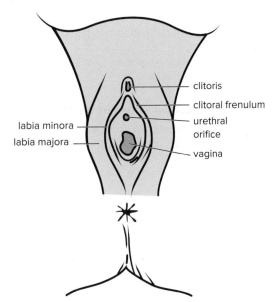

Fig. 4.6 Anatomy of the female perineum

labels: clitoris, clitoral frenulum, urethral orifice, vagina, labia minora, labia majora

Technique

1. Lie the patient down with the thighs apart and the knees comfortably flexed.
2. Cleanse the pubic region, groin, vulva and perineum with antiseptic solution.
3. Separate the labia minora with the thumb and forefinger of the non-dominant hand to expose the vaginal orifice and the urethral opening. Sweep a swab from anterior to posterior across this area and then discard. Repeat with a second swab.
4. Apply a sterile split sheet to expose the vagina and urethral opening, rewash hands and don sterile gloves. Again lightly swab the urethral orifice.
5. Set aside a small amount of lidocaine jelly for lubricating the catheter tip. Introduce the nozzle of the tube of the jelly into the urethra and slowly insert approximately 10 mL. The labia should be kept apart with the V-shaped arrangement of the fingers. Wait at least 5 minutes for local anaesthesia to develop.
6. Expose the tip of the catheter (e.g. 16 FG) from its envelope, dip it in the gel in the sterile bowl and, using a 'no touch' technique, insert the catheter into the urethral opening and guide it in smoothly. It should pass directly without difficulty.
7. Inflate the balloon and connect the catheter to a sterile closed drainage system (if required).

CATHETERISATION IN CHILDREN

The female child should lie with legs apart in the frog leg position. Catheter size guidelines:
• for diagnostic purposes: 5 FG

• for indwelling 0–6 months: 6 FG
• 2 years: 8 FG
• 5 years: 10 FG
• 6–12 years: 12 FG.

LUMBAR PUNCTURE

Main indications

• Diagnostic purposes, e.g. meningitis, MS, Guillain-Barre syndrome, SAH, CNS syphilis
• Introducing contrast media
• Introducing chemotherapeutic agents
In children:
• Febrile, sick infant with no focus of infection
• Fever with meningism
• Prolonged seizure with fever

Contraindications

• *Absolute:* Local skin infection, bleeding diathesis
• *Relative:* Raised intracranial pressure, depressed conscious state, focal neurological signs

Essentials of lumbar puncture 1: Preparation

1. Explain the procedure to the patient.
2. The patient should be in the lateral recumbent position, with the back maximally flexed and vertical to the table (Fig. 4.7). The shoulders and hips must be perpendicular to the bed.
3. The patient should be well immobilised. Avoid slumping.
4. Open the spinal pack, if required, and have three plain sterile tubes and one fluoride tube (for glucose) ready.
5. Adopt the sterile procedure (wash hands, mask, gloves, antiseptic prep).
6. Apply 1% lidocaine to skin and subcutaneous tissue (not necessary in infants). Inject 0.5–1 mL and wait 2 minutes.

Surface anatomy

Imaginary line between tops of iliac crests lies at spinous process of L_4 or between L_3 and L_4.[5] Insert the needle at L_4–L_5 interspace (preferably) or L_3–L_4 (the conus medullaris of the spinal cord ends at L_1–L_2 but finishes near L_3 at birth).

Essentials of lumbar puncture 2: Procedure

1. Use a 21- to 22-gauge LP needle (9 cm) for an average adult; 22–23 gauge × 4 cm for infants, × 5 cm for 4 to 10 years, × 6 cm for older children.
2. Insert the needle at right angles to the skin.
3. Slowly advance slightly cephalad (about 10°: aim for the umbilicus), otherwise perfectly parallel.
4. Keeping the bevel of the needle facing up, advance 1 mm at a time. You will feel a 'give' when the dura is pierced (about 4–7 cm in adults, 2–3 cm in children).

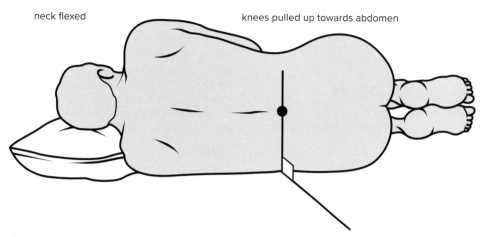

neck flexed   knees pulled up towards abdomen

Fig. 4.7 Lumbar puncture: the patient is placed in the fetal position with the back perpendicular to the bed. A line along the top of the iliac crests will intersect the midline at approximately the interspinous space between L_3 and L_4 (or the L_4 spinous process) in adults.

5. Withdraw the stylus, and wait 30 seconds for CSF flow. Rotating the needle through 90–180° may allow CSF to flow. Measure CSF opening pressure with manometer.
6. If CSF is bloodstained, get three samples.
7. Remove the needle with one quick motion.

Recordings

- CSF pressure with manometer (N < 180 mm).
- CSF biochemistry, microbiology, immunology (oligoclonal bands)
  Note: Don't aspirate CSF

Post-care

Lie flat for at least 1 hour.
Careful observation and bed rest (8 to 12 hours).

LUMBAR PUNCTURE IN CHILDREN

The same principles apply: use the L_3-L_4 or L_4-L_5 space for insertion (provide analgaesia as for venepuncture). Give local anaesthesia to dural level with 1% lidocaine. Have an assistant restrain the child, who should have the spine maximally flexed, in the lateral position on the edge of a flat surface.

TAPPING ASCITES

Abdominal paracentesis is often required as a therapeutic procedure to drain ascitic fluid in patients with terminal malignancy. The method is very simple. Select a site where there is shifting dullness and under which there are no solid organs (including an enlarged spleen). The ideal site is in the left iliac fossa midway between the umbilicus and the anterior superior iliac spine (the LHS equivalent of McBurney's point) and lateral to the line

of the inferior epigastric artery (Fig. 4.8). It is best to have an intravenous line in place.

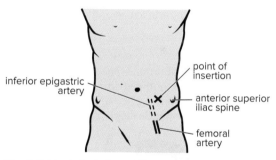

inferior epigastric artery

point of insertion

anterior superior iliac spine

femoral artery

Fig. 4.8 Ideal site to tap ascites

Tip: A PleurX drainage system, which consists of an indwelling catheter and vacuum collection system, is recommended for safe portable drainage, and can be used in the home. It was specifically designed for thoracocentesis.

Method

1. After the bladder is emptied, ask the patient to lie supine.
2. Put on a mask and sterile gloves.
3. Swab the skin with antiseptic.
4. Infiltrate 5 mL of 1% or 2% xylocaine into the anterior abdominal wall down to the parietal peritoneum at the chosen site.
5. Insert a 19-gauge intravenous cannula on a 20 mL syringe. Aspirate gently.
6. When ascitic fluid is obtained, remove the stilette and syringe and connect the plastic indwelling catheter via intravenous tubing to a sterile drainage bag, so that drainage occurs by gravity into a sterile closed drainage system.

7. The rate of flow can be regulated by the control on the IV tubing. It is recommended that the maximum fluid drained is 2000 mL at any one time. Remove after 4–6 hours to help prevent infection.

INSERTING A CHEST DRAIN

The main indications for this are:
- pneumothorax, e.g. large spontaneous, ventilated, tension (Chapter 17)
- malignant pleural effusion
- traumatic haemopneumothorax
- postoperative e.g. thoracotomy.

Location for chest aspiration

The majority of chest aspirations are performed in the 'triangle of safety' (Fig. 4.9), which is a triangle situated in the anterior half of axilla above the level of the fifth intercostal spaces. It contains no important or dangerous structures in the chest wall. The boundaries are:
- anteriorly: the anterior axillary line
- posteriorly: the mid-axillary line
- inferiorly: a horizontal line drawn posteriorly from the level of the nipple in a man or the 4th intercostal space in a woman.

Methods

The method of aspiration of a pneumothorax via the 'triangle of safety' is outlined in Chapter 17 under 'Pneumothorax', and for a pleural effusion, which is performed where it is located in the pleural cavity, as follows.

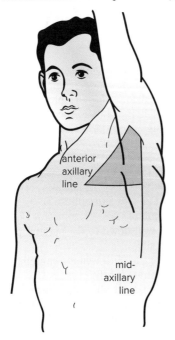

Fig. 4.9 The 'triangle of safety'

anterior axillary line

mid-axillary line

ASPIRATION OF PLEURAL EFFUSION

Use a recent chest X-ray to aid the clinical examination in order to select the best site for aspiration. A common site for a malignant effusion is on the posterior chest wall medial to the angle of the scapula, in the intercostal space below the upper limit of dullness to percussion. Avoid going too low. Beware of pneumothorax either from puncture of the visceral pleura or from air entry via the chest wall or apparatus.

Method

1. Explain the procedure to the patient, who sits on a stool facing the bed and leaning slightly forwards with the arms folded in front resting on a pillow on the bed.
2. Using a sterile procedure with gloves and gown, swab the skin with antiseptic.
3. Infiltrate the overlying skin with 1% lidocaine with adrenaline (25-gauge needle) and change to a 21-gauge needle and two-way or three-way with Leur stop cock or other connectors. Slowly infiltrate the chest wall down to pleura. Fluid appears in the syringe on aspiration (apply steady suction as you advance carefully) after the pleura is penetrated (Fig. 4.10).
4. Aspirate the fluid and by turning the tap, direct the fluid into the collecting container. To aspirate large volumes of fluid insert an intravenous catheter and connect to a three-way tap. This is repeated until all the fluid is tapped. It is normally recommended that no more than 1 to 1.5 L of fluid be removed at any one time.
   Caution: Ensure that air does not enter the pleural space at any stage. Reposition or withdraw the cannula or needle if pain on aspiration or coughing.
5. Upon withdrawing the catheter, immediately apply a sterile collodion dressing. Order a follow-up chest X-ray.

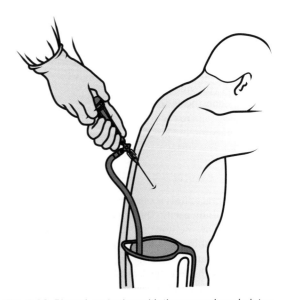

Fig. 4.10 Pleural aspiration with three-way Leur-Lok tap

A simpler technique

This technique is useful for tapping recurrent malignant effusions and can be performed at home. Insert a size 18 intravenous cannula. Withdraw the stilette and connect the plastic cannula to an intravenous tubing set with the end draining into a drainage bag by gravity.

PleurX drainage system

This is ideal to drain malignant effusions when the catheter can be retained for ongoing drainage.

SUBCUTANEOUS FLUID INFUSIONS

Subcutaneous fluids are useful when:
- relatively small amounts of crystalloid are needed (15 mL/kg per 12 hours)
- intravenous access is not required for systemic therapy.

This method of administering fluid has been used for more than 30 years. It can be sited and supervised by the nursing staff.

Complications are rare and usually relate to local oedema, which settles spontaneously once the infusion has been ceased.

Practical aspects

- Access to the subcutaneous space is via a 21-gauge butterfly needle, which is replaced daily.
- One ampoule of hyaluronidase (hyalase) is given prior to infusion and before subsequent bags of crystalloid. (This is necessary when skin elasticity is high, as in children.)
- Crystalloid solution (normal saline or 4% dextrose and 1/5 normal saline) with infusion set is then connected to the butterfly needle.
- The infusion is usually run at a maximum of 15 mL per kg over 4 to 12 hours per 24 hours. (This enables the patient to move about.)
- Most regions are suitable. The more convenient are the abdomen, the anterior thigh and the shoulder.
- The drip rate can be reduced if any discomfort is produced.

CONTINUOUS SUBCUTANEOUS INFUSION OF MORPHINE

When the oral and/or rectal routes are not possible or are ineffective, a subcutaneous infusion of morphine (for terminal pain) with a syringe pump can be used.

It is also useful for symptom control when there is a need for a combination of drugs, e.g. for pain, nausea and agitation. It may avoid the bolus peak effects (sedation, nausea or vomiting) or trough effects (breakthrough pain) found with intermittent parenteral morphine injections.

Practical aspects

- Access to the deep subcutaneous space is via a 21-gauge butterfly needle, which is replaced regularly (1, 2, 3 or 4 days).
- Most regions are suitable. The more convenient are the abdomen, the anterior thigh and the anterior upper arm. (Usually the anterior abdominal wall is used.)
- The infusion can be managed at home.
- About one-half to two-thirds of the 24-hour oral morphine requirement is placed in the syringe.
- The syringe is placed into the pump driver, which is set for 24-hour delivery.
- Areas where oedema is present are not suitable.

INTRAVENOUS IRON INFUSION

Substance: Ferric carboxymaltose (Ferinject) available as 100 mg/2 mL, 500 mg/10 mL ampoules

Criteria: Symptomatic iron deficiency: anaemia (Hb < 100 and ferritin < 20 µg/L)

Failed trial of oral iron for iron deficiency anaemia and persistent anaemia

Anaemia of chronic disease e.g. chronic kidney failure

Precautions: Obtain specialist advice and recommendation

History of allergic disorders

Others—see product information (PI)

Contraindications: Hypophosphataemia

First trimester of pregnancy

Hypersensitivity to the substance or any of its excipients

Other—see PI

Basic equipment requirements:

Tourniquet

0.9% (N) saline 100 mL bags

20 mL ampoule saline flush

Butterfly cannulas 21 and 23 g

Accessories

Note: functional accessible resuscitation equipment, drugs (adrenaline and hydrocortisone) and oxygen

Dosing regimen (simplified):

maximum single dose of Ferinject: patients with body weight < 35 kg—500 mg; body weight ≥ 35 kg—1000 mg

Max. single dose should not exceed 1000 mg (20 mL)/ day nor once a week

Note: If adverse effects develop cease infusion immediately and monitor vital signs

Recommended administration volume time and rate

Iron dose	Amount of N saline	Diluted infusion time
100–200 mg (2–4 mL)	50 mL	3 minutes
200–500 mg (4–10 mL)	100 mL	6 minutes
500–1000 mg (10–20 mL)	150 mL	15 minutes

Therapeutic venesection

Apart from venesection for blood donation, the process is used for treatment of blood disorders.

Indications

Hereditary haemochromatosis; polycythaemia—various especially rubra vera; transfusion-associated overload; porphyria cutanea tarda.

Options

Blood transfusion service; local pathology service; your surgery treatment room (especially rural and remote).

Requirements

Basic training including support staff.

Patient preliminaries

Iron studies, haematocrit, (elevated ferritin and haematocrit is indication), stable vital signs. Must drink ample fluids prior to procedure—the day before and 3 glasses of water prior to the procedure.

Equipment

Venesection kit (needle, collection bag, sampling port); adequate protection equipment; scales.

Method

Under strict asepsis, introduce the needle into a large vein in the cubital fossa (usual site), establish blood flow under gravity into the bag which is placed below the cubital fossa on scales and monitor flow. It is usual to collect 450–500 mL of blood (500 mL weighs about 600 g); it usually takes about 15–30 minutes. Check puncture site to ensure haemostasis, apply sterile cotton wool and tape, then a firm bandage (leave about 2 hours). Discard the bag according to local policies for blood products. Instruct patient to lie down for 15–20 minutes.

References

1. McLaren P. Dilating peripheral veins. Anaesthesia and Intensive Care, 1994; 22: 318.
2. Van der Walt JH. Dilating peripheral veins—another suggestion. Anaesthesia and Intensive Care, 1994; 22: 624.
3. Wishaw KL. Dilating veins, a simple approach. Letter to the editor. Anaesthesia and Intensive Care, 1995; 23: 123.
4. Thomson K, Tey D, Marks M (eds.). Paediatric Handbook (8th edn). Melbourne: Wiley Blackwell, 2009: 32.
5. Chakraverty R, Pynsent P, Issacs K. 'Which spinal levels are identified by palpation of the iliac crests and the posterior iliac spines? J Anat. 2007, February; 210-2: 232-6.

Chapter 5
LEG VEINS AND ULCERS

PERCUTANEOUS LIGATION FOR THE ISOLATED VEIN

This method can be used for the cosmetically unacceptable, isolated varicose vein in the leg, as an alternative to sclerotherapy. A 3/0 polyglycolic acid (Dexon) suture is simply inserted through the skin to encircle and ligate the vein.

Equipment

You will need:
- 3/0 polyglycolic acid suture
- cutting-edge needle
- needle holder and scissors
- local anaesthetic agent.

Method

1. Infiltrate LA around the site or sites of the vein to be ligated:
   - small veins (up to 5–10 cm), a single suture
   - larger veins, multiple sutures, 5–10 cm apart.
2. Using a cutting-edge needle, pass the suture under the vein (Fig. 5.1a).
3. Bring the suture through the skin and then simply tie it tightly to occlude the vein by constriction (Fig. 5.1b). The treated vein thromboses and atrophies after a short period.
4. Review the patient in 4 weeks and remove the suture.

Precautions

Avoid areas near the dorsalis pedis artery and the common peroneal nerve, or other significant arteries, veins or nerves.

(a)

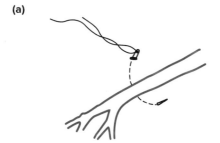

(b)

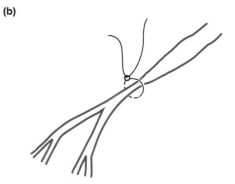

Fig. 5.1 Percutaneous ligation for isolated varicose vein

AVULSION OF THE ISOLATED VEIN

This method can be used to treat the cosmetically unacceptable isolated varicose vein in the leg. It is possible to avulse the vein using local anaesthesia along the length of the varicose vein.

Equipment

You will need:

- local anaesthetic
- no. 15 scalpel blade (and handle if not disposable)
- six small Halsted artery forceps ('mosquitoes')
- self-adhesive closure strips 1.2 cm (Steri-Strips), or nylon suture with cutting edge needle
- non-stick gauze dressing with wool and crepe bandage.

Method

1. Infiltrate LA along the length of varicose vein to be avulsed (up to 20 mL of 1% lignocaine can be used):
   - small vein (up to 5–10 cm): a single incision (5–10 mm) along or across the midpoint of the vein
   - larger veins: multiple incisions 5–10 cm apart, depending on the length of the varicose vein avulsed at first incision (Fig. 5.2a).
2. Locate and identify the vein using an artery forceps, ensuring that it is not a nerve. Grasp the vein with two artery forceps in parallel, then divide between the two with the scalpel (Fig. 5.2b).
3. Avulse the vein on either side by applying further forceps while pulling on the vein (Fig. 5.2c). Provided the length of the varicose vein has been infiltrated with LA, there should be no pain. Apply pressure for 2 to 3 minutes to stop bleeding once the vein has been avulsed.
4. Achieve skin closure by using either self-adhesive closure strips or suture. The suture can be removed in approximately 10 to 14 days.

5. Apply non-stick gauze dressing to the wound, followed by a wool and crepe bandage. The dressing can be left for 3 days and then removed.
6. If multiple avulsions have been carried out, it may be necessary to reapply a crepe bandage for another 2 to 3 days.
7. The patient should be free to do limited walking after the operation, and usually unrestricted walking after 24 hours.

Special precautions

Beware of nerves and arteries, avoiding areas involving the foot and the region of the lateral popliteal nerve where it curves around the neck of the fibula.

ENDOVASCULAR TREATMENT OF VEINS

Endovascular treatment is appropriate for varicose veins and spider veins. It can be managed readily in the GP's office but requires training in a reputable certified course.

The main methods are thermal ablation by radiofrequency or laser energy and injection sclerotherapy.

Radiofrequency ablation

A radiofrequency fibre is inserted into the vein and radiofrequency energy is delivered into the vein to provide heat at about 120°C.

Laser energy ablation

This is a similar method to radiofrequency.

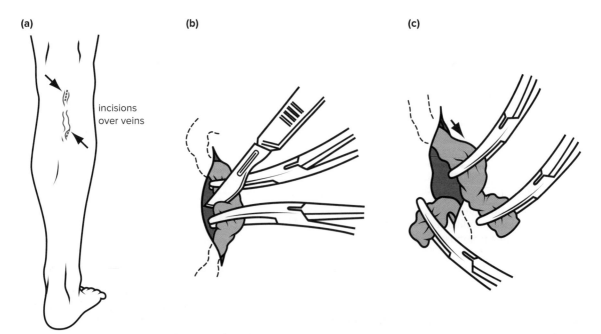

(a) incisions over veins (b) (c)

Fig. 5.2 Avulsion of the isolated varicose vein

Injection sclerotherapy

This is particularly suitable for sapheno-femoral incompetence below the knee. The chemicals can be delivered either as liquid or foam (under ultrasound guidance). Those in common use are sodium tetradecyl sulphate, polidocanol and aethoxysklerol.

It is necessary to wear specially fitted compression stockings for up to 2 weeks after therapy.

TREATMENT OF SUPERFICIAL THROMBOPHLEBITIS

When a large varicose vein becomes thrombosed, a tender, raised nodular cord is formed along the line of the vein. There is thrombosis in the superficial vein with no connection to deeper veins. It is usually a self-limiting disorder.

Clinical features

1. The skin is reddened and the tender nodular cord is palpable (Fig. 5.3a).
2. There is pain and localised oedema.
3. There is no generalised swelling of the limb or the ankle.

Management method

Propagation of thrombus can usually be prevented by uniform pressure over the cord.

1. The whole of the tender cord should be covered by an adhesive pad or a thin strip of foam (Fig. 5.3b) and then a firm crepe bandage applied.
2. The bandage and the pad are left on for 7 to 10 days.
3. Bed rest with leg elevated, if severe; otherwise keep active.
4. Prescribe a non-steroidal anti-inflammatory drug for about 7 days. Anticoagulants are not usually required. However, sometimes a low molecular weight (LMW) heparin (e.g. fondaparinux) is given for up to 45 days if the thrombus involves thigh veins.[1]

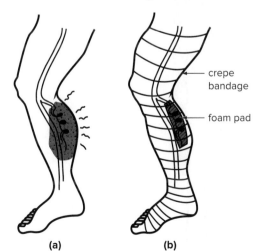

Fig. 5.3 Superficial thrombophlebitis

A specialist opinion should be sought for superficial thrombophlebitis above the knee, as this disorder may require ligation at the saphenofemoral junction.

Finally, one must always bear in mind the association between thrombophlebitis and deep-seated carcinoma elsewhere in the body.

MANAGEMENT OF DEEP VENOUS THROMBOSIS (DVT)

Investigations

- Duplex US: accurate for above-knee thrombosis; improving for distal calf (consider repeating in 1 week if initial test normal).
- Contrast venography, esp. if ultrasound −ve.
- MRI is very accurate.
- D dimer test: useful where probability of DVT is low, as a normal D dimer usually excludes diagnosis, but a positive result doesn't confirm diagnosis.

Management

- Prevention (cases at risk)
- Early and frequent mobilisation
- Elastic or graded compression stockings
- Physiotherapy
- Pneumatic compression
- Electrical calf muscle stimulation during surgery
- Surgery: LMW heparin daily or unfractionated heparin 5000 U (SC) bd *or* tds (LMW heparin for orthopaedic surgery)
- Long flights/sitting: LMW heparin prior to flying and on arrival

Treatment

- Admit to hospital (usually 5–7 days) if any complications, but more often treated as an outpatient
- Collect blood for APTT, INR and platelet count (check kidney function)
- One-way-stretch elastic bandages (both legs to above knees) *or* class II graded compression stocking to affected leg, especially if swelling. Be cautious of the Homan's (dorsiflexion) test as it may dislodge any thrombus
- IV heparin—daily IV injection of LMW heparin e.g. enoxaparin

  or

  unfractionated heparin 380 U/kg SC loading then 250 U/kg SC bd

  or

  5000 U heparin statim bolus IV then infusion in IV saline

  or

  LMW heparin—SC according to weight

- Oral anticoagulant (warfarin) for 6 months (monitor with INR). Avoid aspirin
- Mobilisation upon resolution of pain, tenderness and swelling

Surgery is necessary in extensive and embolising cases.

RUPTURED VARICOSE VEIN

Advice for this potentially dangerous (because of heavy blood loss) problem is often sought over the telephone. Advise local pressure (not proximal) and elevation. Both a proximal and a distal percutaneous suture (Fig. 5.1a, b on p. 79) may be necessary.

VENOUS ULCERS[2]

The area typically affected by varicose eczema and ulceration is shown in Figure 5.4. The secret of treating ulcers due to chronic venous insufficiency is the proper treatment of the physical factors, especially using compression. Removal of fluid from a swollen leg is mandatory; oral frusemide is of benefit where the oedema is due to cardiac failure, but oedema due to venous insufficiency or lymphoedema requires compression.

Most chronic ulcers have a biofilm at the base, which delays healing. Oral and topical antibiotics are best avoided—treatment is via debridement and appropriate antimicrobial dressings.

Mechanically debride using topical anaesthesia (e.g. EMLA cream applied 30 minutes beforehand). An alternative is autolytic debridement using products such as cadexomer iodine, hydrogels or honey products.

Treatment method example

1. Meticulously clean the ulcer with N saline or water. If slough, apply a hydrogel (e.g. IntraSite). If deep or contaminated, instil cadexomer iodine powder or ointment.

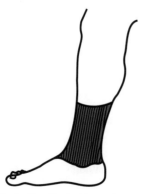

Fig. 5.4 Area typically affected by varicose eczema and ulceration (the 'gaiter' area)

2. Options:
   - A • Cover with an adhesive foam dressing (e.g. Allevyn)
     - Padded dressing (e.g. Velband) is optional
     - Occlusive paste dressing (e.g. Viscopaste) for 7–14 days from base of toe to just below knee
   - B • Cover with Allevyn (or similar)
     - Padded dressing
     - Compression bandage e.g. Eloflex to just below knee
   - C Improvised method:
     - apply paraffin gauze
     - pack defect with sponge rubber (Fig 5.5)
     - apply compression bandage.
3. Consider using a Tubigrip stockinette cover.
4. Insist on as much elevation of the leg as is possible.

Note: Dressings should be changed when they become loose or fall off, or when discharge seeps through. Patients may get ulcers wet and have baths.

Infection in leg ulcers

- Bacteria are often present in chronic leg ulcers, but that doesn't necessitate antibiotics.
- The need for oral antibiotics is based on signs of spreading infection.

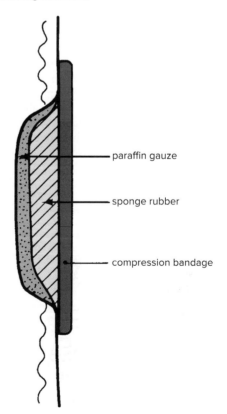

paraffin gauze

sponge rubber

compression bandage

Fig. 5.5 Dressing for venous ulcer

- If a swab is required, use the Levine method to reduce unhelpful positive results—do not swab the exudate or eschar, but clean and debride first, then swab.

APPLYING A COMPRESSION STOCKING

- Inelastic compression works better than elastic, but elastic compression (e.g. Tubigrip) is cheaper, and better than no compression at all.

- Apply three layers of tubular bandage in different lengths; the first reaches to below the knee, then to mid-calf, then to lower calf.
- To facilitate the sliding of a compression stocking over an ulcer on the leg, place a plastic shopping bag firmly over the foot and then slide the stocking over this. Once on, the plastic bag is pulled down and out.

References

1. Di Nisio M, Wichers IM, Middeldorp S. Treatment for superficial thrombophlebitis of the leg. Cochrane Database of Systematic Reviews 2018, Issue 2. Art. No.: CD004982. DOI: 10.1002/14651858.CD004982.pub6

2. Ulcer and wound management [version 2]. In: eTG complete [Internet]. Melbourne: Therapeutic Guidelines Limited; 2015 Jul.

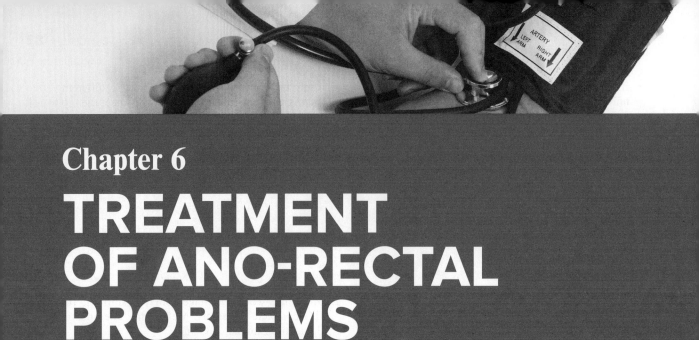

Chapter 6

TREATMENT OF ANO-RECTAL PROBLEMS

PERIANAL HAEMATOMA

This painful condition usually develops with straining to pass stool. Surgical intervention is recommended, especially in the presence of severe discomfort. The treatment depends on the time of presentation after appearance of the haematoma.

Stage 1 treatment: Within 24 hours of onset

While the haematoma is still fluid, the treatment is by simple aspiration of the blood (Fig. 6.1). No local anaesthetic is necessary. If this is unsuccessful, surgical drainage is recommended.

Equipment

You will need a:
- 2 mL or 5 mL syringe
- 19-gauge needle

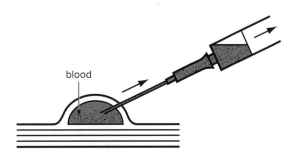

Fig. 6.1 Aspiration of blood for perianal haematoma

Stage 2 treatment: Within 24 hours to 5 days of onset

By now the blood has clotted, and a simple incision over the haematoma to remove the thrombosis followed by deroofing is the most appropriate treatment.

Equipment

You will need:
- 1% lidocaine with adrenaline (1–2 mL)
- a 25-gauge needle and 2 mL syringe
- a no. 15 scalpel blade
- a plain-toothed dissecting forceps (not essential).

Method

1. Swab the perianal area with povidone iodine, then inject 1–2 mL of LA into the pedicle of the skin around the base of the haematoma (Fig. 6.2a). An alternative is to apply a liberal amount of local anaesthetic ointment and wait 20 to 30 minutes.
2. Make a stab incision with the scalpel blade into the skin over the haematoma.
3. Extend the incision along the main axis of the haematoma (Fig. 6.2b).
4. Evacuate the thrombus with gentle, lateral pressure (Fig. 6.2c) or lift out with forceps.
5. An alternative and perhaps better method is to deroof the haematoma with scissors (like taking the top off a boiled egg). Squeeze out the clot.
6. Apply pressure to the incised area with a plain gauze swab to achieve haemostasis.

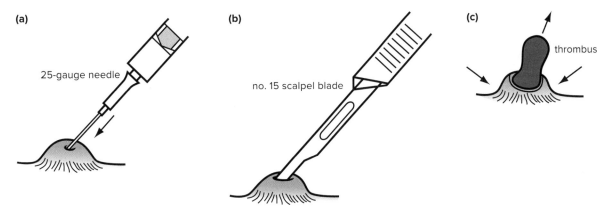

Fig. 6.2 Treatment of perianal haematoma: **(a)** local anaesthetic; **(b)** incision over haematoma; **(c)** thrombus expressed by digital pressure

7. When bleeding has stopped, apply a small dressing of gauze, then a combine (5 cm × 5 cm) folded in half.
8. Retain the dressing with well-fitting underpants (not adhesive), apply an ice pack and rest. Remove the next day.
9. No stitch is required unless haemostasis is a problem.

Stage 3 treatment: Day 6 onwards

The haematoma is best left alone unless it is very painful or (rarely) infected. Resolution is evidenced by the appearance of wrinkles in the previously stretched skin. The haematoma will ultimately become a skin tag.

Note: A gangrenous haematoma or a very large thrombosed pile should be surgically excised. Some surgeons recommend surgical excision for most residual haematoma. The patient should have analgesics and sitz baths.

Sitz bath

A sitz bath is a bath of warm medicated water deep enough to cover the hips. Suitably sized plastic containers may be available at a discount chemist. Add one of the following to the water: 2 teaspoons of salt, 1 teaspoon of baking soda (sodium bicarbonate) or 1–2 teaspoons of Epsom salts (magnesium sulphate).

Follow-up

The patient should be reviewed in 4 weeks for rectal examination and proctoscopy, to examine for any underlying internal haemorrhoid that may predispose to further recurrence. Prevention includes an increased intake of dietary fibre and avoidance of straining at stool.

PERIANAL SKIN TAGS

The skin tag is usually the legacy of an untreated perianal haematoma. It may require excision for aesthetic reasons, for hygiene or because it is a source of pruritus ani or irritation.

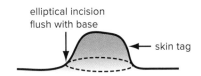

Fig. 6.3 Excision of perianal skin tag

Method

1. Make a simple elliptical excision at the base of the skin under LA (Fig. 6.3). Suturing of the defect is usually not necessary.
2. Apply a light gauze dressing for about 24 hours. The patient is advised to have twice-daily salt baths until healing is complete.

RUBBER BAND LIGATION OF HAEMORRHOIDS

Before the procedure

- Two glycerine suppositories (to empty rectum)
- Paracetamol and codeine oral analgesics

Rubber band ligation of haemorrhoids (best for stages 2 and 3) is a simple technique performed through a lubricated proctoscope which can be held by the patient after insertion (Fig. 6.4a). One or two rubber bands are stretched over the loading cone onto the metal drum of the banding instrument. It is now usually performed at routine colonoscopy. Associated carcinoma has to be considered.

Method

1. Thread the long grasping forceps through the drum of the banding instrument and grasp the haemorrhoid about 1 cm above the dentate line (Fig. 6.4b). (It is important to keep above the dentate line.)

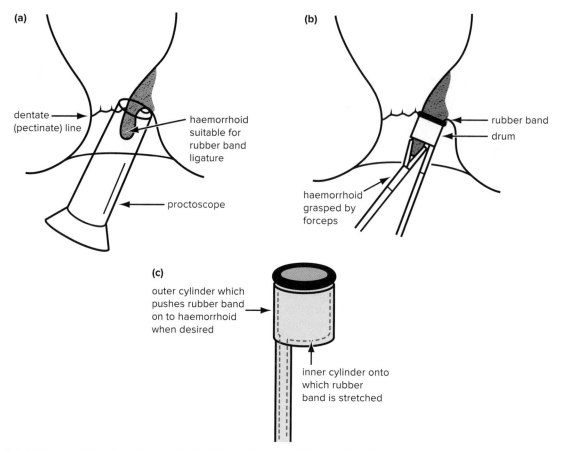

Fig. 6.4 Rubber band ligation of haemorrhoids: **(a)** proctoscope; **(b)** haemorrhoid grasped by forceps; **(c)** operational end of applicator

2. Apply gentle traction to the haemorrhoid to indent its base.
3. Snap the band or bands onto the haemorrhoid by pushing the trigger mechanism (Fig. 6.4c).

Post-procedure

- If possible, avoid a bowel action on day 1.
- Take simple analgesics as necessary.
- Don't drive home (prone to get vasovagal attacks).

INJECTION OF HAEMORRHOIDS

Aims

- To exclude associated tumours (? colonoscopy)
- To produce fibrosis in the submucous layer
- To avoid injection into haemorrhoidal vessels

The procedure is best for small haemorrhoids that bleed frequently. Otherwise it is not favoured practice because of adverse fibrosis.

Equipment

You will need:

- a proctoscope with illumination and lubricant
- a haemorrhoid (Gabriel) injection syringe and needle, or a 10 mL disposable syringe with a 21-gauge needle
- a 5 mL ampoule of sclerosant solution such as 5% phenol in almond oil, hypertonic saline or ALTH (aluminium potassium sulphate and tannic acid)
- a 19-gauge drawing-up needle
- forceps and cotton wool to wipe away faeces.

Method

1. The patient lies in the left lateral position.
2. Insert the lubricated proctoscope to visualise the haemorrhoids.
3. Draw up 5 mL of oily phenol.
4. Aim the injection at the upper end (base) of the haemorrhoid, which should be above the anorectal ring (injections given below this are very painful). Pierce the mucosa with a quick stab.

5. Inject up to 3 mL into the submucous plane. The bevel of the needle should be directed towards the mucosa rather than towards the lumen of the rectum. The injection should be painless (Fig. 6.5). Inject the phenol slowly until an opalescent swelling (blanching) is seen, displaying the vessels in the mucosa more superficially (the 'striate' sign).
6. The amount of phenol injected varies from 1 mL to 5 mL (usually 3 mL).

ANAL FISSURE[1]

The acute fissure

Treatment is with warm saline sitz baths, analgesics and 15 g bran or psyllium fibre orally each day for 3 months.

Milder cases

In a milder case of anal fissure the discomfort is slight, anal spasm is a minor feature and the onset is acute.

Conservative management

- Anaesthetic/corticosteroid suppositories or ointment (e.g. Xyloproct, Proctosedyl)
- High-residue diet (consider the addition of unprocessed bran)
- Avoidance of constipation with hard stools (aim for soft bulky stools)
- Glyceryl trinitrate ointment (Nitro-bid 2%) diluted 1 part with 9 parts white soft paraffin applied to the lower anal canal 2 to 3 times daily. A commercial

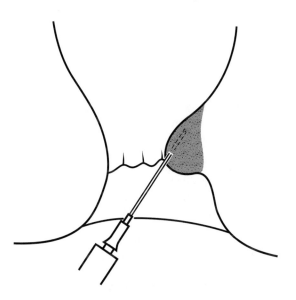

Fig. 6.5 Position of needle for the injection of haemorrhoids

preparation is Rectogesic ointment—apply 3 times daily for 6 weeks or until healed. Warn the patient about headache and lightheadedness
- Some clinics favour the topical application of 2% diltiazem cream for 6–8 weeks.[1]

More severe chronic fissures

The feature here is a hyperactive anal sphincter, and a practical procedure is necessary to solve this painful problem. Methods include:

Method 1: Digital anal dilatation

Under general anaesthesia (or even adequate local anaesthesia), undertake four-finger (maximum) anal dilatation for 4 minutes. This is effective, but is usually followed by a brief period of incontinence.

Anal dilatation under general anaesthesia is a most appropriate treatment for children with anal fissures.

Method 2: Inject botulinum toxin into the sphincter

Several studies indicate excellent results when botulinum toxin is injected into the surrounding internal sphincter. Its availability and considerable cost are limiting factors.

Method 3: Lateral sphincterotomy

The anal sphincter mechanism comprises internal and external sphincters. The spasm of the internal sphincter that occurs because of an anal fissure is relieved by the procedure of lateral sphincterotomy, allowing the fissure to heal in about 2 weeks. The procedure gives dramatic relief; however, the complication of permanent faecal incontinence has to be considered and surgical intervention with excision of the fissure is usually preferred practice.[1]

PROCTALGIA FUGAX

Main features

- Fleeting rectal pain in adults
- Varies from mild discomfort to severe spasm
- Lasts 3 to 30 minutes
- Often wakes patient at night
- Can occur at any time of day
- A functional bowel disorder

Management

- Explanation and reassurance
- Salbutamol inhaler (2 puffs inhaled statim) worth a trial

Alternatives include glyceryl trinitrate spray for the symptom or prophylactic quinine bisulphate at night.

PERIANAL ABSCESS[2]

Clinical features

- Severe, constant throbbing pain
- Fever and toxicity
- Hot, red, tender swelling adjacent to anal margin
- Non-fluctuant swelling

Careful examination is necessary to make the diagnosis. Look for evidence of a fistula-in-ano and an ischio-rectal abscess.

Treatment

Drainage via a cruciate incision over the point of maximal induration (Fig. 6.6a).

Method

1. Infiltrate 10 mL of 1% lidocaine with adrenaline in and around the skin overlying the abscess (in some people a general anaesthetic may be preferable).
2. Make a cruciate incision.
3. Insert artery forceps to open the abscess cavity and evacuate the pus.
4. Excise the corners of the cruciate incision to produce a circular skin defect (about 2 cm in diameter) (Fig. 6.6b).
5. Dress the wound with gauze soaked in a mild antiseptic.

(a)

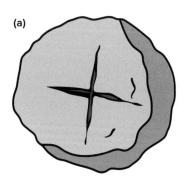

(b)

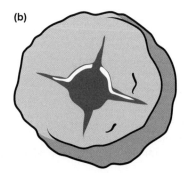

Fig. 6.6 Perianal abscess: **(a)** cruciate incision over abscess; **(b)** extension of cruciate incision

Post-procedure

- Change gauze dressings twice daily.
- Have warm saline sitz baths prior to new dressing.
- If undue bleeding occurs, pack the cavity for 24 hours and add covering dressings.

Antibiotics

If a perianal or perirectal abscess is recalcitrant or spreading with cellulitis, use metronidazole 400 mg (o) 12 hourly for 5–7 days plus cephalexin 500 mg (o) 6 hourly for 5–7 days.

PILONIDAL CYST ± ABSCESS

Incise and drain as for an abscess. Use a microbiological swab stick to break down abscess loculations and send it off for micro and culture. Pack the wound. Refer for excision of the extensive presacral sinus network.

ANAL FISTULA

Specialist referral is appropriate to determine the tracts. A modern method is the Seton management whereby thin silicone, silk or latex slings are inserted into the tracts under general anaesthetic by a surgeon. The method is particularly important for high tracts.

PERIANAL WARTS

It is important to distinguish the common viral warts from the condylomata lata of secondary syphilis. Counselling and support are necessary. Not all warts are sexually transmitted.

Treatment

The warts may be removed by chemical or physical means. The simplest and most effective treatment for readily accessible warts is:

- podophyllotoxin 5% paint (a more stable preparation than podophyllin)
  - Apply bd with plastic applicator for 3 days.
  - Repeat in 4 days if necessary (may need four treatments).

or

- podophyllin 25% solution in tinct benz co
  - Apply with a cotton wool swab to each wart.
  - Wash off in 4 hours, then dust with talcum powder.
  - Repeat once weekly until warts disappear.

or

- imiquimod (Aldara) cream
  - Apply 3 times weekly until resolved.

ANAL FIBRO-EPITHELIAL POLYPS

These polyps are usually overgrown anal papillae that present as an irritating prolapse. They are removed by infiltrating the base with local anaesthetic, crushing it with artery forceps and applying a ligature. They are benign but the removed lesion should undergo histological examination if there is any doubt.

PRURITUS ANI

In addition to the usual measures, consider cleaning the anus (after defaecation) with cotton wool dampened in warm water. Cotton wool is less abrasive than paper, and soap also irritates the problem.

General measures

- Stop scratching.
- Bathe carefully: avoid hot water, excessive scrubbing and soaps.
- Use bland aqueous cream, Cetaphil lotion or Neutrogena soap.
- Keep the area dry and cool.
- Keep bowels regular and wipe with cotton wool soaked in water.
- Wear loose-fitting clothing and underwear.
- A folded square of toilet paper separating the buttocks provides temporary partial relief.
- Avoid local anaesthetics and antiseptics.

If still problematic and a dermatosis is probably involved, use:
- hydrocortisone 1% cream, or
- hydrocortisone 1% cream with clioquinol 3% to 5% (most effective).

If an isolated area and resistant, infiltrate 0.5 mL of triamcinolone intradermally.

If desperate, use fractionated X-ray therapy.

RECTAL PROLAPSE

In the emergency situation it may be possible to reduce the swelling and thence the prolapse by covering the prolapse with a liberal sprinkling of fine crystalline sugar (common table sugar).

CAUTIONARY POINTS REGARDING ANO-RECTAL DISORDERS

- Every patient who presents with ano-rectal problems should undergo a digital rectal examination for detection of possible ano-rectal cancers.
- Practitioners need to be properly trained in techniques such as sclerosant injections and rubber band ligation in order to reduce the likelihood of complications.
- Be aware of the association of haemorrhoids and colorectal carcinoma.

References

1. Schlichtemeter S., Engel A. Anal fissure. Aust Prescr, 2016; 39: 14–17.

2. Daniel WJ. Anorectal pain, bleeding and lumps. Aust Fam Physician, 2010; 39: 376–81.

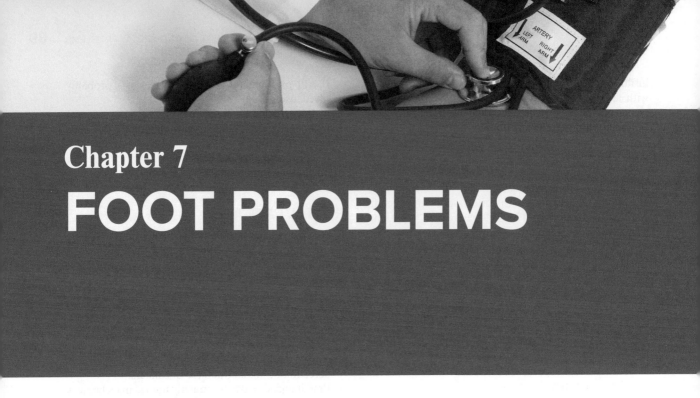

Chapter 7
FOOT PROBLEMS

CALLUSES, CORNS AND WARTS

The diagnosis of localised, tender lumps on the sole of the foot can be difficult. The differential diagnosis of callus, corn and wart is aided by an understanding of their morphology and the effect of paring these lumps (Table 7.1).

A callus (Fig. 7.1) is simply a localised area of hyperkeratosis related to some form of pressure and friction.

A corn (Fig. 7.2) is a small, localised, conical thickening, which may resemble a plantar wart but which gives a different appearance on paring.

A wart (Fig. 7.3) is more invasive, and paring reveals multiple small, pinpoint bleeding spots.

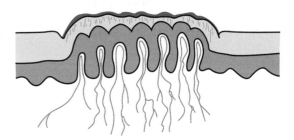

Fig. 7.3 Wart

TREATMENT OF PLANTAR WARTS

There are many treatments for this common and at times frustrating problem. A good rule is to avoid scalpel excision, diathermy or electrocautery because of the problem of scarring. One of the problems with the removal of plantar warts is the 'iceberg' configuration (Fig. 7.4) and not all may be removed. Pare the wart with a scalpel or file with a pumice stone or emery board prior to treatment.

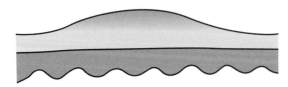

Fig. 7.1 Callus

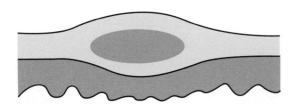

Fig. 7.2 Corn

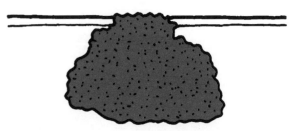

Fig. 7.4 'Iceberg' configuration of plantar wart

Table 7.1 Comparison of the main causes of a lump on the sole of the foot

	Typical site	Nature	Effect of paring
Callus	where skin is normally thick: beneath heads of metatarsals, heels, inframedial side of great toe	hard, thickened skin	*normal skin*
Corn	where skin is normally thin: on soles, fifth toe, dorsal projections of hammer toes	white, conical mass of keratin, flattened by pressure	*exposes white, avascular corn with concave surface*
Wart	anywhere, mainly over metatarsal heads, base of toes and heels; has bleeding points	viral infection, with abrupt change from skin at edge	*exposes bleeding points*

Liquid nitrogen

1. Pare wart to level of tolerance.
2. Apply liquid nitrogen (use double freeze–thaw cycle).
3. Repeat every 2 weeks until resolved.

Can be painful and results are often disappointing.

Topical chemotherapy

1. Pare wart (particularly in children).
2. Apply Upton's paste to wart each night and cover.
3. Review as necessary.
4. If preferred, apply topical anaesthetic cream (e.g. EMLA) an hour prior to each episode of paring.

(Upton's paste comprises trichloroacetic acid 1 part, salicylic acid 6 parts, glycerine to a stiff paste. It is available on the PBS as an extemporaneous prescription.)

Topical chemotherapy and liquid nitrogen

1. Pare wart (a 21-gauge blade is recommended).
2. Apply paste of 70% salicylic acid in raw linseed oil. This can be done by placing a corn pad over the wart and filling the central hole with the paste. Protect the surrounding skin with nail polish (acetone) or strapping tape (e.g. Sleek tape).
3. Occlude for 1 week.
4. Pare on review, then curette or apply liquid nitrogen and review.

Other combo methods

- 70% salicylic acid in linseed oil paste for 2 to 3 days followed by 40% salicylic acid in white soft paraffin 2 to 3 times weekly.

Curettage under local anaesthetic

1. Pare the wart vigorously to reveal the extent of the wart.
2. Thoroughly curette the entire wart with a dermal curette.
3. Hold the foot dependent over a kidney dish until the bleeding stops (this always stops spontaneously and avoids a bleed later on the way home).
4. Apply 50% trichloroacetic acid to the base.

Occlusion with topical chemotherapy

A method of using salicylic acid in a paste for the treatment of plantar warts is described here.

Equipment

You will need:
- 2.5 cm (width) elastic adhesive tape
- 30% salicylic acid in Lassar's paste. (Ask the chemist to prepare a thick paste, like plasticine.)

(Lassar's paste comprises zinc oxide, starch and salicylic acid, dispersed in white petrolatum.)

Method

1. Cut two lengths of adhesive tape, one about 5 cm and the other shorter.
2. Fold the shorter length in half, sticky side out (Fig. 7.5a).
3. Cut a half circle at the folded edge to accommodate the wart.
4. Press this tape down so that the hole is over the wart.
5. Roll a small ball of the paste in the palm of the hand and then press it into the wart.
6. Cover the tape, paste and wart with the longer strip of tape (Fig. 7.5b).
7. This paste should be reapplied twice daily for 2 to 3 weeks.
8. The reapplication is achieved by peeling back the longer strip to expose the wart, adding a fresh ball of paste to the wart weekly and then recovering with the upper tape.

The plantar wart invariably crumbles and vanishes. If the wart is particularly stubborn, 50% salicylic acid

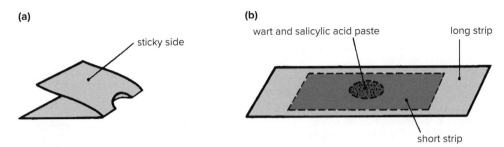

Fig. 7.5 **(a)** 'Window' to fit the wart is cut out of shoulder strip of elastic adhesive tape; **(b)** larger strip covers the wart and shoulder strip

can be used. For finger warts use 20% salicylic acid. This method should not be used for vaginal, penile or eyelid warts.

Alternative chemicals

- Formalin: Wearing gloves, syringe a small amount out of a specimen jar and place in a test tube. Upturn the test tube on the wart and leave in place for 5 minutes. Repeat daily and pare the wart weekly. Formalin is toxic: use with caution and keep in a locked cabinet.
- Salicylic acid 17%, lactic acid 17% in collodion (Dermatech Wart Treatment).
- Paste of trichloroacetic acid 1 part, salicylic acid 6 parts, glycerine 20 gm (Upton's paste).
- Salicylic acid, lactic acid in collodion (Duofilm).
- DCP ointment (see Chapter 3).

Poultice of aspirin and tea tree oil[1]

Method

1. Place a non-effervescent 125–300 mg soluble aspirin tablet on the centre of the wart and dampen it with 15% tea tree oil in alcohol.
2. Cover with a cotton pad and tape firmly with Micropore. Allow it to get wet to encourage dissolution.
3. After one week remove the dressing and debride or curette the friable slough.
4. Repeat if necessary.

Dr Scholl's corn pads

Apply pad with 40% salicylic acid daily for 2 days then according to response.

Simple (and unusual) treatments

The banana skin method

1. Cut a small disk of banana skin to cover the wart.
2. Apply the inner soft surface of the banana skin to the wart and cover with tape.
3. Perform this daily for a few weeks or as long as necessary.

The citric and acetic acid method

Soak pieces of lemon rind in vinegar for 3 to 4 days and then apply a small piece to the wart each day and cover with tape. The crumbling slough can usually be curetted out after 2 to 3 weeks.

TREATMENT OF CALLUSES[2]

- No treatment is required if asymptomatic.
- Remove the cause.
- Proper footwear is essential—wide shoes and cushioned pads over the ball of the foot.
- Provide paring with a scalpel blade (the most effective) or file with callus files.
- If severe, daily applications of 10% salicylic acid in soft paraffin or Eulactol Heel Balm with regular paring.

Paring method

Hold a no. 10 scalpel blade with the bevel almost parallel to the skin and shave the lines of any cracks with small, swift strokes (Fig. 7.6). Scrape along the lines of any cracks, not into them. Be careful not to draw blood.

TREATMENT OF CORNS

Hard corns (e.g. outside of toes)

- Remove the cause of friction and use wide shoes.
- Soften the corn with daily applications of 15% salicylic acid in collodion and then pare when soft.

An alternative is to apply commercial medicated disks (e.g. 40% salicylic acid) on a daily basis for about 4 days, then pare.

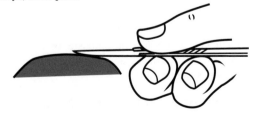

Fig. 7.6 Method of using a scalpel or similar knife to shave off a callus

Soft corns in webbing of toes

For soft corns between the toes (usually the last toe-web), treat in the same way, but keep the toe-webs separated with lamb's wool at all times, or use cigarette filter tips (these can be purchased at tobacco stores) separately and dust with a foot powder.

'CRACKED' HEELS

Method 1

- Soak the feet for 30 minutes in warm water containing an oil such as Alpha-Keri or Derma Oil.
- Pat dry, then apply a moisturising cream such as Nutraplus (10% urea) or Eulactol Heel Balm.
- Apply twice daily and keep covered at night e.g. with cotton socks.

Method 2

Consider applying medical skin glue, e.g. Histoacryl or even superglue, to neatly fill a dry crack and leave, with review in 4 days. This provides instant pain relief and often good healing.

PLANTAR FASCIITIS

Plantar fasciitis is a very common and surprisingly debilitating condition that may take 12 to 36 months (typically 2 years) to resolve spontaneously.

Features

- Pain:
  - under the heel (about 5 cm from end of heel)
  - can be diffuse over heel
  - when first step out of bed
  - relieved by walking around after shower
  - increasing towards the end of the day
  - worse after sitting
  - felt as a severe throbbing while sitting.
- Minimal signs—often local tenderness over anterior calcaneus.
- X-ray (usually unnecessary) may reveal a calcaneal spur.

Patient advice

- Avoid standing for long periods if possible.
- Rest from long walks and running.
- Try to cope without injections.
- Keep the heel 'cushioned' by wearing comfortable shoes and/or inserts in shoes.
- Surgery is rarely required and is not usually recommended. Excision of the calcaneal spur is advised against.

Footwear and insoles

Obtain good, comfortable shoes with a cushioned sole (e.g. Florsheim 'Comfortech'; sporting 'runners').
Examples of orthotic pads:
- Viscospot® orthotic
- Rose insole
- an insole tailored by a podiatrist
- a pad made from sponge or sorbo rubber placed inside the shoe to raise the heel about 1 cm. A hole corresponding to the tender area can be cut out of the pad to avoid direct contact with the sole (Fig. 7.7).

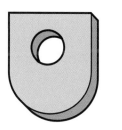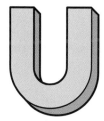

Fig. 7.7 Types of insole heel pads made from sponge or sorbo rubber

Hydrotherapy

The following tips have proved very useful.

Hot and cold water treatment

The patient places the affected foot in a small bath of very hot water and then a small bath of cold water for 20 to 30 seconds each time. This is continued on an alternating basis for 15 minutes—preferably twice a day and best before retiring at night.

Therapeutic foot massage

Commercial electrical foot hydro-massagers are available at low cost and are recommended for patients with plantar fasciitis.

Exercises[3,4]

Most foot surgeons now recommend regular stretching exercises as the basis of effective treatment. The aim is to allow the plantar fascia to heal at its 'natural length'. Stretching should be performed at least 3 times or more if manageable a day. It is recommended to perform at least two of the following exercises.

Exercise 1: sitting position stretch

1. Sit on a bed with both legs straight out in front of you and your hands on your knees.
2. Using a rope towel or cord looped around the foot, pull the foot back and point your toes towards your

head, bending the foot upwards at the ankle (Fig. 7.8a). The more effort you put into the motion, the better the stretch will be.

3. Hold the position for as long as possible (at least 30 seconds). Repeat several times.

Exercise 2

1. Stand on a stair, with the ball of your foot (or feet) on the edge of the stair, and keep your knees straight.
2. Holding the rails for balance, let your heels gently drop as you count to 20. Do not bounce (Fig. 7.8b). You should be relaxed, and no active muscle contraction should be necessary in your leg.
3. Lift your heels and count to 10.
4. Repeat the cycle twice. You will feel tightness both in the sole or heel of the foot, and at the back of the leg (as the Achilles tendon is also stretched).

Exercise 3

1. Stand against a solid wall with your painful foot behind you and the other foot closer to the wall (Fig. 7.8c).
2. Point the toes of the affected foot towards the heel of the front foot. Keep the knee of the painful leg straight and the painful heel on the floor.
3. Bend the front knee forward—you will feel the Achilles tendon in the painful foot grow tight.
4. Count to 20, then relax for a count of 10.

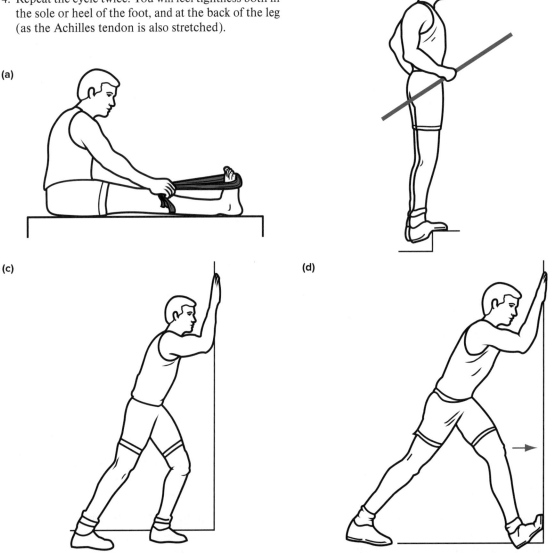

(a)   (b)   (c)   (d)

Fig. 7.8 Exercises for plantar fasciitis: **(a)** exercise 1; **(b)** exercise 2; **(c)** exercise 3 (right foot affected); **(d)** exercise 4 (left foot affected)

5. Repeat the cycle twice.
6. Change over the position of each foot and repeat the program to stretch the opposite Achilles tendon.

Exercise 4

You must be wearing flexible sole shoes for this exercise.
1. Stand against the wall with your good foot behind you and the painful foot jammed into the juncture of the wall and floor (Fig. 7.8d).
2. Bend the knee of the front leg, which will bring it towards the wall. You will feel that both the Achilles tendon and the tissue on the sole of the foot (plantar fascia) are being stretched by this exercise.
3. Count to 20, then relax for a count of 10.
4. Repeat the cycle twice.
5. Change over the position of each foot and repeat the program to stretch the opposite side.

Strapping for plantar fasciitis

Strapping of the affected foot can bring symptomatic relief for the pain of plantar fasciitis. A few strapping techniques can be used but the principle is to prevent excessive pronation, create a degree of inversion and reduce tension on the origin of the plantar fascia by compressing the heel. Use non-stretch sticking tape about 3–4 cm wide.

Method

- Start with the tape on the lateral side of the dorsum of the foot (Fig. 7.9a).
- Run the tape in a figure-of-eight configuration to include the sides of the heel but squeeze the heel from the sides to make a 'pad' immediately before applying and fixing the tape.
- Repeat twice (Fig. 7.9b).

If reinforcement is desired, a U-shaped strip of tape can be applied to the sides of the foot—from the neck of the metatarsals on one side to the other. Also, a strip of holding tape can encircle the foot.

Other tips

Manual massage

Massage the sole of the foot (particularly the tender area) over a wooden foot massager, a bottle filled with water or a frozen water bottle, or even a golf ball for 5 minutes, preferably 3 times daily.

Course of NSAIDs

It is worthwhile to conduct a trial of a 3-week course of NSAIDs during the time when there is most pain (about 4 to 7 weeks after the problem commences). It can be continued if there is a good response.

Injection

An injection of corticosteroid mixed with local anaesthetic can be very effective during the period of severe discomfort (Fig. 2.30.) The relief usually lasts for 2 to 4 weeks during this difficult period. However, injections are generally avoided.

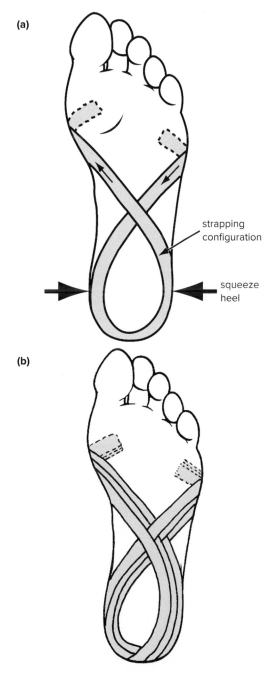

(a)

strapping configuration

squeeze heel

(b)

Fig. 7.9 Strapping for plantar fasciitis: **(a)** first application; **(b)** final appearance

MORTON'S INTERDIGITAL NEUROMA

The diagnosis is made on clinical grounds but an ultrasound examination may detect the neuroma, which is usually located between the third and fourth metatarsal heads. Early diagnosed problems should be treated conservatively by wearing loose wide shoes with a low heel and using a sponge rubber metatarsal pad (Fig. 7.10). If excessive pronation is present, an orthosis with a dome under the affected interspace to help spread the metatarsal heads is appropriate. Other possible treatments for chronic discomfort include an injection of corticosteroid and local anaesthetic into the neuroma, preferably under ultrasound guidance (if available), or radiofrequency ablation of the nerve. Some clinics use alcohol instead of corticosteroid. However, most will eventually require surgical excision, preferably with a dorsal approach. This results in permanent numbness of the innervated area and the patient needs to be forewarned.

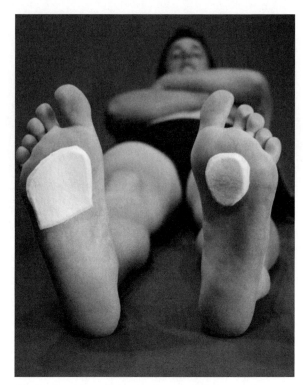

Fig. 7.10 Plantar metatarsal padding

Source: P. Brukner & K. Khan, *Brukner & Khan's Clinical Sports Medicine, Volume 1: Injuries* (5th Edn), McGraw-Hill, Sydney, 2017.

References

1. Györy AE. A duct tape-free wart remedy. Complementary Medicine, 2003; Sept/Oct: 4.
2. Warren G. Controlling callus. Medicine Today, 2003; 4(4): 95–7.
3. DiGiovanni BF, Nawoczenski DA, Lintal ME et al. Tissue-specific plantar fascia-stretching exercise enhances outcomes in patients with chronic heel pain: a prospective, randomized study. J Bone Joint Surg, 2003; 85-A: 1270–7.
4. RACGP. HANDI project. Stretching exercises: plantar faciitis. www.racgp.org.au/your-practice/guidelines/handi/about/the-handi-project, viewed 23 May 2016.

Chapter 8
NAIL PROBLEMS

SPLINTERS UNDER NAILS

Foreign bodies, mostly wooden splinters, often become deeply wedged under fingernails and toenails (Fig. 8.1a). Efforts by patients to remove the splinters often aggravate the problem. Methods of effective removal are outlined here.

The needle lever method

Take a sterile hypodermic needle, or any household needle that can be sterilised in a gas jet flame, and insert it just underneath the splinter, parallel to the nail through the entry tract. Then push the protruding end of the needle downwards. Since the needle spears the splinter, the lever effect drags out the splinter.

The V-cut out method

Equipment

You will need:
- needle, syringe and 1% lidocaine
- small scissors
- splinter forceps or small-artery forceps.

Method

1. Perform a digital nerve block to anaesthetise the involved digit (may not be necessary in rugged individuals or fairly distal splinters).
2. Using small but strong scissors, cut a V-shaped piece of nail from over the end of the splinter (Fig. 8.1b). It is important to leave sufficient splinter exposed so that a good grip can be obtained. (A poor grip can result in fragmentation of the splinter.)

3. Obtain a good grip on the end of the splinter with the splinter or small-artery forceps, and remove with a sharp tug in the axis of the finger (Fig. 8.1c).

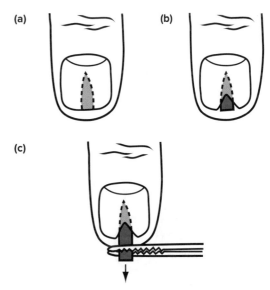

Fig. 8.1 Shows: **(a)** splinter under nail; **(b)** V-shaped incision; **(c)** tug with forceps

The 'paring' method

Use a no. 15 scalpel blade to gradually pare the nail overlying the splinter to create a window so that the splinter can be lifted out (Fig. 8.2). This is painless since the nail itself has no innervation.

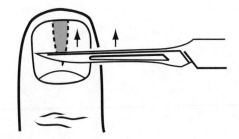

Fig. 8.2 Method of paring over a nail splinter using light shaving strokes

ONYCHOGRYPHOSIS

Onychogryphosis, or irregular thickening and overgrowth of the nail, is commonly seen in the big toenails of the elderly (Fig. 8.3). It is really a permanent condition, not infrequently misdiagnosed as onychomycosis and given futile antifungal treatment. Simple removal of the nail by avulsion is followed by recurrence some months later. Softening and burring of the nail gives only temporary relief, although burring sometimes provides a good result. The powder from burring can be used as culture for fungal organisms.

Permanent cure requires ablation of the nail bed after removal of the nail. Two methods of nail bed ablation are:

- total surgical excision
- cauterisation with pure phenol.

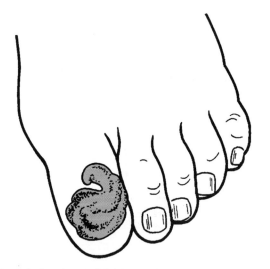

Fig. 8.3 Onychogryphosis

Adapted from A. Forrest et al., *Principles and Practice of Surgery*, Churchill Livingstone, Edinburgh, 1985, with permission.[1]

Cauterisation method

1. Apply a tourniquet to the toe after administering ring block.
2. Remove the nail by lifting it away from the nail bed and then grasping the total nail or two halves (after it is cut down the middle) with strong artery forceps and using a combination of rotation and traction.
3. Paint the nail bed and germinal layer with pure phenol on a cotton bud, with special attention to the groove containing the nail matrix. Leave the phenol on for 2 to 3 minutes, flush it with alcohol (e.g. methylated spirits) to neutralise it, mop dry and apply a dressing. Pack a small piece of chlorhexidine (Bactigras) tulle into the wound and then cover with sterile gauze and a bandage.

Caution:

- Avoid spilling pure phenol onto normal skin. Phenol is toxic and must be stored safely.
- Remember to remove the tourniquet. Start winding on the dressing bandage first, to control blood seepage.

ONYCHOMYCOSIS

Obtain fungal microscopy and culture before treatment, because antifungal medications can remain in the nail for many months, impeding the accuracy of subsequent testing. Be generous with the nail sample from affected areas: clippings, scrapings and crumbling debris from under the nail. Antifungal treatment will be unsuccessful if there is another cause for the nail deformity—commonly onychogryphosis in older people.

Cure usually requires an oral antifungal agent for a few months: griseofulvin or terbinafine for dermatophytes, or the 'azoles' if candida is present as well.

To reassure the frustrated patient, scrape a horizontal groove along the proximal edge of the nail before treatment and explain that as this line 'grows out', the new nail behind it will look clean.

MYXOID PSEUDOCYST

There are two types of digital myxoid pseudocysts (also known as mucous cysts) appearing in relation to the distal phalanx and nail in either fingers or toes (more common) (Fig. 8.4). One type occurs in relation to, and often connecting with, the distal interphalangeal joint and the other occurs at the site of the proximal nail fold.

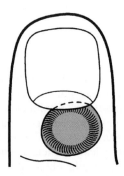

Fig. 8.4 Myxoid pseudocyst: typical position of the cyst

The latter (more common) is translucent and fluctuant, and contains thick clear gelatinous fluid, which is easily expressed after puncture of the cyst with a sterile needle. Osteoarthritis of the DIP is associated with leakage of myxoid fluid into the surrounding tissue to form the cyst.

Some pseudocysts resolve spontaneously. If persistent and symptomatic attempt:

- repeated aspiration (aseptically) at 4–6 weekly intervals
  or
- cryosurgery
  or
- puncture, compression, then infiltration intralesionally with triamcinolone acetonide (or similar steroid).

Pseudocysts tend to persist and recur; if so, refer to surgery for total excision of the proximal nail fold and/or ligation of the communicating stalk to the DIP.

SUBUNGUAL HAEMATOMA

The small, localised haematoma

There are several methods of decompressing a small, localised haematoma under the fingernail or toenail that causes considerable pain. The objective is to release the blood by drilling a hole in the overlying nail with a hot wire or a drill/needle, without the need for local anaesthetic.

Method 1: The sterile needle

Simply drill a hole by twisting a standard disposable hypodermic needle (21- or 23-gauge) into the selected site. Some practitioners prefer drilling two holes to facilitate the release of blood.

Method 2: The hot paper clip

Take a standard, large paper clip (Fig. 8.5a) and straighten it. Grasping the clip with insulation or forceps, heat one end until it is red hot in the flame of a spirit lamp (Fig. 8.5b). Immediately transfer the hot wire to the nail, and press the point lightly on the nail at the centre of the haematoma. After a small puff of smoke, an acrid odour and a spurt of blood, the patient will experience immediate relief (Fig. 8.5c).

Method 3: Electrocautery

This is the best method. Simply apply the hot wire of the electrocautery unit to the selected site (Fig. 8.6). It is very important to keep the wire hot at all times and to be prepared to withdraw it quickly, as soon as the nail is pierced. It should be painless.

Method 4: Algerbrush II

A gentler method suitable for children is the Algerbrush II, used by ophthalmologists to remove rust rings from

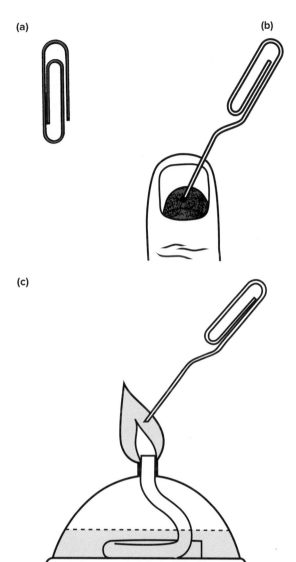

Fig. 8.5 (a) A standard paper clip; **(b)** the end of the paper clip is heated in the flame of a spirit lamp; **(c)** the point of the clip is pressed lightly on the nail at the centre of the haematoma

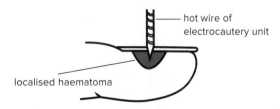

Fig. 8.6 Electrocautery to subungual haematoma

the cornea. It resembles a small dental burr, is battery operated and gently drills through the fingernail.

Important precautions

- Reassure patients that the process will not cause pain; they may be alarmed by the preparations.
- The hot point must quickly penetrate, and go no deeper than the nail. The blood under the nail insulates the underlying tissues from the heat and, therefore, from pain.
- The procedure is effective for a recent traumatic haematoma under tension. Do not attempt this procedure on an old, dried haematoma, as it will be painful and ineffective.
- Advise the patient to clean the nail with spirit or an antiseptic and cover with an adhesive strip to prevent contamination and infection.
- Advise the patient that the nail will eventually separate and a normal nail will appear in 4 to 6 months.

The large haematoma

Where blood occupies the total nail area, a relatively large laceration is present in the nail bed. To permit a good, long-term functional and cosmetic result, it is imperative to remove the nail and repair the laceration (Fig. 8.7). The rule is if > 50% of the nail area, remove the nail.

Method

1. Apply digital nerve block to the digit.
2. Remove the nail.
3. Repair the laceration with 4/0 absorbable sutures.
4. Replace the fingernail, which acts as a splint, and hold this in place with a suture for 10 days. A false acrylic nail is an alternative.

It takes 4 months to grow a new fingernail.

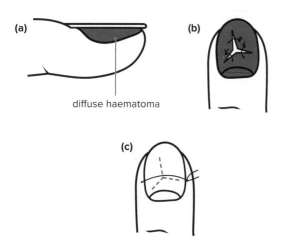

Fig. 8.7 Shows **(a)** diffuse haematomas; **(b)** sutures to laceration; **(c)** fingernail as splint

INGROWING TOENAILS (ONYCHOCRYPTOSIS)

There are a myriad methods to treat ingrowing toenails. Some very helpful ones are presented here.

Cautionary note

Treatment of ingrowing toenails is a potential legal 'minefield', especially with wedge resection.

Keep in mind the following:

- Full and detailed discussion with the patient about the procedure used and its risks is recommended.
- Avoid adrenaline with the local anaesthetic, especially if there is any peripheral vascular compromise—use plain lidocaine or bupivacaine.
- Avoid prolonged use of a tourniquet and do not forget to remove a rubber band if used.
- Avoid tight circumferential dressings.
- Be careful with people with diabetes or peripheral vascular disease.
- Avoid excessive use of phenol for nail bed cautery.
- Give clear post-operative instructions.
- It is best to treat when the infection settles.

Prevention

It is important to fashion the toenails so that the corners project beyond the skin (Fig. 8.8). Then each day, after a shower or bath, use the pads of both thumbs to pull the nail folds as indicated.[2]

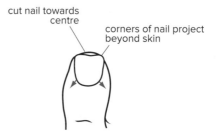

Fig. 8.8 Stretch nail folds with thumb daily

The spiral tape method

This simple technique involves the application of strong adhesive tape such as Elastoplast or Leukosilk 12.5 mm to retract the skin off the ingrowing nail. At first use the thumb pads, despite the discomfort, to retract the skin. The tape is then passed around the plantar surface to anchor the tape in loops around the proximal aspect of the toe (Fig. 8.9). The application of Friar's Balsam to the distal 'anchor' gives a better grip. This process is repeated 2 to 4 times weekly until the problem settles.[3]

Central thinning method

An interesting method for the prevention and treatment of ingrowing toenails is to thin out a central strip of the

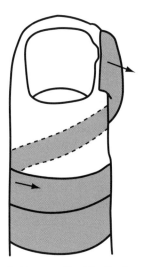

Fig. 8.9 The spiral tape method for the ingrowing toenail

nail plate. This is usually performed with the blade of a stitch remover or a no. 15 scalpel blade.

The central strip is about 5 mm wide and is thinned out on a regular basis (Fig. 8.10).

Patients can thin their own nail using a pumice stone if preferred.

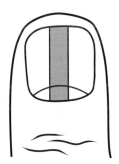

Fig. 8.10 Illustrating strip of nail plate to thin out

Excision of ellipse of skin

Figure 8.11 shows the toe in extremis. The procedure transposes the skinfold away from the nail. The skin heals, the nail grows normally and the toe retains its normal anatomy.

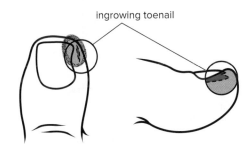

ingrowing toenail

Fig. 8.11 Ingrowing toenail

Method

1. An elliptical excision is made after a digital block (Fig. 8.12a). The width of the excision depends on the amount of movement of the skinfold required to fully expose the nail edge.
2. The skinfold is forced off the nail (Fig. 8.12b). Any blunt instrument can be used for this purpose. The wound closure holds the fold in its new position.
3. Any granulation tissue and debris should be removed with a curette. The toe heals well, and there are usually no recurrences of ingrowing.

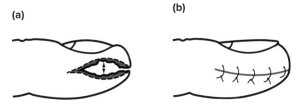

(a)

(b)

Fig. 8.12 Excision of ellipse of skin

Electrocautery

If the nail is severely ingrown, causing granulation tissue or infection of the skin or both, a most effective method is to use electrocautery to remove a large wedge of skin and granulation tissue so that the ingrown nail stands free of skin (Fig. 8.13).

This is performed under digital block. The toe heals surprisingly quickly and well (with minimal pain). The long-term result is excellent, because the nail that is not cut in this procedure can grow (and be trimmed) free of flesh.

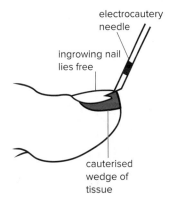

electrocautery needle

ingrowing nail lies free

cauterised wedge of tissue

Fig. 8.13 Electrocautery to wedge of tissue

BLOODLESS FIELD IN A DIGIT

Procedures on digits are ideally suited to creating a bloodless field using a tourniquet after completing a ring block with LA.

- Dip a thick rubber band in sterilising solution and wrap it multiple times around the base of the digit. Optionally, clip the final loop with mosquito forceps.
- A finger of a surgical glove held by forceps makes a rubber band substitute.
- Or instead use the whole glove, as follows: snip off the very tip of a glove finger and 'wear' the glove on the finger or toe, with the digit tip poking out through the hole. Roll the latex tightly down to the base of the digit. Potential disaster awaits if the post-operative dressing is applied without remembering to remove the tourniquet.

WEDGE RESECTION

The aim is to remove about one-quarter of the nail. Excise en bloc the wedge of nail, nail fold, nail wall and nail bed. Then back cut and curette out the lateral recess to ensure that the spicule of germinal matrix is removed.

Phenolisation

This method uses 80% phenol (pure solution) to treat the nail bed after simply removing the wedge of nail. It is not necessary to perform a standard wedge resection of the ingrown nail and nail bed. The success rate is better than curetting, at almost 100%.[4]

Method

1. Perform a ring block with plain local anaesthetic.
2. Apply a tourniquet so that a bloodless field is obtained.
3. Using scissors, mobilise the nail on the affected side and excise the nail sliver for about one-quarter of its width.
4. Curette the nail sulcus to remove any debris from the area.
5. Lift the nail fold and insert a cotton bud soaked (not saturated) in 80% phenol onto the corresponding nail bed (Fig. 8.14).
6. Leave the bud in place for 1½ to 2 minutes.
7. Remove and wash out the nail fold area with an alcohol swab or methylated spirits.
8. Apply a dressing and review as necessary.

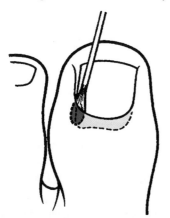

Fig. 8.14 Phenolisation method: lift the nail fold and apply the phenol on a stick

Cautionary tale

Pure phenol is a cytotoxic agent that causes a chemical burn and can be destructive to skin, causing a nasty slough. Several doctors using this excellent method claim that its value has been spoilt by causing severe burns to the surrounding skin. This has occurred because the swab had excess phenol that spilt onto the surrounding skin. This must be avoided with carefully controlled application, and if spillage occurs it must be washed off immediately with alcohol.

Wedge resection of nail with delayed nail fold excision

This method works very well where there is infection with swollen tissue.

Method

1. Perform a digital block.
2. Cut a standard wedge of ingrown nail (as for previous method). No further tissue is removed (Fig. 8.15a).
3. Dress and leave for 2 to 3 months.
4. After this time, perform a linear elliptical excision of the nail fold skin for the length of the nail extending to almost the tip of the toe. This should be about 3–4 mm from the nail margin to ensure skin necrosis does not occur. Suture and allow to heal (Fig. 8.15b).

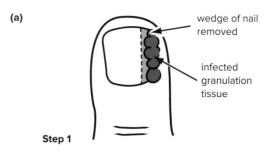

(a)

wedge of nail removed

infected granulation tissue

Step 1

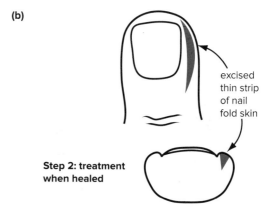

(b)

excised thin strip of nail fold skin

Step 2: treatment when healed

Fig. 8.15 Wedge resection of nail with delayed nail fold excision

THE ELLIPTICAL BLOCK DISSECTION OPEN METHOD

This method, described by Chapeski, is claimed to cure all cases of ingrown toenails and the wound, if performed aseptically and dressed properly, will not get infected. The wound heals in about 4 weeks.

Method

1. Perform a digital block.
2. Place an elastic band around the toe and wait 5 minutes.
3. An incision is made at the base of the nail, about 3–4 mm from the edge, and then continued towards the side of the nail in an elliptical sweep to end up under the tip of the nail about 3–4 mm from the edge.
4. The ingrown skin (about 10 × 20 mm) is thus removed along with subcutaneous tissue (it is important that none of the skin remains around the edge of the nail) (Fig. 8.16).

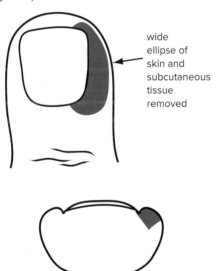

wide ellipse of skin and subcutaneous tissue removed

Fig. 8.16 Elliptical block dissection open method

5. Cauterise any bleeding points, e.g. with a silver nitrate stick.
6. A 3 mm thick Sofra-Tulle square is then placed directly over the wound, followed by a single gauze square (to wrap the toe), then a simple 25 mm Elastoplast pressure dressing.

Note: Bleeding can be a problem when the patient walks, so place a small plastic bag over the foot before pulling on the shoe. The patient should elevate the foot at home for an hour or so.

Follow-up

- Next day, the patient should soak the foot in lukewarm water for 15 to 20 minutes, gradually peel off the old dressing and then apply several layers of fine mesh gauze and tape them into place.
- Repeat the soaking procedure religiously 3 times daily for 20 minutes.
- Follow up the patient weekly for 4 weeks—cauterise any granulation tissue (a sign of poor compliance) with silver nitrate and dress.

The 'plastic gutter' method

This simple method separates the ingrowing nail from the skin to allow healing.[4]

Method

1. Cut a length (to match the nail) of tubing from a scalp vein plastic cannula and cut it down the middle to form a hemi-cylinder.
2. Under suitable local anaesthetic lift the skin around the ingrowing toenail with forceps and insert the tubing (Fig. 8.17). Leave it in place for 1 week covered with a dressing. It can be stitched to the skin.
3. Repeat if necessary.

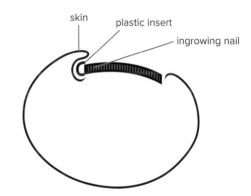

skin   plastic insert   ingrowing nail

Fig. 8.17 Illustration of the 'plastic gutter' method

TIP FOR POST-OPERATIVE PAIN RELIEF

Procedures on the toe, especially for ingrown toenails, can be very painful, especially during the night after the surgery.

Plan these procedures as the final appointment for the day and use the long-acting local anaesthetic bupivacaine 0.5% (Marcaine).

PARONYCHIA

The extent of the procedure depends on the extent of the infection (Fig. 8.18). For all methods anaesthetise the finger or toe with a digital block.

Method 1: Lateral focus of pus

1. With a size 11 or 15 scalpel blade incise over the focus of pus (Fig. 8.19a).
2. Probe deeply until all pus is released.
3. Insert a small wick into the wound and allow to heal.

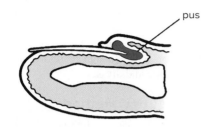

Fig. 8.18 Paronychia

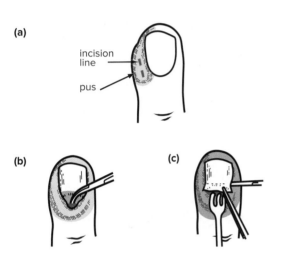

Fig. 8.19 Treatment of paronychia: **(a)** incision for lateral focus of pus; **(b)** elevation of eponychial fold; **(c)** excision of proximal end of nail

Reproduced from A. Forrest et al., *Principles and Practice of Surgery,* Churchill Livingstone, Edinburgh, 1985, with permission.[1]

Method 2: Central focus of pus

Elevate the eponychial fold with a pair of fine artery forceps (Fig. 8.19b). This will release the pus.

Method 3: Infection adjacent to nail

Gently pack a fine wisp of cotton wool or gauze into the space between the paronychia and the nail and apply povidone-iodine. Dry and repeat as necessary. It should be relatively painless.

Method 4: Extensive infection under nail

1. If the infection extends under the nail, this fold should be pushed back proximally with a small retractor to expose the nail base.
2. Elevate the nail base bluntly and excise the proximal end of the nail with sharp scissors (Fig. 8.19c). (Alternatively, the nail can be removed.)
3. Apply petroleum jelly gauze dressing and use a light splint for 3 days.
4. The patient should be encouraged to wear gloves to keep the area dry.

EXCISION OF NAIL BED

Method

1. Apply a tourniquet after digital or ring block.
2. Make skin incisions (Fig. 8.20a).
3. Avulse the nail using strong artery forceps.
4. Elevate the skin flaps (Fig. 8.20b).
5. Excise the nail bed carefully, including the undersurface of the overhanging skin (Fig. 8.20c).
6. Scrape the bone with a Volkman's spoon to ensure that no parts of the nail root remain.

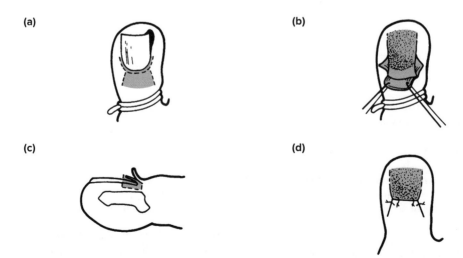

Fig. 8.20 Excision of nail bed: **(a)** skin incisions; **(b)** elevation of skin flap; **(c)** excision of nail bed; **(d)** suturing of skin flaps

Reproduced from A. Forrest et al., *Principles and Practice of Surgery,* Churchill Livingstone, Edinburgh, 1985, with permission.[1]

7. Apply the phenolisation method also at this stage (with caution).
8. Suture the skin flaps (Fig. 8.20d).

NAIL AVULSION BY CHEMOLYSIS

Indication

Dystrophic toenails (e.g. from chronic fungal infection) in patients with peripheral vascular disease or other conditions where surgery is inadvisable.

Equipment

You will need:
- 40% salicylic acid ointment
- plastic 'skin'.

Method

1. Apply plastic 'skin' spray to the skin around the nail to prevent possible skin maceration.
2. Apply 40% salicylic acid ointment to the nail. Use a liberal application, but confine it to the nail.
3. Cover with plastic kitchen wrap.

Post-procedure

- Reapply the ointment every 2 days.
- Maintain for about 4 weeks.
  This treatment will soften and destroy the nail.

TRAUMATIC AVULSED TOENAIL

If a toenail, particularly of the great toe, is torn away, it is appropriate to reapply it as a splint, secure it with stay sutures (e.g. chromic catgut) and apply continuing dressings (Fig. 8.21). This provides protection and promotes healing.

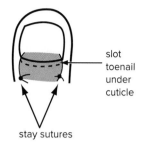

Fig. 8.21 Traumatic avulsed toenail

LONGITUDINAL TRAUMATIC NAIL LACERATION

An example is laceration through the nail bed of the thumb. Primary suture including the nail, preferably under antibiotic cover, is appropriate and can give a good outcome while preserving the small piece of nail (Fig. 8.22).

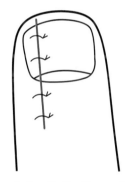

Fig. 8.22 Suture of a longitudinal traumatic nail laceration

References

1. A. Forrest et al., *Principles and practice of surgery,* Edinburgh: Churchill Livingstone, 1985.
2. Gregson H. Ingrowing toenails: prevention. Aust Fam Physician, 1989;18:11;143.
3. Babbage NF. Ingrowing toenails. Aust Fam Physician, 1985;14:8;768.
4. Buckley J. Ingrowing toenails: the phenolisation method. Aust Fam Physician 1989;18:1;33.

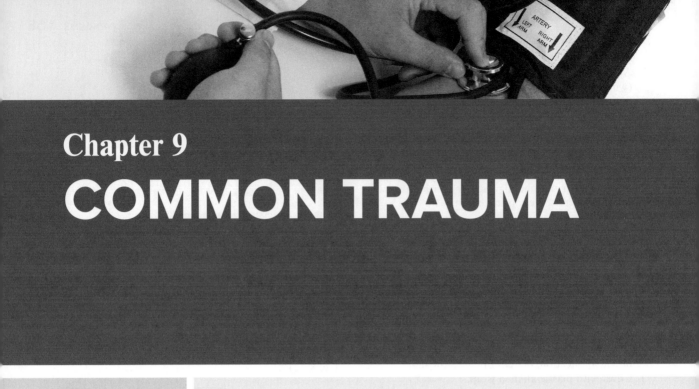

Chapter 9
COMMON TRAUMA

General

ESSENTIAL TIPS FOR DEALING WITH TRAUMA

Common traps

- Failure to diagnose a foreign body
- Failure to diagnose a ruptured tendon
- Exposed joint capsule in the fist
- Beware of bites, high pressure guns and puncture wounds
- Be cautious of fractures and dislocations around the elbow in children

Stab wounds

Always assume (and look for) the presence of nerve, tendon or artery injury.

Foreign bodies

Buried wooden splinters, gravel and slivers of glass are old traps—if suspected and not found on simple exploration, order high-resolution ultrasound, which is good at detecting wood and glass. CT is best.

Falling on the outstretched hand

Consider the following fractures: Colles and Smith (distal radius); scaphoid; radius and ulna shafts; head of radius; Bennett's fracture (carpo-metacarpal joint of thumb); supracondylar (children); neck and shaft of humerus, clavicle and the dislocations—lunate and shoulder.

Jumping or falling from a substantial height onto feet

Always consider a fractured calcaneum, talus, spine (especially lumbar) or pelvis and central dislocation of hip. Concussion can follow.

Vascular complications of fractures and dislocations

Upper limb: supracondylar fracture of humerus (brachial artery); compartment syndrome of flexor muscles.

Lower limb: supracondylar fracture of femur (popliteal vessels); dislocation of knee; disruption of pelvis (up to 5000 mL of blood).

Cut finger or toe

Always look for a peripheral nerve injury.

Finger tourniquet

If using a small tourniquet such as a rubber band for haemostasis, clip on a small artery forceps so it is not forgotten when you finish.

OTHER CAUTIONARY TIPS

- You can get concussion from a heavy fall onto the coccyx/sacrum.
- Think of a sewing needle in the knee or in the feet of children for unexplained pain.

- Treat (evacuate) haematomas of the nasal septum and ear because they can collapse cartilage.
- Beware of pressure gun injuries into soft tissue, especially those involving oil and paint.

- Beware of a painful immobile elbow in a child—look for a fracture that can cause trouble later.
- Beware of the scaphoid fracture after a fall onto an outstretched hand. Examine the snuffbox.

Finger trauma

Finger injuries can be treated by simple means, providing there are neither tendon nor nerve injuries complicating the lacerations or compound fractures involved.

FINGER TIP LOSS

Not all finger tip loss demands an immediate graft or tidy-up amputation. If there is no exposed phalanx tip and the area of exposed subdermal tissue is small, conservative management is best. Remember that a grafted finger tip is insensate. If the amputated skin tip is available, it should be replaced (use Steri-Strips or a couple of small sutures), as it may take as a graft or merely act as a good biological dressing.

Large skin loss

Apply a split skin graft, preferably using a Goulian knife with three spacing devices.

AMPUTATED FINGER

In this emergency situation, instruct the patient to place the severed finger directly into a fluid-tight sterile container, such as a plastic bag or sterile specimen jar. Then place this 'unit' in a bag containing iced water with crushed ice.

Note: Never place the amputated finger directly in ice or in fluid such as saline. Fluid makes the tissue soggy, rendering microsurgical repair difficult.

Care of the finger stump

Apply a simple, sterile, loose, non-sticky dressing and keep the hand elevated.

FINGER TIP DRESSING

A method of applying a dressing (using an adhesive dressing strip) for an injured finger tip is described.

Method

1. Cut a suitable length of the dressing strip almost as long as the finger.
2. Cut through the adhesive margins to the central non-adhesive dressing about 1–1.5 cm from the top (Fig. 9.1).
3. Remove the backing from the lower larger segment and apply to the injured side of the finger. Wrap the adhesive part around the circumference of the finger.

Cut a suitable length of a dressing strip. Cut through the adhesive to the dressing strip—1–1.5 cm from the top.

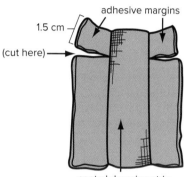

Remove the backing from the lower segment and apply to the injured side of the finger.

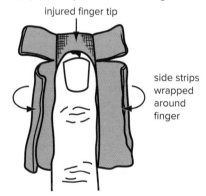

Remove the backing from the upper segment and fold it backward over the tip.

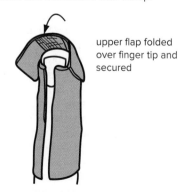

Fig. 9.1 Applying a finger tip dressing

4. Now remove the backing from the upper segment and fold it backwards over the tip, with the adhesive margins wrapped around the finger to provide the most effective dressing. Alternatively, the upper dressing can be folded over the fingertip first while the crossbar side flaps wrap around the base of the tip to secure the dressing.

Abrasions

Abrasions or 'gravel rash' vary considerably in degree and potential contamination. They are common with bicycle or motorcycle accidents and skateboard accidents. Special care is needed over joints such as the knee or elbow.

MANAGEMENT (SEE CHAPTER 1)

- Clean meticulously, remove all ground-in dirt, metal, clothing and other material.
- Scrub out dirt with sterile normal saline under anaesthesia (local infiltration or general anaesthesia for deep wounds). Adequate local anaesthesia may also be achieved by coating the wound liberally with Xylocaine jelly 2% and leaving for 10 minutes.
- Treat the injury as a burn.
- When clean, apply a protective dressing (some wounds may be left open).
- Use paraffin gauze and non-adhesive absorbent pads such as Melolin.
- Ensure adequate follow-up.
- Immobilise a joint that may be affected by a deep wound.

Haematomas

HAEMATOMA OF THE PINNA ('CAULIFLOWER EAR')

When trauma to the pinna causes a haematoma between the epidermis and the cartilage, a permanent deformity known as 'cauliflower ear' may result. The haematoma, if left, becomes organised and the normal contour of the ear is lost.

The aim is to evacuate the haematoma as soon as practicable and then to prevent it re-forming. One can achieve a fair degree of success even on haematomas that have been present for several days.

Method

1. After cleansing the pinna with a suitable solution (e.g. cetrimide), insert a 25-gauge needle into the haematoma and aspirate the extravasated blood.
2. Position the needle at the lowest point while pressing the upper border of the haematoma gently between finger and thumb (Fig. 9.2a).
3. Apply a padded test tube clamp or clothes line peg or any similar plastic clamp (preferable) to the haematoma site and leave on for 30–40 minutes. The test tube clamp has large jaws that allow it to be placed over the haematoma site (Fig. 9.2b).

Generally, daily aspirations and clamping are sufficient to eradicate the haematoma completely.

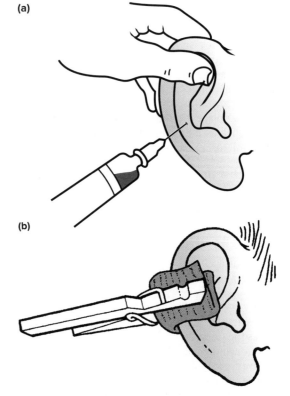

(a)

(b)

Fig. 9.2 Treatment of cauliflower ear

HAEMATOMA OF THE NASAL SEPTUM

Septal haematoma following injury to the nose can cause total nasal obstruction. It is easily diagnosed as a marked swelling on both sides of the septum when inspected through the nose (Fig. 9.3). It results from haemorrhage between the two sheets of mucoperiosteum covering the septum. It may be associated with a fracture of the nasal septum.

Note: This is a most serious problem as it can develop into a septal abscess. The infection can pass readily to the orbit or the cavernous sinus through thrombosing veins and may prove fatal, especially in children. Otherwise it may lead to necrosis of the nasal septal cartilage followed by collapse and nasal deformity.

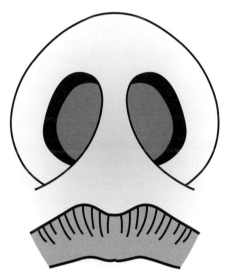

Fig. 9.3 Inferior view of nasal cavity showing bilateral swelling of septal haematoma

Treatment

- Remove the blood clot on both sides through an incision, under local anaesthetic. This must be done within 2 hours of injury.
- Prescribe oral antibiotics, e.g. penicillin or erythromycin.
- Treat as a compound fracture if an X-ray reveals a fracture.

PRETIBIAL HAEMATOMA

A haematoma over the tibia (shin bone) can be persistently painful and slow to resolve. An efficient method is, under very strict asepsis, to inject 1 mL of 1% of lidocaine and 1 mL of hyaluronidase and follow with immediate ultrasound. This may disperse or require drainage.

ROLLER INJURIES TO LIMBS

A patient who has been injured by a wheel or by rollers passing over a limb can present a difficult problem. An arm caught in the wringers of an old-fashioned washing machine used to be a common example, but a more likely problem now is the wheel of a vehicle passing over a limb, especially a leg.

A freely spinning wheel is not so dangerous, but more serious injuries occur when a non-spinning (braked) wheel passes over a limb. This leads to a 'degloving' injury due to shearing stress. The limb may look satisfactory initially, but skin necrosis will follow.

To manage a 'wheel over the limb' injury, treat it as a serious problem and admit the patient to hospital for observation. Surgical intervention with removal of necrotic fat may be essential. Fasciotomy with open drainage may also be an option.

Fractures

TESTING FOR FRACTURES

This method describes the simple principle of applying axial compression for the clinical diagnosis of fractures of bones. It applies especially to suspected fractures of bones of the forearm and hand, but also applies to all bones of the limbs.

Many fractures are obvious when applying the classic methods of diagnosis: pain, tenderness, loss of function, deformity, swelling and sometimes crepitus. It is sometimes more difficult if there is associated soft-tissue injury from a blow or if there is only a minor fracture such as a greenstick fracture of the distal radius.

If the bone is compressed gently from end to end, a fracture will reveal itself and the patient will feel pain. A soft-tissue injury of the forearm will show pain, tenderness, swelling and possibly loss of function. It will, however, not be painful if the bone is compressed axially—that is, in its long axis.

Walking is another method of applying axial compression, and this is very difficult (because of pain) in the presence of a fracture in the weight-bearing axis or pelvis. Hence, every patient with a suspected fracture of the lower limb should be tested by walking.

Method

1. Grasp the affected area both distally and proximally with your hands.
2. Compress along the long axis of the bones by pushing in both directions, so that the forces focus on the affected area (fracture site; Fig. 9.4a). Alternatively, compression can be applied from the distal end with stabilising counterpressure applied proximally (Fig. 9.4b).
3. The patient will accurately localise the pain at the fracture site.

(a)

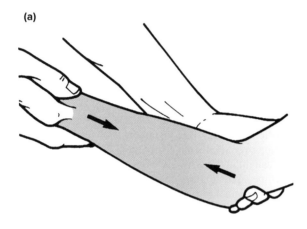

(b)

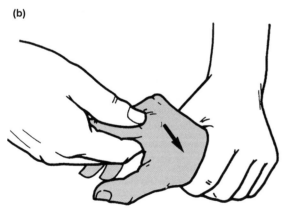

Fig. 9.4 Testing for fractures: **(a)** axial compression to detect a fracture of the radius or ulnar bones; **(b)** axial compression to detect a fracture of the metacarpal

SPATULA TEST FOR FRACTURE OF MANDIBLE

A simple office test for a suspected fractured mandible is to get the patient to bite on a wooden tongue depressor (or similar firm object).

Ask them to maintain this bite as you twist the spatula (Fig. 9.5). If they have a fracture, they cannot hang on to the spatula because of pain.

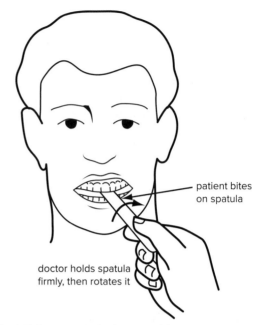

patient bites
on spatula

doctor holds spatula
firmly, then rotates it

Fig. 9.5 Spatula test for fracture of the mandible

FIRST AID MANAGEMENT OF FRACTURED MANDIBLE

- Check the patient's bite and airway.
- Remove any free-floating tooth fragments and retain them.
- Replace any avulsed or subluxed teeth in their sockets. *Note:* Never discard teeth.
- First aid immobilisation with a four-tailed bandage (Fig. 9.6).

Treatment

Refer for possible internal fixation.

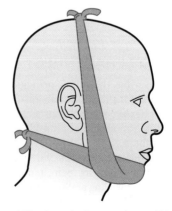

Fig. 9.6 Immobilisation of a fractured mandible in a four-tailed bandage

A fracture of the body of the mandible will usually heal in 6 to 12 weeks (depending on the nature of the fracture and the fitness of the patient).

FRACTURED CLAVICLE

There is a history of a fall onto the outstretched hand or elbow. The patient has pain aggravated by shoulder movement and usually supports the arm at the elbow and clasped to the chest. The most common fracture site is at the junction of the outer and middle thirds, or in the middle third.

Treatment

- St John elevated sling to support the arm—for 3 weeks.
- Figure-of-eight bandage (used mainly for severe discomfort).
- Early active exercises to elbow, wrist and fingers.
- Active shoulder movements as early as possible.

Special problem

Fracture at the lateral end of the bone. Consider referral for open reduction.

Healing time

4 to 8 weeks.

The healing times for uncomplicated fractures are presented in Table 9.1, page 111.

BANDAGE FOR FRACTURED CLAVICLE

A figure-of-eight bandage can be made simply by inserting pads of cotton wool into pantyhose or stockings.

FRACTURED RIB

A simple rib fracture can be extremely painful. The first treatment strategy is to prescribe analgesics such as paracetamol, and encourage breathing within the limits of pain.

If pain persists in cases of single or double rib fracture with no complication, application of a rib support is most helpful.

The universal rib belt

A special elastic rib belt can provide thoracic support and mild compression for fractured ribs (Fig. 9.7). Despite its flexibility it gives excellent support and symptom relief while permitting adequate lung expansion.

The elastic belt is 15 cm wide and has Velcro grip fastening, so it can be applied to a variety of chest sizes.

Healing time

3 to 6 weeks.

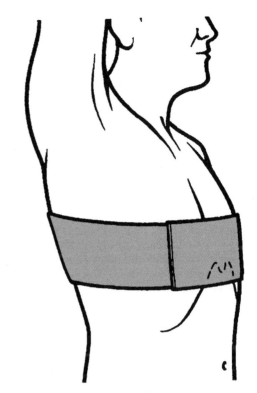

Fig. 9.7 Method of application of rib belt

Towel or pillow method

The patient can wrap a standard-sized towel (folded lengthwise to a third of its width) around the chest and secure it with a large safety pin. When the patient is about to cough, the towel can be pulled tight by the patient. An alternative is to clutch a pillow to the affected side of the chest while coughing.

PHALANGEAL FRACTURES

These fractures require as near perfect reduction as possible, careful splintage and, above all, early mobilisation once the fracture is stable—usually in 2 or 3 weeks.

Early operative intervention should be considered if the fracture is unstable.

Angulation is usually obvious, but it is most important to check for rotational malalignment, especially with torsional fracture. A simple method is to get the patient to make a fist of the hand and check the direction in which the nails are facing. Furthermore, each finger can be flexed in turn and checked to see if the fingertips point towards the tubercule of the scaphoid (palpable halfway along the base of the thenar eminence and 1.5 cm distal to the distal wrist crease).

The phalanges

- Distal phalanges: usually crush fractures; generally heal simply unless intra-articular.

- Middle phalanges: tend to be displaced and unstable—beware of rotation.

- Proximal phalanges: are the greatest concern, especially of the little finger; intra-articular fractures usually need internal fixation.

Treatment of uncomplicated fractures

For non-displaced phalanges with no rotational malalignment, strap the injured finger to the adjacent normal finger with an elastic garter or adhesive tape for 2 to 3 weeks, i.e. 'buddy strapping' (Fig. 9.8). A strip of gauze between the two fingers may prevent chaffing. Start the patient on active exercises.

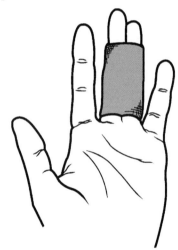

Fig. 9.8 Treatment of non-displaced phalanges by 'buddy strapping': the fractured finger is strapped to an adjacent healthy finger

If pain and swelling is a problem, splint the finger with a narrow dorsal or anterior slab (a felt-lined strip of malleable aluminium can be used) (Fig. 9.9). An alternative is to bandage the hand while the patient holds

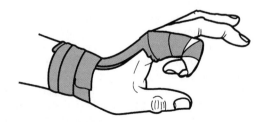

Fig. 9.9 Method of splinting a phalangeal fracture of the index finger by a posterior plaster slab

a tennis ball or appropriate roll of bandage in order to maintain appropriate flexion of all interphalangeal joints.

SLINGS FOR FRACTURES

There are three slings in common use in first aid:

Sling	Main indications
Collar and cuff	Fractured humerus
Broad arm	Fractured forearm
St John	Fractured clavicle
	Dislocated acromioclavicular joint
	Subluxed acromioclavicular joint
	Infected or fractured hand

Collar and cuff sling

This is useful for the patient with a fractured humerus, including an undisplaced supracondylar fracture, because it allows gravity to realign the distal and proximal parts of the fractured bones.

Method

1. Using a narrow bandage, make a clove hitch (Fig. 9.10a). The clove hitch is made by fashioning two loops—one towards your body and the other away, leaving one end of the bandage longer than the other. Now place your fingers under the loops and bring them together.
2. Slide the loops over the wrist of the injured arm with the knot of the clove hitch on the thumb side of the wrist.
3. Gently flex the elbow and elevate the injured arm so that the fingers point towards the opposite shoulder (Fig. 9.10b).
4. Place the long end of the bandage around the neck and tie the bandage, using a reef knot (Fig. 9.10c).

The broad arm sling

This has multiple uses but is used mainly for injuries to the forearm and wrist.

Method

1. Place an open triangular bandage over the patient's chest, with the point of the triangle stretching beyond the elbow of the injured side. Place the flexed forearm over the bandage as shown (see Fig. 9.11a).
2. Carry the upper end of the bandage over the shoulder on the uninjured side, around the back of the neck. Ensure that the injured arm lies slightly above the horizontal position.
3. Tie the long ends of the bandage in the hollow above the collar bone of the injured side (see Fig. 9.11b).
4. Fold the corner adjacent to the injured elbow and secure it with a safety pin.

(a)

(b)

(c)

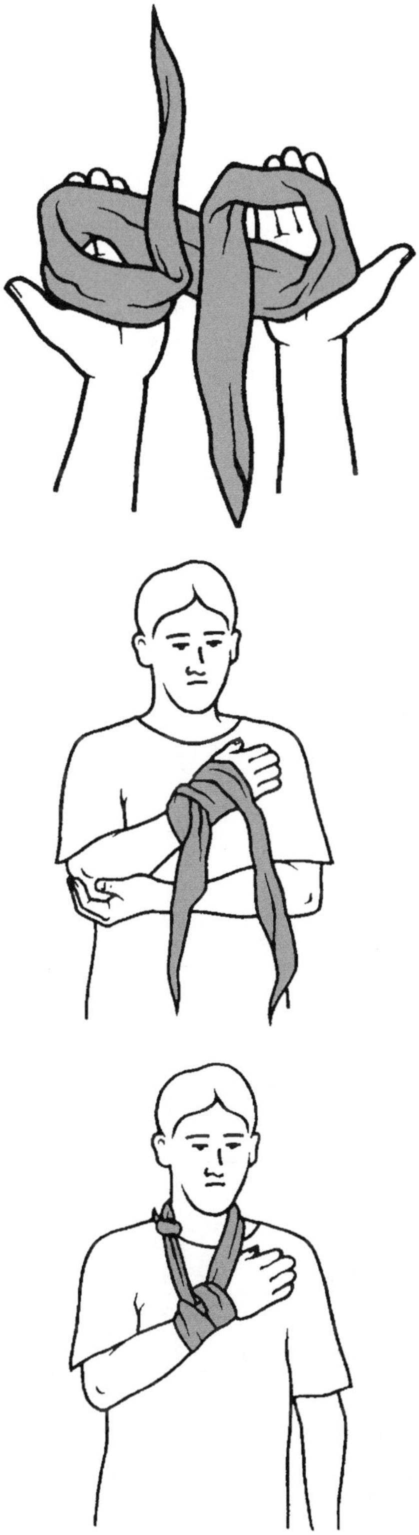

Fig. 9.10 (a) Preparing a clove hitch; **(b)** flex the elbow and elevate the injured arm; **(c)** applying a collar and cuff sling

(a)

(b)

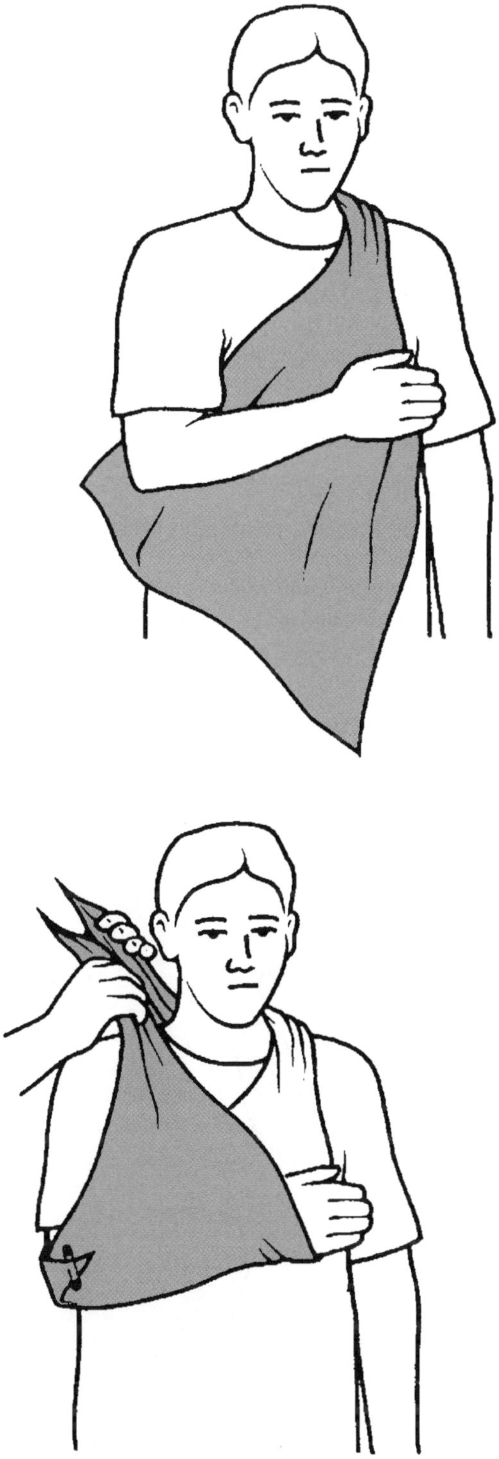

Fig. 9.11 (a) The broad arm sling: first step; **(b)** the broad arm sling

The St John sling

This sling, used for a fractured clavicle, dislocated acromioclavicular joint, or fractured or infected hand, supports the elbow and keeps the hand in elevation resting comfortably on the shoulder of the uninjured side.

Method

1. Place an open triangular bandage over the patient's forearm and hand with the point of the triangle to the elbow and the upper end over the far shoulder.
2. Tuck the long edge of the bandage under the whole forearm to make a supporting trough (Fig. 9.12a).
3. Convey the lower dependent end around the patient's back to the front of the far shoulder.
4. Tie the ends as close to the fingers as possible (Fig. 9.12b).
5. Tuck the triangular point firmly in between the forearm and the bandage.
6. Secure the fold with a safety pin when the sling is firm, comfortable and at the correct elevation.

(a)

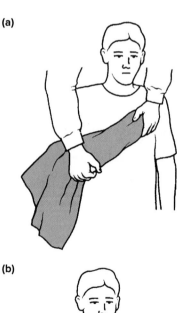

(b)

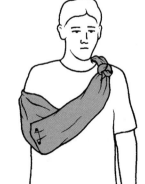

Fig. 9.12 The St John sling: **(a)** first step; **(b)** the St John sling

Table 9.1 Healing of uncomplicated fractures (adults)

Fracture	(Approximate) average immobilisation time (weeks)
Rib	3–6 (healing time)
Clavicle	4–8 (2 weeks in sling)
Scapula	weeks to months
Humerus	
• neck	3–6
• shaft	8
• condyles	3–4
Radius	
• head of radius	3
• shaft	6
• Colles' fracture	4–6
Radius and ulna (shafts)	6–12
Ulna—shaft	8
Scaphoid	8–12
Metacarpals	
• Bennett's #	6–8
• other	3–4
Phalanges (hand)	
• proximal	3
• middle	2–3
• distal	2–3
Pelvis	Rest in bed 2–6
Femur	
• femoral neck	according to surgery
• shaft	12–16
• distal	8–12
Patella	3–4
Tibia	12–16
Fibula	6
Both tibia and fibula	12–16
Potts fracture	6–8
Lateral malleolus avulsion	3
Calcaneus	
• minor	4–6
• compression	14–16
Talus	12
Tarsal bones (stress #)	8
Metatarsals	4
Phalanges (toes)	0–3
Spine	
• spinous process	3
• transverse process	3
• stable vertebra	3
• unstable vertebra	9–14
• sacrum/coccyx	3

The makeshift sling

An effective sling can be made with a large jumper or windcheater.

Method

1. Place the sleeves of the jumper around the neck and knot the ends.
2. Guide the affected arm into the sleeve until a suitable recess is found.

IMPORTANT PRINCIPLES FOR FRACTURES

- Plain X-rays often unnecessary for some fractures e.g. 'greenstick' of arm, clavicle.
- Children under 8 years usually take half the time to heal.
- Have a check X-ray in 1 week (for most fractures).
- Radiological union lags behind clinical union.

Other trauma

PRIMARY REPAIR OF SEVERED TENDON

Immediate repair of cut tendons by primary suture is important (certainly within 72 hours), preferably by an experienced surgeon. Partial ruptures usually require no active surgery, although primary repair is recommended if greater than 40% of the tendon diameter is severed.

Method for totally cut tendon

1. Debride the wound.
2. Pass a loop suture of 3/0 monofilament nylon on a straight needle into the tendon through the cut surface close to the edge to emerge 5 mm beyond and then construct a figure-of-eight suture as shown in Fig. 9.13a–c.
3. Pull the two ends of the suture to take up the slack without bunching the tendon (Fig. 9.13d).
4. Repeat this with the other end of the tendon (Fig. 9.13e).
5. Tie the corresponding suture ends together in order to closely approximate the cut ends of the tendon (Fig. 9.13f).
6. Bury the knots deep between the tendon and cut the sutures short (Fig. 9.13g).

Post-operation

Hold the repaired tendons in a relaxed position with suitable splintage for 3 to 4 weeks.

BURNS AND SCALDS

Burns can be caused by flame/fire, hot liquids, hot objects such as irons and heaters, ultraviolet radiation, electricity and certain chemicals. Scalds are burns from hot liquids, hot food or steam.

First aid, including safety rules

The immediate treatment of burns, especially for smaller areas, is immersion in cold running water such as tap water, for a minimum of 20 minutes. Do not disturb charred adherent clothing but remove wet clothing.

- Ensure you and the burnt person are safe from further injury or danger.
- Cool a burnt or scalded area immediately for at least 20 minutes with cool to cold (around 15°C; preferably running) water.

Safety first rules

- Stop the burning process and remove any source of heat, if possible.
- *Flames:* Smother with a blanket (preferably a 'fire blanket' if available).
  - Direct flames away from the head or douse with water.
  - Roll person on ground if clothing still burning: 'stop, drop and roll'.
  - Remove clothes over the burnt area IF not stuck to skin.
- *Scalds:* Remove clothing that has been soaked in boiling water or hot fat.
  - Remove clothing carefully only if the skin is not blistered or stuck to it.
  - Cool with cool or tepid water for at least 20 minutes.
- *Chemical burns:* Remove affected clothing.
  - Wash or irrigate the burn for at least 30 minutes.
  - Do not try to neutralise the chemical.
- *Electrical:* Disconnect the person from the electrical source.
  - Use a wooden stick or chair to remove person if you cannot switch off the electricity. (Don't approach if connected to high-voltage circuit.)

Some useful rules

- It is best to cut clothing with sharp scissors, especially from limbs.
- Remove possible constricting items, e.g. bracelets, watches, rings.
- Cover the burn with plastic cling wrap (discard the first 6 cm). Apply this in strips and not wrapped circumferentially.

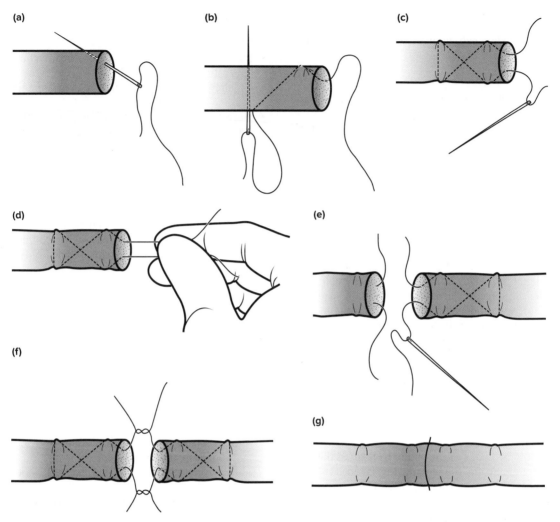

Fig. 9.13 Primary suture of a cut tendon: **(a–c)** inserting figure-of-eight suture; **(d)** pulling the two ends of the suture; **(e)** inserting a similar suture in the other end of the tendon; **(f)** tying the sutures and burying the knots; **(g)** suture is completed

- A burnt hand can be placed in a plastic bag.
- Give basic analgesics for small burns e.g. paracetamol.
- Cool running water is useful for 3 hours after a burn.
- Cool the burn; warm the patient.

Some don'ts

- Prick blisters (leave this decision to experienced medical attendants).
- Apply creams, ointments, grease, lotions.
- Apply adhesive, sticky or fluffy cotton dressings.
- Put butter, oils, ice or ice water on burns on anyone, especially children.
- Apply hydrogel products as initial first aid.

Types of burns

There are three levels of burns.

- *Superficial*—affects only the top layer of skin. The skin will look red and is painful e.g. sunburn.
- *Partial thickness*—causes deeper damage. The burn site will look red, blistered, peeling and swollen with yellow fluid oozing and is very painful. This is further classified as epidermal or, if deeper, dermal.
- *Full thickness (deep dermal)*—damages all layers of the skin. The burn site will look white or charred black. There may be little or no pain. Hypertrophic scarring is highly likely.

Remember

Consider your own safety as you stop the burning process:
- if on fire—stop-drop-roll
- if chemical—flush with copious water
- if electrical—turn off power.

Refer the following burns to hospital:
- > 9% surface area, especially in a child
- > 5% in an infant
- all deep burns
- burns of difficult or vital areas (e.g. face, hands, perineum/genitalia, feet)
- burns with potential problems (e.g. electrical, chemical, circumferential)
- suspicion of inhalational injury
- suspicion of non-accidental injury in children or vulnerable people
- burns in the elderly, children < 12 months and pregnant women.

Always give adequate pain relief. During transport, continue cooling by using a fine mist water spray.

Major burns

A major burn is an injury to more than 20% of the total body surface for an adult and more than 10% for children. As a guiding rule, one arm is about 9%, one leg 18%, face 7% in adults and 16% in toddlers. The surface area of burns for a child is shown in Figure 9.14, which includes the useful Lund–Browder chart for estimating the extent of the burn.

Major burns are a medical emergency and require urgent treatment: call triple zero (000) or your local emergency number. Expect deterioration.

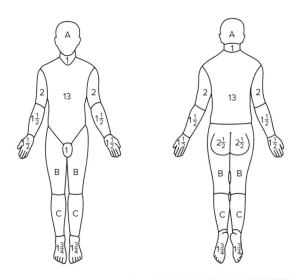

Area	Age 0	1	5	10	15	Adult
A = ½ of head	9½	8½	6½	5½	4½	3½
B = ½ of one thigh	2¾	3¼	4	4¼	4½	4¾
C = ½ of one leg	2½	2½	2¾	3¼	3¼	3½

Fig. 9.14 Lund and Browder chart: estimation of extent of burns in children

Guidelines for going straight to hospital (burns unit)

- Full thickness burns—adults over 10% and children over 5% of body surface
- Burns including partial thickness burns to difficult and vital areas—hands, feet, face, joints, perineum and genitalia
- Circumferential burns—those that go right around a limb or the body
- Respiratory/inhalation burns (effects may be delayed for a few hours)
- Electrical burns
- Chemical burns

Commonly used appropriate burns dressings

- Open weave retention stretch adhesive material (e.g. Acticoat, Fixomull, Mefix). Requires daily or twice daily cleansing of the serous ooze and reapplication of outer bandage. Useful for irregular surfaces such as hands. Leave 7 days. Remove after soaking in a little cooking oil to negate the adhesive.
- Semipermeable transparent (e.g. Opsite, Tegaderm)
- Hydrocolloids (e.g. Comfeel, Duoderm)
- Paraffin impregnated gauze (e.g. Jelonet, Unitulle)

Treatment

1. *Very superficial—intact skin:* Can be left with an application of a mild antiseptic only. Review if blistering.
2. *Superficial—blistered skin:* Apply a dressing to promote epithelialisation (e.g. hydrocolloid sheets, hydrogel sheets) covered by an absorbent dressing (e.g. paraffin gauze or Melolin™)
or
a retention stretch adhesive material (e.g. Fixomull, Mefix, Opsite) with daily or twice daily cleaning of the serous ooze and reapplication of outer bandage. Leave 7 days.

Acticoat™

A silver impregnated dressing favoured by several burns units including Royal Perth Hospital. Preferred for deeper superficial wounds. Main indications—acute burns, partial thickness and infected or contaminated wounds.[1]

Method for acute burns—after first aid (for first 48 hours)

- Apply Acticoat dressing over cleansed burnt area with dark side facing wound. Moisturise the silver dressing with sterile water.
- For a secondary dressing, apply two layers of Jelonet, followed by dry gauze or padding.

- Secure with loose bandages or loose stretch netting. If wound bed is dry, apply gel (e.g. IntraSite gel) over the wound before applying Acticoat.
  Rule: Wound must be kept moist otherwise skin damage and delayed healing occurs.

Guidelines to patient for retention dressings

- First 24 hours: keep dry. If there is any ooze coming through the dressing, pat dry with a clean tissue.
- From day 2: wash over dressing twice daily. Use gentle soap and water, rinse then pat dry. Do not soak. Rinse only. Do not remove the dressing as it may cause pain and damage to the wound. If the wound becomes red, hot or swollen or if pain increases, return to the clinic.
- From day 7: return to the clinic for removal of the dressing. Two hours prior to coming into the clinic, soak the dressing with olive oil, then cover with Glad Wrap.
  Note: Dressing must be soaked off with oil (e.g. olive, baby, citrus or peanut). Debride 'popped blisters'. Only pop blisters that interfere with dermal circulation.
3. *Deep burns.* If considerable ooze, apply the following in order.
   - hydrogel (SoloSite gel, Solugel or similar)
   - non-adherent neutral dressing (e.g. Melolin)
   - layer of absorbent gauze or cotton wool (larger burns).
   Change every 2 to 4 days with analgesic cover. Surgical treatment, including skin grafting, may be necessary.

Exposure (open method)

- Keep open without dressings (good for face, perineum or single surface burns).
- Renew coating of antiseptic cream every 24 hours.

Dressings (closed method)

- Suitable for circumferential wounds.
- Cover creamed area with non-adherent tulle (e.g. paraffin gauze).
- Dress with an absorbent bulky layer of gauze and wool.
- Use a plaster splint if necessary.

Burns to the hand

For superficial blistered burns to the hand or similar 'complex' shaped parts of the body apply strips of the retention stretch adhesive dressings as described above. They conform well to digits. Apply an outer bandage. At 7 days soak the dressings in oil for 2 hours prior to coming into the clinic.

Severe burns and escharotomy

Be aware of the potential for full thickness burns to lead to contractures. Surgical full thickness incision of the tough leathery burn eschar of a circumferential burn may be essential to release pressure and restore blood flow to unburned skin, especially when considering transport of a burns patient. This is a high-risk procedure and consultation with a burns specialist is advisable. The incisions usually follow the LAID rule: Longitudinal incisions, Axial planes, Into normal skin and Down to subcutaneous fat (Fig. 9.15).

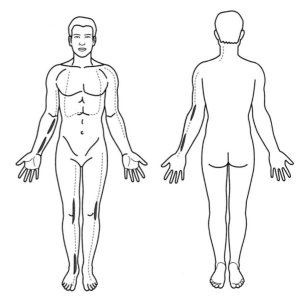

Fig. 9.15 Escharotomy incision lines and typical incision sites (avoid nerves)

RAPID TESTING OF THE HAND FOR NERVE INJURY

Following an injury to the arm or hand that has the potential for a nerve injury, it is important when one examines a hand to have a knowledge of simple tests that detect injuries to the three main nerves—the median, the ulnar and the radial.

The 'quick' hand test for nerve injury

Get the patient to make the following configurations:
- '4-fingered cone' (Fig. 9.16a)—if the patient can do this, the ulnar nerve is intact
- '5-fingered cone' and ability to approximate the thumb (Fig. 9.16b)—success means the median nerve is intact
- 'trigger test' for the thumb—that is, extension—if normal, the radial nerve is intact (Fig. 9.16c).

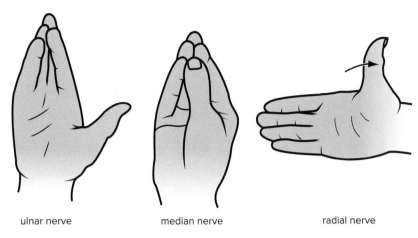

ulnar nerve   median nerve   radial nerve

Fig. 9.16 Rapid testing of the hand for nerve injury

Summary of arm nerve injuries

- Ulnar nerve—inability to abduct little finger
- Median nerve—inability to abduct thumb
- Radial nerve—inability to extend thumb

Froment's sign

Ask the patient to grip a sheet of paper forcefully between the thumbs and index fingers while the examiner tries to pull the paper away. A positive Froment's sign is a weak pinch with marked flexion of the interphalangeal joint of the thumb. This occurs because of loss of action of adductor pollicis caused by injury to the deep branch of the ulnar nerve. Flexor pollicis longus overcompensates.

References

1. Fong J, Wood F, Fowler B. A silver coated dressing reduces the incidence of early burn wound cellulitis and associated costs of inpatient treatment. Burns, 2005; 31: 562–7.

2. Douglas HE, Wood F. Burns dressings. Australian Fam Physician, 2017, 46(3): 94–7.

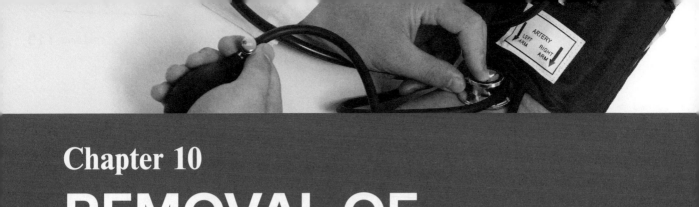

Chapter 10
REMOVAL OF FOREIGN BODIES

General

CAUTIONARY NOTE

Failure to diagnose the presence of a foreign body has emerged as a common cause of malpractice actions against general practitioners. It is particularly important to locate and remove foreign bodies, especially splinters in children, glass slivers after motor vehicle accidents and pub brawls, and metal objects such as needles in the feet of children.

REMOVAL OF MAGGOTS

The larvae of the common blowfly can find their way into the most unexpected corners of the body, and can be extremely difficult to remove.

This unusual problem is more likely to occur in unkempt people, such as those who are homeless or have alcohol addiction, and in those with exposed wounds. Examples of sites that can become infested are the eye, the ear, traumatic wounds in comatose victims, and rodent ulcers.

The eye

The presence of maggots should be suspected when an unkempt person presents with a red eye and with marked swelling (Fig. 10.1). When disturbed, the maggots crawl for cover and are difficult to see and remove.

Method

1. Instil LA (e.g. amethocaine).
2. Instil two drops of eserine (physostigmine) or pilocarpine to 'paralyse' the maggots.

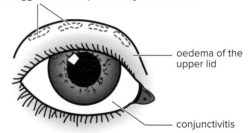

Fig. 10.1 Maggots in the eye

3. Remove the maggots with fine forceps or flush out.

Wounds

A writhing mass of maggots can be a difficult problem, and has to be rendered inactive. The old 'trick' was to use chloroform, but ether is just as effective.

Method

1. Irrigate the infested wound with the anaesthetic until the activity ceases.
2. Carefully remove all the intruders.

Using dextrose

Apply 10% dextrose to the maggots. If unsuccessful apply 50% dextrose.

REMOVAL OF SUBCUTANEOUS FLY LARVAE (CUTANEOUS MYIASIS)

The cutaneous lumps of larvae (maggots) of flies tend to present as itchy 'boils'. These are usually seen in travellers to tropical areas whereby the flies can introduce the larvae through a skin bite. Examples are the bot fly of Central and South America and the Tumbu fly of Africa. The simplest treatment is lateral pressure and tweezer extraction through the small circular hole or placing of petroleum jelly (Vaseline) or thick ointment over the lesion to induce emergence by oxygen restriction, then apply a topical antibiotic. A similar principle is to tape strips of plastic over the lesion, then bandage as appropriate. Leave for 2 days and then carefully squeeze out the maggot by lateral compression.

REMOVAL OF LEECHES

There are several varieties of leeches in this country, but the most troublesome are the small, black leeches that inhabit the damp forests of New South Wales, Victoria and Tasmania. The major problem is the difficulty of removing a parasite adhering firmly to such awkward anatomical sites as the eye, ear canal or the urethral meatus in men.

No attempt should be made to extract the leech manually. There are several methods of inducing leeches to 'jump off' rapidly:
- application of hot objects
- application of salt
- application of a detergent
- application of toothpaste
- slicing the leech in half with a knife.

Method

1. With extreme care, apply a hot object near the end of the leech. The object could be the hot tip of a snuffed-out match (Fig. 10.2) or the heated end of a paper clip. Best avoided if another method is available.
2. The leech soon lets go!

EMBEDDED TICKS

Some species of ticks, notably the paralysis tick (*Ixodes holocyclus*), can be very dangerous to human beings, especially to children. If they attach themselves to the head and neck, a serious problem is posed. As it is impossible to distinguish between dangerous and non-dangerous ticks, early removal is mandatory. Severe toxicity may require assisted ventilation. The tick should be totally removed, and the mouthparts of the tick must not be left behind. Do not attempt to grab the tick by the body and tug. This is rarely successful in dislodging the tick, and more toxin is thereby injected into the host.

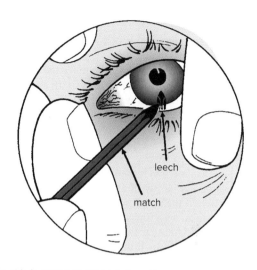

Fig. 10.2 Removal of leech from the eye

As an office procedure, many practitioners grasp the tick's head as close to the skin as possible with fine forceps or tweezers, and pull the tick out sideways with a sharp rotatory action. There are proprietary tick removal devices that may be effective. This is acceptable, but not as effective as the methods described here.

First aid bush removal method

1. Saturate the tick with petrol, kerosene or insect repellent such as Rid, and leave for 3 minutes.
2. Loop a strong thread around the tick's head as close to the skin as possible, and pull sharply.

Alternative methods

- Apply tea tree oil 12 hourly—leave 24 hours and remove.
- Apply 5% acetic acid firmly onto the tick with a cotton bud. Wait 30 seconds, then slowly turn the end of the bud anticlockwise until the tick is dislodged.

Shock freezing

Freeze the tick with liquid nitrogen and remove it *in toto*.

Lidocaine anaesthetic method

Infiltrate 1% lidocaine under and around the head of the tick. It should then be easily extracted because of immobilisation and eversion of the mouth parts. If not, move on to the office procedure.

Loop of suture material method

1. Select a long length of 3/0 nylon or silk or dental floss.
2. Loop it over the tick and tie a single knot.
3. Holding the nylon flush with the skin, slowly tighten the knot over the neck of the tick.
4. Pull off the tick with a sharp rotatory action.

Office procedure

1. Infiltrate a small amount of LA in the skin around the site of embedment.
2. With a no. 11 or 15 scalpel blade make the necessary very small excision, including the mouth parts of the tick to ensure total removal (Fig. 10.3).
3. The small defect can usually be closed with a Bandaid or Steri-Strips.

Punch biopsy method

A very practical method is to inject local anaesthetic and then use a punch biopsy of appropriate size to remove the entire tick. If the punch will not fit over the tick, cut it behind its head with fine scissors and then punch out the head parts. Use a cross pulley stitch (Fig. 1.14) to close the wound. A punch is the most practical method of removing residual embedded mouthparts after a failed tick removal.

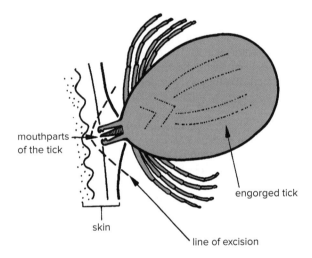

mouthparts of the tick

engorged tick

skin

line of excision

Fig. 10.3 Removing the embedded tick

REMOVAL OF RING FROM FINGER

From time to time one is faced with the need to remove a ring from a swollen finger. Destruction of a possibly valuable piece of jewellery can often be avoided by the following.

Method

1. Using a needle, bent paper clip or bobby pin, pass a length of dental tape (the best), cord or string (or Mersilk) under the ring (Fig. 10.4a). The ring should be over the narrowest part of the phalanx for this.
2. Liberally apply petroleum jelly or moistened soap paste to the finger, distal to the ring. Wind about six turns of the string around the finger close to and immediately distal to the ring (Fig. 10.4b).

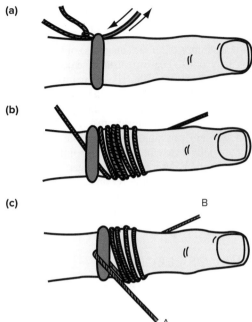

(a)

(b)

(c)

B

A

Fig. 10.4 Removal of ring from finger: **(a)** thread string through bobby pin or needle passed under ring; **(b)** wind string firmly round finger after liberally applying Vaseline; **(c)** hold firm at B and pull and unwind at A

3. While holding the end (B) of the cord firmly, pull the proximal end (A) over the ring, roughly parallel to the long axis of the finger, unwinding it steadily in the same direction in which the distal coils were wound originally (Fig. 10.4c). The pressure of the cord is thus applied successively around the periphery of the ring, forcing it distally. The distal cords, by applying pressure, also help to reduce the oedema of the finger.

In many cases the ring slides off with little or no discomfort and without damage to ring or finger.

Sometimes a digital block may be necessary.

SPLINTERS UNDER THE SKIN

The splinter under the skin is a common and difficult procedural problem. Instead of using forceps or making a wider excision, one method is to use a disposable hypodermic needle to 'spear' the splinter (Fig. 10.5) and then use it as a lever to ease the splinter out through the skin.

Reactive objects such as thorns, spines and wood should be removed as soon as possible.

Superficial horizontal splinters

These are usually readily palpated under the skin. Apply antiseptic and infiltrate with local anaesthetic (sometimes

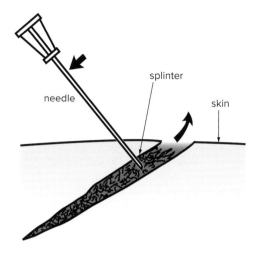

Fig. 10.5 Removal of splinters

unnecessary if very superficial). Incise the skin over the length of the splinter using a no. 15 scalpel blade, to completely expose the splinter. Lift it out with the scalpel blade or with forceps.

Alternatively, the overlying skin can be deroofed with a sterile 19-gauge needle in a feathering motion and then speared out with the aid of fine forceps.

The vertical splinter[1]

This is more difficult but can be removed by making a superficial circular excision over the splinter followed by a deeper encircling incision to undermine the sides of the wound. The smallest available punch biopsy (usually 2 mm) may be used to pierce through the dermis. The free central block of tissue containing the object can be picked out with fine forceps (Fig. 10.6).

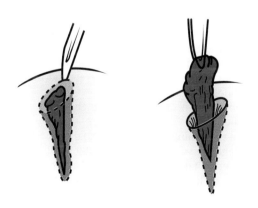

Fig. 10.6 Method of removal of the vertical splinter

REMOVING SPINES OF PRICKLY PEAR, CACTUS AND SIMILAR PLANTS FROM THE SKIN

Gently apply an adhesive dressing such as Fixomull or Mefix. Then remove the prickles by pulling in the direction that they are pointing out of the skin with the grain, otherwise they will break at skin level. Hair removal waxing methods provide an alternative.

DETECTING FINE SKIN SPLINTERS— THE SOFT SOAP METHOD

Problem

Finding fine foreign bodies in the skin that are difficult to see, such as cactus spurs and glass slivers.

Method

1. Spread soft soap very lightly over the skin. The soap permits easier identification of the foreign bodies.
2. If wooden or plant material, paint the skin with tincture of iodine and wipe off the excess; the wood stains red.
3. Remove the foreign bodies with splinter (or other types) forceps.

DETECTING SKIN SPLINTERS

High-resolution ultrasound imaging by experienced operators can assist in both the diagnosis and removal of these foreign bodies. Table 10.1 shows the comparative efficacy of X-rays and ultrasound.

CT scans are also very effective.

Table 10.1 Efficacy of X-ray and ultrasound

Material	Plain X-ray	Ultrasound
Wood	Poor	Good
Glass	Good	Good
Metal	Good	Good
Plastic	Moderate	Good
Plant (e.g. thorns)	Poor	Good

REMOVING THE IMPLANON ROD

Identify the 4 cm long rod in the subcutaneous tissue by palpation and the insertion scar. (If not palpable, arrange ultrasound examination.) The rod usually develops a fibrous capsule, which may eventually require dissecting away from the tip of the rod. Infiltrate around the rod with LA. Palpate to identify one end of the rod with your finger. Then manipulate and depress it so that the opposite end 'tents' the skin. Make an incision over this pointing end and then blunt dissect around the rod until it is sufficiently exposed to remove with forceps.

- The direction of the incision should be parallel to the implant (not perpendicular).
- When placing the incision, err on the side of being just proximal to the tenting.
- For a tough fibrous capsule, use a size 2 biopsy punch to snare the rod after locating the end. (Punch the subcutaneous tissue, not skin.)
- To prevent the rod slipping away under pressure from the scalpel, skewer the LA needle horizontally underneath and at right angles to the rod.

DETECTING METAL FRAGMENTS

A simple tip for detecting subcutaneous metal pieces is to use a magnet and run it over the skin (the larger the magnet the better). If the metal 'tents' the skin, this is the site to make the incision.

If a needle is buried vertically in the skin, don't squeeze the skin in order to try to 'pop it out'. Instead, stretch the skin tight and the tip may protrude enough to be grasped.

EMBEDDED FISHHOOKS

Six methods of removing fish hooks are presented here, some relying on removal in a direction continuous with their direction of entry to conform with the nature of the barb, others requiring removal in the reverse direction, against the barb. Method 4 or 5 is recommended as first-line management.

Method 1

1. Inject 1–2 mL of LA in front of and then below the hook.
2. Cut the shank with wire cutters or pliers below the needle's eye (Fig. 10.7a). Alternatively, repeated bending (using two holders) at this point will cause the shank to snap.
3. With a needle holder grasp the shank, press the point of the barb through the skin and remove.

Method 2

1. After anaesthetising, a sharp pull in the direction shown (Fig. 10.7b) will in most cases make the barb continue on its natural path and come out through the skin.
2. The barb can then be cut off easily and the rest of the hook extracted.

No surgical instruments are required, simply a pair of pliers or wire cutters, but all personnel present should close their eyes when the barb is cut off. If the available instruments are incapable of cutting through a thick hook, an alternative is to crush the barb flat and withdraw the hook back through its entry point.

Method 3

1. Inject 1–2 mL of LA around the fish hook.
2. Grasp the shank of the hook with strong artery forceps.
3. Slide a D11 scalpel blade in along the hook, sharp edge away from the hook, to cut the tissue and free the barb (Fig. 10.7c).
4. Withdraw the hook with the forceps.

Method 4

This method, used by some fishermen, relies on a loop of cord or fishing line to forcibly disengage and extract the hook intact. It requires no anaesthesia and no instruments—only nerves of steel, especially for the first attempt.

1. Take a piece of string about 10–12 cm long and make a loop. One end slips around the hook as a double loop, the other hooking around one finger of the operator.
2. Depress the shank with the other hand in the direction that tends to disengage the barb.
3. At this point give a very swift, sharp tug along the cord. (Some find that using a ruler in the loop to flick out the hook is ideal.)
4. The hook flies out painlessly in the direction of the tug (Fig. 10.7d).

Note: You must be bold, decisive, confident and quick, as half-hearted attempts do not work.

For difficult cases, some local anaesthetic infiltration may be appropriate. Instead of a short loop of cord, a long piece of fishing line double-looped around the hook and tugged by the hand will work.

Method 5

This method, regarded by some as the best, involves 'flicking' the hook out by traversing its path of entry into the skin. It is a variant on method 4.

1. Loop a length of fishing tackle around the eye of the hook.
2. Loop a length of string around the front curve of the hook.
3. Keep the fishing tackle taut by holding it firmly in a straight line with the non-dominant hand.
4. Now pull sharply outwards with the dominant hand so that it flicks the hook out (Fig. 10.7e).

Caution: Take care not to let the hook fly off uncontrollably.

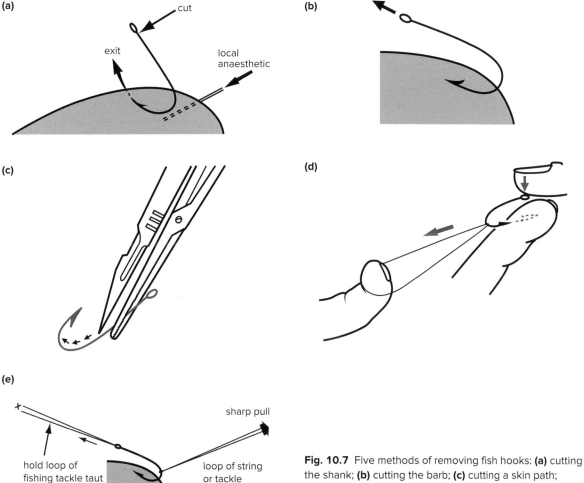

Fig. 10.7 Five methods of removing fish hooks: **(a)** cutting the shank; **(b)** cutting the barb; **(c)** cutting a skin path; **(d)** intact removal; **(e)** using double-string method

Method 6: The Irish (Castletownbere) method

Principle

Cover the barb of the hook with the bevel of the needle, which must be large enough (e.g. 17G, 19G) to accommodate the tip of the barb. There is then no resistance to its removal.

Method

1. Inject 0.5 to 1 mL of local anaesthetic using an insulin-type syringe into the actual puncture wound, wait 10 minutes.
2. Insert a 19-gauge needle into the entrance wound and feed it along the hook until it is stopped by the barb (ensure that the bevel of the needle is directed towards the hook). The sharp tip of the hook is now inside the lumen of the needle (Fig. 10.8a).

3. Reverse out the hook and needle. Withdrawal is easy as the barb is covered by the stylus of the needle and there is no resistance to bringing it out (Fig. 10.8b).

Helpful tips

- Some barbs are deflected slightly to one side (left or right) on the way back. It is helpful if the patient can bring a sample of the fish hook.
- It can help to practise on a cooked sausage first to convince you how easy it is.

PENETRATING GUN INJURIES

Injuries to the body from various types of guns present decision dilemmas for the treating doctor. The following tips represent guidelines including special sources of danger to tissues from various foreign materials discharged by guns.

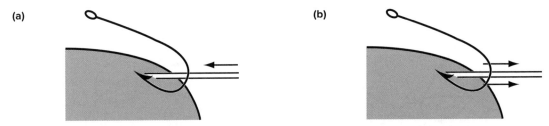

Fig. 10.8 (a) Needle bevel engages barb; **(b)** fish hook removed with needle

Gunshot wounds

Airgun

The rule is to remove subcutaneous slugs but to leave deeper slugs unless they lie within and around vital structures (e.g. the wrist). A special, common problem is that of slugs in the orbit. These often do little damage and can be left alone, but referral to an ophthalmologist would be appropriate.

0.22 rifle (pea rifle)

The same principles of management apply but the bullet must be localised precisely by X-ray. Of particular interest are abdominal wounds, which should be observed carefully, as visceral perforations can occur with minimal initial symptoms and signs.

0.410 shotgun

The pellets from this shotgun are usually dangerous only when penetrating from a close range. Again, the rule is not to remove deep-lying pellets—perhaps only those superficial pellets that can be palpated.

12-gauge shotgun

This powerful gun can produce extensive damage at a range of several metres and is difficult to deal with. Stray pellets are a common finding in rural patients and can be left.

Pressure gun injuries

Injection of grease, oil, paint and similar substances from pressure guns (Fig. 10.9) cause very serious injuries, requiring decompression and removal of the substances.

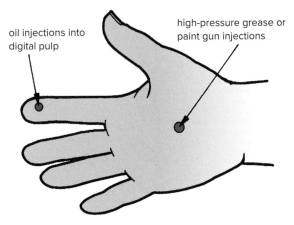

oil injections into digital pulp

high-pressure grease or paint gun injections

Fig. 10.9 Dangerous accidental injections into the hand

Grease gun and paint gun

High-pressure injection of paint or grease into the hand requires urgent surgery if amputation is to be avoided. There is a deceptively minor wound to show for this injury, and after a while the hand feels comfortable. However, ischaemia, chemical irritation and infection can follow, with gangrene of the digits resulting in, at best, a claw hand due to sclerosis. Treatment is by immediate decompression and meticulous removal of all foreign material and necrotic tissue.

Oil injection

Accidental injection of an inoculum in an oily vehicle into the hand also creates a serious problem with local tissue necrosis. If injected into the digital pulp, this may necessitate amputation. Such injections are common on poultry farms, where many fowl-pest injections are administered.

Ear, nose and throat

REMOVAL OF VARIOUS FOREIGN BODIES

Removal of foreign bodies (FBs) from the nose in children is a relatively urgent procedure because of the risks of aspiration. The same mechanical principles of removal apply to the ear.

The nose should be examined using a nasal speculum under good illumination. The tip of the nose should be raised and pressed with the tip of a thumb. Do not attempt to remove FBs from the nose by grasping with 'ordinary' forceps.

Summary of methods of removal

1. It is best to pass an instrument behind the FB and pull it forward. Examples of instruments are:
   - a eustachian catheter (Fig. 10.10a)
   - a probe to roll out the FB, e.g. bent wax curette
   - a bent hairpin
   - a bent paper clip.
2. Snaring the FB is the method most suitable for soft foreign bodies (e.g. paper, foam rubber, cotton wool). It is more applicable to the nose. Examples of instruments are:
   - a foreign-body remover (Fig. 10.10b)
   - crocodile forceps (Fig. 10.10c).
3. Application of suction that uses instruments such as:
   - a rubber catheter
   - a fine sucker.
4. Irritation of FBs in nose (e.g. white pepper sprinkled in nose to induce sneezing).
5. Blowing techniques.

Soft foreign bodies

The snaring technique is most suitable for soft objects such as paper, foam rubber and cotton wool.

Method

Under good light and being careful not to push the object further back into the nose, snare the material with either crocodile forceps or an FB remover and gently remove.

Probe technique

The method shown in Figure 10.11 simply requires good vision, using a head mirror or head light and a thin probe.

Method

1. Insert the probe under and just beyond the FB (Fig. 10.11a).
2. Lever it in such a way that the tip of the probe 'rolls' the FB out of the obstructed passage (Fig. 10.11b, c).

This technique seems to be successful with both hard and soft FBs.

Bent hairpin technique

This method requires an old-fashioned hairpin (the type with crinkly edges) bent to an angle of about 30°.

Method

1. Push the pin back beyond the FB.
2. Depress the pin to ensnare the object.
3. Gently withdraw the FB (Fig. 10.12).

(a)

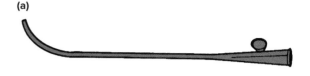

(b)

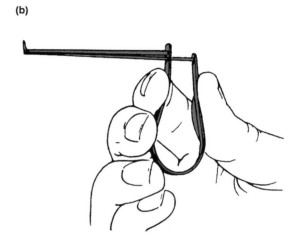

(c)

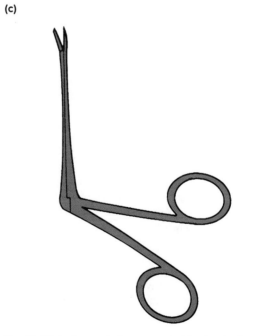

Fig. 10.10 Instruments for removal of foreign bodies: **(a)** eustachian catheter; **(b)** foreign-body remover; **(c)** crocodile forceps

(a)

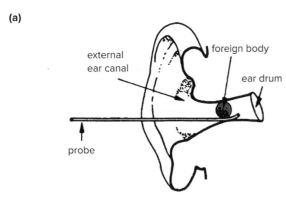

(b)

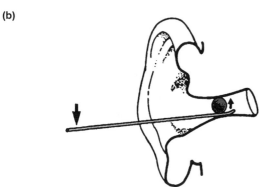

(c)

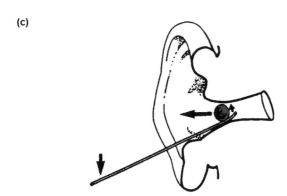

Fig. 10.11 Removal of foreign body from ear: **(a)** probe inserted under foreign body; **(b)** tip of probe is lifted by depressing outer end of probe; **(c)** continuing levering 'rolls' the foreign body out

This method is relatively painless and highly effective; other methods of removing FBs may push them deeper into the nares.

Bent paper clip technique

A simple, effective and disposable instrument can be made with a paper clip.

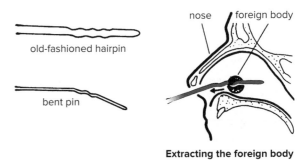

Extracting the foreign body

Fig. 10.12 Extracting the foreign body using a hairpin

Method

1. As demonstrated in Figure 10.13, open the paper clip with the hairpin bends at both ends intact.
2. Angulate the smaller end of the clip. The sharp ends of the hairpin bends should be bent towards the straight stems of the clip so that they do not cause trauma. The degree of angulation can be increased by the use of small-artery forceps if desired. The larger loop acts as a handle to get an effective grip.
3. The angulated end, passed gently over the FB in the nose or ear canal, acts as a scoop to remove the foreign body.

Note: It is important to remember that only FBs that can easily be seen in the ear or nose could be removed by this method. The paper clip instrument is not suitable for the removal of deeper FBs. Patient cooperation is also very important.

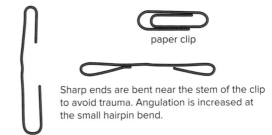

Paper clip opened with hairpin bends at both ends intact

Fig. 10.13 Extracting the foreign body using a bent paper clip

Hooked needle technique

The sharp point of a hooked needle makes it a more effective, albeit riskier, removal tool than a paper clip. With practice, it works well for any FB that can be pierced (e.g. tissue, cotton wool, Blu Tac, organic objects). Avoid this technique in wriggling children.

Method

1. Grasp the tip (1 mm proximal to the bevel) of a 23-gauge needle with forceps and bend it at right angles.

2. To create a thin handle, tightly wedge a cotton bud or insulin syringe into the needle hub.
3. Lie the patient on the bed with the relevant ear upwards.
4. Using an otoscope with a sliding lens, half-open the lens—the gap allows the needle through, with still enough lens for focus. Use a large (adult) otoscope disposable earpiece (Fig. 10.14).
5. Visualise the FB then carefully slide the needle through the earpiece, keeping the hooked bevel pointing away from the wall of the ear canal.
6. Pierce the FB from the side, then slowly lift out the entire contraption from the ear canal in one piece—don't attempt to withdraw the needle back through the otoscope.

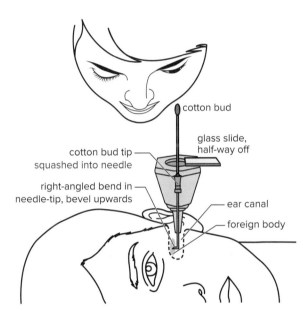

Fig. 10.14 Hooked needle through an auriscope: an effective method for difficult foreign body removal

Rubber catheter suction technique

The following is a relatively simple and painless way of removing FBs from the ears and noses of children.

The only equipment required is a straight rubber rigid catheter (large type) and perhaps a suction pump. The procedure causes minimal distress to a frightened child, avoids the need for a general anaesthetic, and is less traumatic than mechanical extraction for objects such as a round bead.

Method

1. Cut the end of the catheter at right angles (Fig. 10.15a).
2. Smear the rim of the cut end with petroleum jelly.
3. Apply this end to the FB and then apply suction.

Oral suction may be used for a recently placed or 'clean' object, but gentle pump suction, if available, is preferred (Fig. 10.15b).

It is advisable to pinch closed the suction catheter until close to the FB, as the hissing noise may frighten the child.

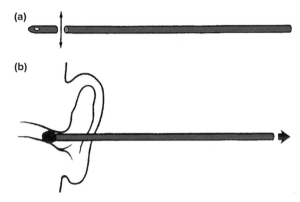

Fig. 10.15 Extracting the foreign body using a rubber catheter: **(a)** catheter cut straight across near its extremity; **(b)** application of suction (orally or by pump)

Pneumatic otoscopic attachment vacuum technique

The following method is ideal for the removal of an FB from the nose or ear of a child where it can be very difficult to extract without the use of a general anaesthetic. The method is similar to using a rubber catheter with the end cut off, and applying it to the FB using oral suction.

Method

- Use the pneumatic otoscope attachment by removing the end fitting.
- Squeeze the bulb to create a vacuum effect.
- Place the end of the rubber tubing against the FB (Fig. 10.16).
- Release the hand-squeeze on the bulb in order to create suction.
- Extract the object.

This method works very well for smooth, round FBs such as beads.

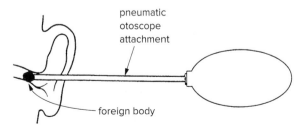

Fig. 10.16 The rubber tubing is placed against the foreign body

Tissue glue and plastic swab technique

Method

This technique employs the simple method of applying a rapidly setting adhesive to bond the FB to the extracting probe. It works best in dry conditions and for a smooth non-impacted FB. Have acetone available.

1. Apply a thin coat of cyanoacrylate or tissue glue to the end of a hollow plastic swab stick or orange stick.
2. Insert the stick into the ear canal (or nostril) to allow the glue to bond with the FB (if clearly accessible and suitable) for about 1 minute.
3. Remove the FB using gentle traction, perhaps assisted by external pressure from the fingers.

Caution: Avoid touching the skin or mucous membrane.

If glue is accidentally applied to the skin, dissolve the glue with acetone.

First-line blow technique

Press the 'normal' (not affected) nostril and encourage a seated cooperative child to blow out (snort) from the nose. They may feel less inhibited blowing outside the surgery onto the ground.

The 'kiss and blow' or 'mother's kiss' technique

This method, also known as the 'mother's kiss' technique, is used for a cooperative child with a firm, round FB such as a bead or hard pea impacted in the anterior nares.[2,3]

Method

1. Gently occlude the normal nostril with a finger. Place the mouth over the child's mouth, blowing into the mouth until a slight resistance is felt. (This indicates that the glottis is closed.)
2. Then give a sharp high velocity blow (exhalation) to cause the foreign body to 'pop out'.

To encourage cooperation with the technique the child can be asked to give the doctor a 'kiss' (or any ruse to allow placement of the lips over the child's open mouth). Better still, explain the technique to the child's parent and encourage the parent to perform it.

On all occasions that this technique has been used (adapted from an article in *The New England Medical Journal*), the FBs 'popped out' after two attempts, thus avoiding general anaesthetic with intubation.

If stubborn:

- instil nasal decongestants in the nose, leave 20 minutes and try again.

Cautionary tips:

- Beware of a disc (button) or battery and refer for expert management.
- Be mindful of the risk of aspiration of the FB.

GENERAL PRINCIPLES ABOUT A FOREIGN BODY IN THE EAR

The main danger of an FB in the ear lies in its careless removal.

Syringing is very effective and safe for small FBs.

Vegetable FBs, e.g. peas, swell with water and are better not syringed.

Insects commonly become wedged in the meatus, especially in the tropics. They can be syringed or removed with forceps under vision.

Maggots cause a painful ear and their removal is difficult—manual extraction is preferred first line. Insufflation of eserine (phytostigmine) followed by normal saline is usually effective treatment.[4]

INSECTS IN EARS

Live insects should be enticed out or killed by first instilling warm water (first option), saline or olive oil, then syringing the ear with warm water if necessary. The neatest method is to gently drip 4–5 mL of warm water or saline into the ear canal with a syringe, and then snare the insect with forceps as it crawls to the opening. Dead flies that have originally been attracted to pus are best removed by suction. Maggots are best killed by eserine (phytostigmine) drops, although other fluids should work. Syringing the ear is then appropriate.

Note: 2 mL of 1% lidocaine introduced by the blunt end of a syringe or via a cut-off 'butterfly' needle (or other piece of plastic tubing) is also effective.

Note: The ingredients in Waxsol drops can be a problem. Olive oil can be difficult to syringe so water or saline is preferable.

A moth in the ear

This is a very distressing sensation for the patient, who invariably telephones urgently at night with the problem.

First aid method at home

Instruct the patient to insert drops of lukewarm water, olive oil or a similar preparation into the ear to immobilise the moth (Fig. 10.17a).

Note: Ideally, olive oil should be gently warmed, e.g. by placing the bottle under running hot water from a tap for a short while.

Office procedure

Simply syringe the moth out of the ear with tepid water (Fig. 10.17b).

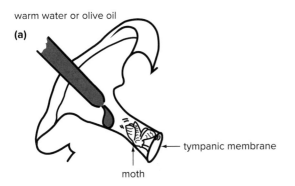

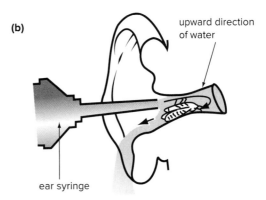

Fig. 10.17 Insect in ear: **(a)** first aid; **(b)** office procedure

COTTON WOOL IN THE EAR

A common problem is the finding of the cotton wool tip of a 'cotton bud' that has become dislodged from injudicious self ear toilet. It can be seen deep in the ear canal.

Method

Use the hooked needle technique (see Fig. 10.14) or obtain a dental broach and fashion a very small hook on the end. When inserted in the ear canal under vision, this hook can easily engage some threads of cotton and then extraction of the FB is simple (Fig. 10.18).

FISH BONES IN THE THROAT

Take a history to include the type of fish (cod bones are dangerous!), whether the meal was subsequently finished, if the pain is localised and can the patient swallow (water and/or dry bread) without severe pain. After spraying the throat with local anaesthetic, use a frontal mirror and dental mirror to find the bone.

A fish bone usually lodges in the tonsil or at the base of the tongue, in which case it can be seen on oral examination. If it cannot be seen, more thorough examination by nasopharyngoscopy is required.

To overcome the difficulty of not having a spare hand to remove the bone, use a laryngoscope, having localised the bone, and remove with packing forceps or intubation forceps.

If there is severe pain and muscle spasm, or a positive X-ray (not all fish bones are radiopaque), give an intramuscular antibiotic and refer to an ENT service.

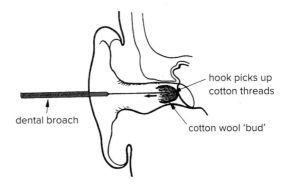

Fig. 10.18 Removal of cotton wool bud from ear

Genital and anal

EXTRICATING THE PENIS FROM A ZIPPER

The patient has accidentally entrapped the foreskin of his penis in his 'fly' zipper. He will already have tried to extricate himself, and further manoeuvring will not only be painful but will continue to impact the skin. It is worthwhile initially to lubricate the zipper with mineral oil and make one attempt to unzip it.

The following are simple and effective techniques, which free the skin but ruin the zipper.

Simple 'first pass' method

Grasp the upper free zip lines with each hand, then rapidly and forcefully separate them outwards and downwards. The zipper usually falls down and releases the entrapped foreskin. It is usually quite painless.

Instrumental methods

Method A

1. Cut the zipper from the trousers for access.
2. Infiltrate LA beneath the entrapped foreskin, or infiltrate the skin at the base of the penis (ring block).
3. Grasp the zip fastener with pliers or any similar 'crushing clamp'. Apply pressure until the zip breaks and the skin is freed (Fig. 10.19a).

Method B

Alternatively, cut across the closed section of the zipper, keeping as close as possible to the fastener (Fig. 10.19b), with a suitable instrument such as a sharp scalpel, and the zipper will fall apart.

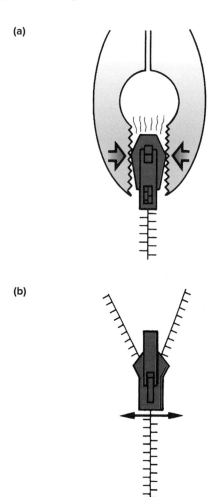

Fig. 10.19 Extracting penis from zipper

Method C

After infiltrating the area with LA, obtain a diagonal type wire cutter and cut the median bar on the top of the zipper slider (Fig. 10.20). The slider then falls apart into two pieces and the zipper teeth can be readily separated.[5]

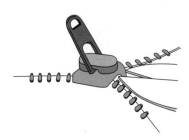

Fig. 10.20 Removing a zipper from penile skin by cutting the median bar

REMOVAL OF IMPACTED VAGINAL TAMPON

The problem associated with this procedure is the unpleasant odour that envelops the surgery, causing considerable embarrassment to both patient and doctor.

Management

Under good vision, the tampon is seized with a pair of sponge-holding forceps and quickly immersed under water. A bowl of water (an old ice-cream container is suitable) is kept as close to the introitus as possible. This results in minimal malodour.

Method

1. *Inspection:* usually in the Sims position with a Sims speculum (other positions can be used).
2. *Removal:* the tampon is grasped with a sponge-holding forceps (dorsal position; Fig. 10.21a).
3. *Disposal:* the tampon is quickly plunged under water without releasing the forceps (Fig. 10.21b). The tampon can be disposed of in the usual sanitary disposal container and the water can be flushed down the toilet.

It may be preferable to use another disposal method, such as taking the forceps and tampon outside and inserting the tampon into a self-sealing plastic bag.

Note: The Master Plumbers Association warns against flushing tampons down toilets because of their tendency to block systems.

Gloved and extraction method

The tampon can be grasped with the gloved hand and then invaginated into the glove, which acts as a receptacle for disposal.

(a)

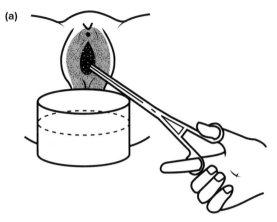

Fig. 10.21 Removal of tampon

(b)

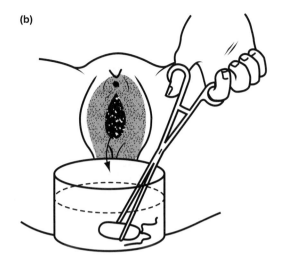

FAECAL IMPACTION

Faecal impaction, manifested as an aggregation of hard faeces in the rectum on rectal examination and associated with constipation or spurious diarrhoea, can be a difficult problem. It often presents in children and the elderly.

Before resorting to a good, old-fashioned '3H' enema (hot water, high, and a hell of a lot), use a Microlax 5 mL enema. This can be carried in the doctor's bag, is very easy to insert and most effective.

Manual disimpaction

Rarely, one has to resort to manual disimpaction, which is a most offensive procedure for all concerned. However, the procedure can be rendered virtually odourless if the products are milked or scooped directly into a pan or preferably a container of water with a fragrant disinfectant such as Pine O Clean. A large plastic cover helps to restrict permeation of the smell.

Discomfort and embarrassment are reduced by this and adequate premedication (e.g. intravenous diazepam, or even IV morphine if hard faecoliths are present).

REMOVAL OF VIBRATOR FROM VAGINA OR RECTUM

Manual removal of a vibrator or similar object from the vagina usually presents no problem, but removal from the rectum (if high) can be difficult without general anaesthesia.

Other objects may be the subject of requiring removal from these cavities; to facilitate manual removal, place the patient in a favourable position such as lithotomy, and provide generous lubrication. For vaginal removal, grasp the object with gloved fingers and apply inferior gradual constant slow traction. If unsuccessful, refer to a surgical unit.

References

1. Chan C, Salem G. Splinter removal. American Fam Physician, 2003; 67: 2557–62.
2. Cook SC, Burton DM & Glasziou P. Efficacy and safety of the 'mother's kiss' technique: a systematic review of the case reports and case series. CMAJ 2012. DOI:10.1503/cmaj.111864
3. Purohit N, Ray S, Wilson T & Chawla OP. The 'parent's kiss': An effective way to remove paediatric nasal foreign bodies. Ann R Coll Surg Engl. 2008 July; 90(5): 420–2.
4. Herdiana F & Nurdian Y. Myiasis of ears and nose are dangerous because of the capability of the larva to penetrate into the brain and the tissue damage due to inflammatory reaction and secondary bacterial infection. ResearchGate. 2017.
5. Porter RS, Kaplan JL. *The MERCK manual of diagnosis and therapy* (19th edn). New Jersey: Merck Research Laboratories, 2011: 3239.

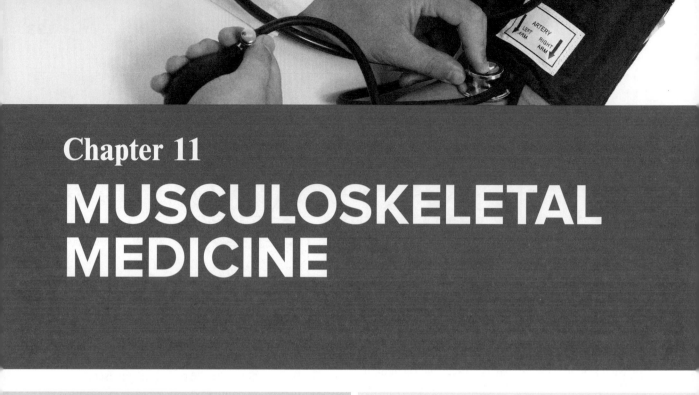

Chapter 11

MUSCULOSKELETAL MEDICINE

Temporomandibular joint

TEMPOROMANDIBULAR DYSFUNCTION

A tender and perhaps clicking temporomandibular joint (TMJ) is a relatively common problem presenting to the general practitioner. In the absence of obvious malocclusion and organic disease, such as rheumatoid arthritis, simple exercises can alleviate the annoying problem in about 2 weeks. Three methods are described as alternatives to splint therapy.

Method 1

1. Obtain a cylindrical (or similar-shaped) rod of soft wooden or plastic material, approximately 15 cm long and 1.5 cm wide. An ideal object is a large carpenter's pencil or piece of soft wood.
2. Instruct the patient to position this at the back of the mouth so that the molars grasp the object with the mandible thrust forward.
3. The patient then rhythmically bites on the object with a grinding movement (Fig. 11.1) for 2 to 3 minutes at least 3 times a day.

Method 2

1. Instruct the patient to rhythmically thrust the lower jaw forward and backward in an anterior–posterior direction with the mouth slightly open, rather like a cheeky schoolchild exposing the bottom lip (Fig. 11.2).
2. This exercise hurts initially but should soon lead to relief of the uncomplicated TMJ syndrome.

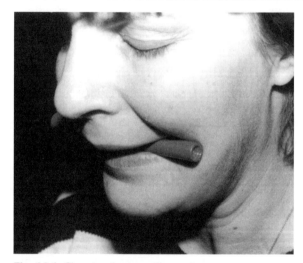

Fig. 11.1 Chewing the 'pencil' exercise

Method 3: The 'six-by-six' program

This is a specific program (separate from the previous exercises) recommended by some dental surgeons. The six exercises should be done 6 times each time, 6 times a day. It takes 1 minute to do them. Instruct the patient as follows:

1. Hold the front one-third of your tongue to the roof of your mouth and take six deep breaths.
2. Hold the tongue to the roof of your mouth and open your mouth 6 times. Your jaw should not click.

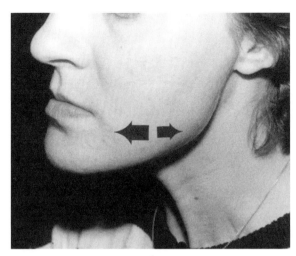

Fig. 11.2 The lower jaw-thrust exercise

3. With your mouth slightly open, hold your chin with both hands, keeping the chin still for these resistance exercises. Without letting your chin move, push it with your hands; up, down and to each side.
4. Hold both hands behind your neck and use your jaw muscles to pull the chin in.
5. Push on the upper lip so as to push the head straight back.
6. Pull your shoulders back as if to touch the shoulder blades together.
   Repeat each exercise 6 times, 6 times a day.
   Note: Patients should use a visual cue to remind them to do the exercises.
   These exercises should be pain-free. If they hurt, do not push patients to the limit until the pain eases.

Method 4: Resisted 'jaw' opening

For this isometric contraction method the patient grasps the jaw mainly on the jaw angle and strongly resists opening of the jaw. This simple exercise is repeated many times a day.

THE TMJ 'REST' PROGRAM

This program is reserved for an acutely painful TMJ condition.
- When eating, avoid opening your mouth wider than the thickness of your thumb and cut all food into small pieces.
- Do not bite any food with your front teeth—use small bite-size pieces.
- Avoid eating food requiring prolonged chewing, e.g. hard crusts of bread, tough meat, raw vegetables.
- Avoid chewing gum.

- Always try to open your jaw in a hinge or arc motion. Do not protrude your jaw.
- Avoid protruding your jaw, e.g. talking, applying lipstick.
- Avoid clenching your teeth together—keep your lips together and your teeth apart.
- Try to breathe through your nose at all times.
- Do not sleep on your jaw: try to sleep on your back.
- Practise a relaxed lifestyle so that your jaws and face muscles feel relaxed.

DISLOCATED JAW

The patient may present with a unilateral or bilateral dislocation. The jaw will be 'locked' and the patient unable to articulate.

Method

1. Get the patient to sit upright with the head against the wall.
2. Wrap gauze around both thumbs and place the thumbs over the last lower molar teeth, with the fingers firmly grasping the mandible on the outside.
3. Firmly thrusting with the thumbs, push downward towards the floor and at the same time press upwards on the chin with the fingers (Fig. 11.3).

This action invariably reduces the dislocation, with the reduction being reinforced by the fingers rotating the mandible upward as the thumbs thrust downward.

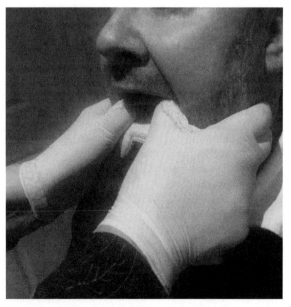

Fig. 11.3 Method of reduction of dislocated jaw

The spine

RECORDING SPINAL MOVEMENTS

Method 1

Simple diagrams obviate the need for copious notes when recording the range of movement of the cervical spine. They are of particular value to the 'whiplash' accident patient, who requires repeated assessment and accurate recording. Done serially, the diagrams are an excellent guide to progress, and assist in the compilation of medicolegal reports.

The neck movement grid (Fig. 11.4a) provides a two-dimensional field on which to record movements of the neck as viewed when standing behind and above the patient (looking down on the patient's head). Not only is the range of movement written on the grid, but pain can be recorded also.[1] If drawing is difficult on medical software, use a pre-formatted table and insert the percentages into the blank squares.

Table 11.1 shows the movements recorded for the patient in Fig. 11.4b.

Table 11.1 'Whiplash' accident patient: Neck movement record

Flexion	full and pain free
Extension	50% (of normal), painful through range
Left rotation	40%, painful at end of range
Right rotation	60%
Left lateral flexion	40%
Right lateral flexion	70%

Method 2

One can use a special direction of movement (DOM) diagram to record movements for all spinal levels. Figure 11.4c illustrates restricted and painful movements (blocked, indicated by II) in flexion, left lateral flexion and left rotation but pain-free extension, right lateral flexion and right rotation (free movements).

SPINAL MOBILISATION AND MANIPULATION

Spinal mobilisation and manipulation are examples of physical therapy that can be very beneficial in many spinal conditions where hypomobility that causes pain and stiffness is present.[1]

These therapies improve the range of joint movement, decrease stiffness and reduce pain. Mobilisation of the

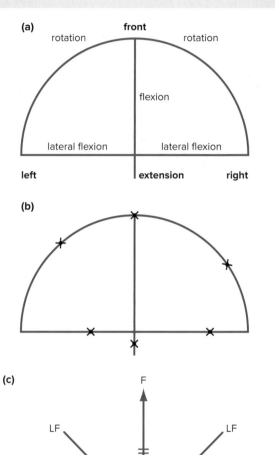

Fig. 11.4 The neck movement grid (viewed from above the patient)

Part 11.4(c) Reproduced from C. Kenna & J. Murtagh, *Back Pain and Spinal Manipulation*, Butterworths, Sydney, 1989, with permission.[1]

spine is a safe procedure but manipulation can have serious sequelae, especially if given inappropriately to the cervical spine. For the cervical spine, mobilisation is a relatively simple and most effective technique, with a similar outcome to manipulation (evidence-based). Manipulation should be left to the experts and is best avoided if possible.

Key concepts

- Mobilisation is a gentle, coaxing, repetitive, rhythmic movement within the range of movement of the joint (Fig. 11.5).
- Manipulation is a high-velocity thrust at the end range (Fig. 11.5).
- If in doubt, use mobilisation in preference to manipulation.
- Always mobilise or manipulate in the direction of no pain.
- Manipulation is generally more effective and produces a faster response, but requires accurate diagnosis and greater skill, and can aggravate some spinal problems.

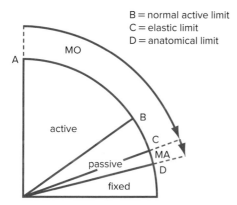

Fig. 11.5 Schematic representation of movement (by rotation) of a joint: mobilisation (MO), A–C; manipulation (MA), C–D

Important contraindications to spinal manipulation

- Disease of the spine (e.g. osteoporosis, neoplasm, rheumatoid arthritis).
- Neurological changes.
- Evidence of nerve root compression (e.g. sciatic pain in the leg, pain extending to the forearm or below the knee).
- Instability of spine following trauma.
- Cerebrovascular disease (for neck).
- Anticoagulation therapy.
- The elderly patient (my rule: avoid > 65 years).
  A golden rule: Opposite movement, no pain. This generally means that manipulation achieves a gapping or opening up of the painful side.

Anterior directed gliding—an example of spinal mobilisation

The technique of anterior directed gliding, also termed posterior–anterior mobilisation, can be applied directly to the spinous process centrally (Fig. 11.6) or over tender points unilaterally. It is a very simple technique, directed either with the thumbs (placed side by side) or the pisiform process of the leading hand (for central mobilisation only). This method is suitable for anywhere along the spine, but particularly for the cervical spine and more so at lateral tender points.

Method (using thumbs)

1. The patient lies prone, with head turned to one side and arms by the side.
2. For the thoracic and lumbar spines, stand at the patient's side and place your thumbs over the tender area. For the cervical spine, stand behind the patient's head.
3. Lean over the patient with your arms perfectly straight and head and shoulders over the treatment area.
4. Obtain an oscillatory movement by gently rocking the upper trunk up and down, with pressure being transmitted to your thumbs by your shoulders and arms.
5. Go as deeply as possible without causing pain.
6. Provide a small-amplitude, controlled oscillation at the rate of one to two per second. Maintain this for about 30 to 60 seconds, with two or three repeats in one treatment session.

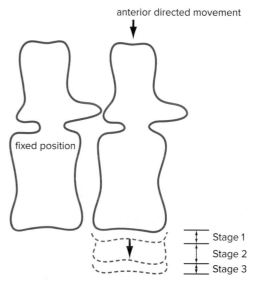

Fig. 11.6 Anterior directed central gliding mobilisation, illustrating the three stages of mobilisation

Reproduced from C. Kenna & J. Murtagh, *Back Pain and Spinal Manipulation*, Butterworths, Sydney, 1989, with permission.[1]

Cervical spine

CLINICAL PROBLEMS OF CERVICAL ORIGIN

Pain originating in the cervical spine is commonly, although not always, experienced in the neck. The patient may complain of headache, or pain around the ear, face, shoulder, arm, scapulae or upper anterior chest.

If the cervical spine is overlooked as a source of pain, the cause of symptoms will remain masked and mismanagement will follow.

Possible symptoms

- Neck pain
- Neck stiffness
- Headache
- Migraine-like headache
- Arm pain (referred or radicular)
- Facial pain
- Ear pain (periauricular)
- Scapular pain
- Anterior chest pain
- Torticollis

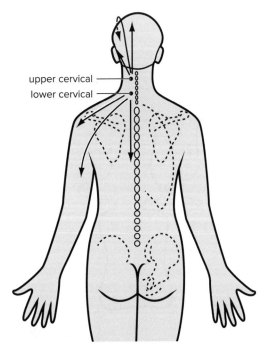

upper cervical
lower cervical

Fig. 11.7 Possible common directions of referred pain from the cervical spine

Reproduced from C. Kenna & J. Murtagh, *Back Pain and Spinal Manipulation*, Butterworths, Sydney, 1989, with permission.[1]

- Dizziness/vertigo
- Visual dysfunction

Figure 11.7 indicates the typical directions of referred pain. Surprisingly, headache, which is commonly caused by cervical problems, is often not considered by clinicians.

Pain in the arm (brachialgia) is common, and tends to cover the shoulder and upper arm area indicated in Figure 11.7. This is the zone of referred pain that is not caused by nerve root compression. It can be a difficult diagnostic dilemma, because pain reference from the fifth cervical nerve segment (C_5) involves musculoskeletal, neurological and visceral structures. Virtually all shoulder structures are innervated by C_5. See dermatome chart (Fig. 11.20).

The practitioner must first determine whether the pain originates in the cervical spine or the shoulder joint, or in both simultaneously, or some other structure. The often missed diagnosis of polymyalgia rheumatica should be considered in the elderly patient presenting with pain in the zone indicated, especially if bilateral.

LOCATING TENDERNESS IN THE NECK

Palpation of the neck to determine the precise level of pain or tenderness can be difficult; however, if the surface anatomy of the neck is clearly defined, the affected level can easily be determined.

Method

1. The patient lies prone on the examination couch with hands (palms up) resting on the forehead. The shoulders should be relaxed.
2. Systematically palpate the spinous processes of the cervical vertebrae:
   - C_2 (axis) is the first spinous process palpable beneath the occiput
   - C_7 is the largest 'fixed' and most prominent process at the base of the neck
   - C_6 is also prominent and easily palpable, but usually 'disappears' under the palpating finger with extension of the neck
   - the spinous process of C_1 (atlas) is not palpable, but the tip of the transverse process is: it lies between the angle of the jaw and the mastoid process
   - the spinous processes of C_3, C_4 and C_5 are difficult to palpate because of cervical lordosis, but their level can be estimated (see Fig. 11.8).

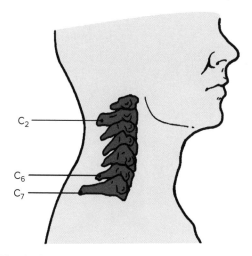

Fig. 11.8 Relative sizes of spinous processes of cervical spine

ACUTE TORTICOLLIS[1]

An amazingly effective treatment for an acute wry neck is muscle energy therapy, which relies on the basic physiological principle that the contracting and stretching of muscles leads to the automatic relaxation of agonist and antagonist muscles.

Note: Lateral flexion or rotation or a combination of movements can be used, but treatment in rotation is preferred. The direction of contraction can be away from the painful side (preferred) or towards the painful side, whichever is most comfortable for the patient.

Method

1. Explain the method to the patient, with reassurance that it is not painful.
2. Rotate the patient's head passively and gently towards the painful side to the limit of pain (the motion barrier).
3. Place your hand against the head on the side opposite the painful one. The other (free) hand can be used to steady the painful level—usually C_3–C_4.
4. Ask the patient to push the head (in rotation) as firmly as possible against the resistance of your hand. The patient should therefore be producing a strong isometric contraction of the neck in rotation away from the painful side. Your counterforce (towards the painful side) should be firm and moderate (never forceful), and should not 'break' through the patient's resistance. To reinforce the effect of this contraction (although not essential), you can ask the patient to inhale and hold the breath and also to look upward in the direction of the contracting muscles (Fig. 11.9a).

5. After 5 to 10 seconds (average 7 seconds) ask the patient to relax; then passively flex the neck gently towards the patient's painful side. During this phase the patient is asked to exhale slowly and to look downward to that side (Fig. 11.9b).
6. The patient will now be able to turn the head a little further towards the painful side.
7. This sequence is repeated at the new and improved motion barrier. Repeat 3 to 5 times until the full range of movement returns.
8. Ask the patient to return the following day for another treatment, although the neck may now be almost normal.

The patient can be taught self-treatment at home using this method.

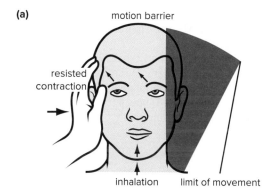

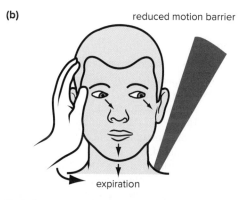

Fig. 11.9 Acute torticollis: **(a)** isometric contraction phase for problem on left side; **(b)** relaxation phase towards the affected (left) side

Reproduced from C. Kenna & J. Murtagh, *Back Pain and Spinal Manipulation*, Butterworths, Sydney, 1989, with permission.[1]

A SIMPLE TRACTION TECHNIQUE FOR THE CERVICAL SPINE

This technique demonstrates the use of longitudinal traction of the neck, especially for the upper cervical spine, as a muscular energy therapy. Coordination of breathing is considered to be a most effective facilitator of this method. It is very safe and gentle, and particularly helpful in the elderly with painful dysfunctional necks.

Method

1. The patient sits on the chair (sitting is preferable to lying supine), with the head in a 'neutral' position.
2. Stand behind the patient and place the palms of your hands on the sides of the patient's face (to spread the pressure evenly around the face and not in one or two sites).
3. Ask the patient to simultaneously breathe in and look upwards (without extending the neck).
4. Hold the patient's neck in a fixed position with very slight traction during this inspiration phase (Fig. 11.10a). The neck muscles will contract during this phase.
5. Ask the patient to then exhale while looking down. Apply a gentle but firm upward stretch (Fig. 11.10b). Maintain this traction for about 7 seconds.
6. Repeat this procedure about 4 times, applying traction during each expiration phase.

NECK ROLLS AND STRETCHES

Indications

Dysfunction of neck, including tenderness and stiffness, usually following injury.

Method

The objective is to produce a smooth, circular motion to the end range in all directions so that stretching occurs at the end range.

1. Patients are instructed to 'draw circles in the air' (Fig. 11.11a) or 'roll their head around their halo'. A wide arc of movement is not necessary, provided that stretch is obtained.
2. The roll is performed at a slow to medium pace, so that tender or painful areas can be avoided by moving just short of this level. As stretch is obtained, these areas become less painful, allowing further stretching.
3. Patients can be taught to stretch the neck themselves (Fig. 11.11b), including the use of a muscle energy technique. No matter how stiff the neck initially, it is surprising how much immediate improvement can be obtained from simple, gentle, lateral stretching.

Patients should be instructed to train themselves into a permanent daily habit of rolling the neck to assess flexibility.

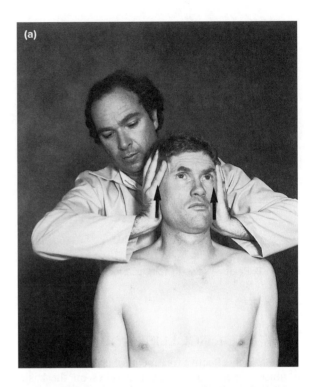

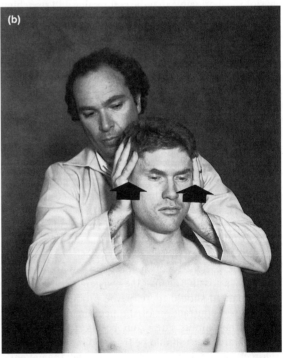

Fig. 11.10 Simple traction technique: **(a)** the therapist applies slight traction during inspiration and upward gaze; **(b)** the therapist applies firm traction during expiration and downward gaze

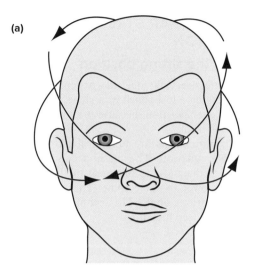
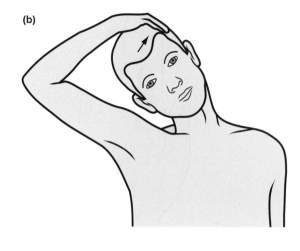

Fig. 11.11 Exercises for the dysfunctional neck: **(a)** the slow neck roll; **(b)** stretching neck into lateral flexion
Reproduced from C. Kenna & J. Murtagh, *Back Pain and Spinal Manipulation*, Butterworths, Sydney, 1989, with permission.

Thoracic spine

ANTERIOR DIRECTED COSTOVERTEBRAL GLIDING

This unilateral mobilisation method is directed at the tender costotransverse joint of the thoracic spine. The joint, which is about 4–5 cm from the midline, is arguably the most common source of musculoskeletal pain in the thoracic spine. The tender area determined by palpation is the target for mobilisation.

Method

1. With the pad of the thumbs applied over the rib (Fig. 11.12), apply a rhythmic oscillating movement (about two per second) at right angles.
2. Maintain this for 30 to 60 seconds with as much pressure as possible without causing discomfort.

THORACIC SPINAL MANIPULATION

A note of caution: Take care in patients with 'red flags' such as previous malignancy and cerebrovascular disease. Avoid manipulation in these patients using the following two techniques and ensure that the neck is not extended. Direct thrust techniques can be dangerous in women over 55, especially in the presence of risk factors for osteoporosis.

Manipulation for the mid-thoracic spine[1]

Of the dozens of manipulative thrusts for dysfunction of the thoracic spine (T_3–T_8), the most effective is the

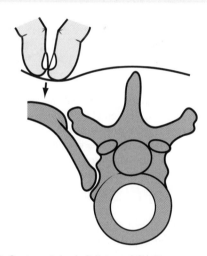

Fig. 11.12 Costovertebral gliding mobilisation
Reproduced from C. Kenna & J. Murtagh, *Back Pain and Spinal Manipulation*, Butterworths, Sydney, 1989, with permission.[1]

postero–anterior indirect thrust, using the underlying hand as a block over the affected area.

Method

1. The patient lies supine on a low couch, with a pillow supporting the head.
2. The patient folds the arms across the body with hands resting on opposite shoulders, the uppermost forearm being the one furthest from you.

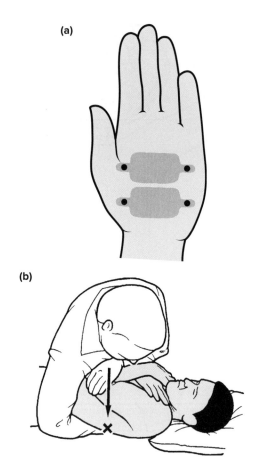

(a)

(b)

Fig. 11.13 Mid-thoracic manipulation: **(a)** cupped hand position, showing position of the vertebrae on the hand—note how the spinous processes run along the long axis and occupy the hollow of the hand; **(b)** manipulation to mid-thoracic spine—note the direction of the applied force (X indicates blockage with the hand)

Reproduced from C. Kenna & J. Murtagh, *Back Pain and Spinal Manipulation*, Butterworths, Sydney, 1989, with permission.[1]

3. Roll the relaxed patient towards you.
4. Place your cupped hand (Fig. 11.13a) on the spine at the painful level, with this level in the palm.
5. Roll the patient back onto the hand, which should feel comfortable (if not, readjust).
6. Lean well over the patient, placing your forearm directly on theirs, and grasp the patient's far elbow with your hand.
7. Rest your chest on your uppermost arm.
8. Ask the patient to inhale and exhale fully.
9. As the patient commences to exhale, lean down to take up the slack on your bottom hand.
10. Towards the end of exhalation, apply a sharp downward thrust (but not too forcefully) with your chest and upper arm directly through the patient's chest onto your hand (Fig. 11.13b).

THORACOLUMBAR STRETCHING AND MANIPULATION

Rotation in the sitting position

In this very effective technique, the patient fixes the pelvis by straddling a low couch or a chair; the couch provides the better position, because it allows greater flexibility of the trunk.

The main indications are unilateral pain at the thoracolumbar junction. The method can be used also for pain (unilateral and bilateral) of the lumbar spine and the lower thoracic spine. The usual rules and contraindications apply. The technique must be coordinated with deep breathing.

Method

1. The patient straddles the end of the couch and sits firm and erect. Alternatively the patient can straddle a chair, facing the back of the chair with a pillow used against the chair to protect the thighs. It must be a standard, open chair, with a carpeted floor.
2. The patient crosses the arms over the chest so that the hands rest on the opposite shoulders. They should be comfortable throughout the procedure, and proper padding should rest against the inner thighs.
3. Stand directly behind the patient. Adopt a firm, wide-based stance.
4. Grasp the patient's shoulders with your hands.
5. Ask the patient to take a deep breath in, exhale fully and relax.
6. When you feel the patient relax, grasp the shoulders and rotate the patient's trunk steadily and firmly, away from the painful side, to the limit of rotation. Before rotation is attempted the patient must be at the absolute limit of stretch. Gently oscillate the trunk at this position of full stretch.
7. If any sharp pain is reproduced at this end range, abandon the treatment.

Mobilisation: Consists of performing a gentle, repetitive, oscillatory rotation of the trunk at this end range for up to 30 seconds.

Manipulation: Consists of a sharp, well-controlled rotation.

Variations of this technique

An alternative and better strategy is to 'hug' the patient's trunk, using the arm that embraces the trunk to grasp the arm near the elbow on the side to be rotated. The thrusting hand can be applied to a specific area of the back corresponding to the level of pain. Thus, a type of 'push–pull' manoeuvre can be achieved, with the embracing arm pulling into rotation and the other hand pushing to achieve a complementary smooth rotation of the trunk. Coordinate this with breathing so the rotation only occurs during the relaxed exhaled stage.

(a)

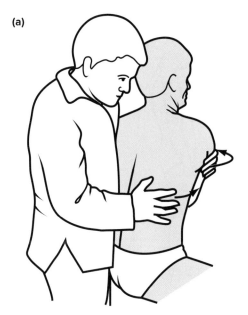

(b)

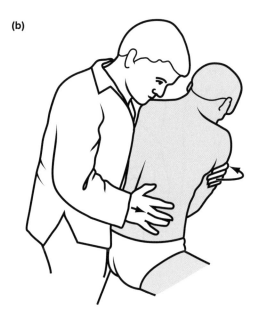

Fig. 11.14 Thoracolumbar manipulation: **(a)** rotation in sitting technique for thoracolumbar region (right-sided problem); **(b)** rotation in sitting technique for lumbar spine (right-sided problem)

Reproduced from C. Kenna & J. Murtagh, *Back Pain and Spinal Manipulation,* Butterworths, Sydney, 1989, with permission.[1]

Figure 11.14a demonstrates the technique for a right-sided problem at the thoracolumbar junction, while Figure 11.14b demonstrates the technique for low lumbar pain. Both rotations are to the left, since rotation to the right reproduces pain.

Lumbar spine

REFERENCE POINTS IN THE LUMBAR SPINE

A working knowledge of the bony landmarks of the lumbar spine is vitally important for determining the level of the spinal pain and for procedures such as epidural injections and lumbar punctures.

This anatomical knowledge is readily determined by using the iliac crests as the main reference point.

Method

1. For the examination the adequately exposed patient should be relaxed, lying prone, with the arms by the sides.
2. Standing behind and below the patient, place your fingers on the top of the iliac crests and your thumbs at the same level on the midline of the back. This level will correspond with the third and fourth lumbar interspace, or slightly higher at the fourth lumbar spinous process.
3. Consequently, the thumbs will either feel the L_3–L_4 gap or the L_4 spinous process.

(When inspecting X-rays of the lumbar spine, it becomes apparent that the upper limits of the iliac crest usually lie opposite the L_3–L_4 interspace.)[2]

The reference points should be marked and the level of each lumbar spinous process can then be identified.

TESTS FOR NON-ORGANIC BACK PAIN

Several tests are useful in differentiating between organic and non-organic back pain (e.g. that caused by depression or complained of by a known malingerer).

Magnuson method (the 'migratory pointing' test)

1. Request the patient to point to the painful sites.
2. Palpate these areas of tenderness, and nearby non-tender areas, on two occasions separated by an interval of several minutes, and compare the sites.

Between the two tests divert the patient's attention from his or her back by another examination.

Burn 'kneeling on a stool' test

1. Ask the patient to kneel on a low stool, lean forward and try to touch the floor.

(a)

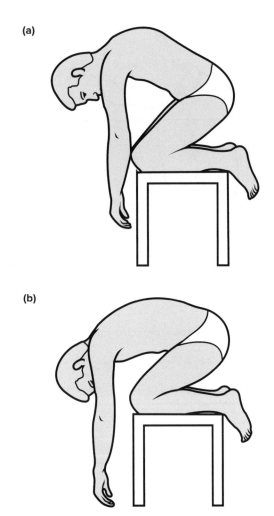

(b)

Fig. 11.15 Back pain tests: **(a)** abnormal attempt to kneel on a stool; **(b)** normal attempt to kneel on a stool

2. The person with non-organic back pain will usually refuse on the grounds that it would cause great pain or that he or she might overbalance in the attempt. Patients with even a severely herniated disc usually manage the task to some degree (Fig. 11.15a, b).

The 'axial loading' test

1. Place your hands over the patient's head and press firmly downward (Fig. 11.16).
2. This will cause no discomfort to (most) patients with organic back pain.

The 'hip and shoulder rotation' test

1. Examine for pain by rotating the patient's hips and shoulders while the feet are kept in place on the floor (Fig. 11.17).

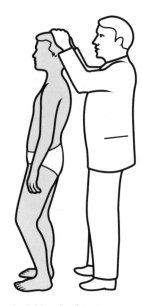

Fig. 11.16 The 'axial loading' test

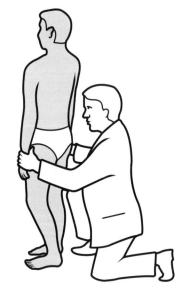

Fig. 11.17 The 'hip and shoulder rotation' test

2. The manoeuvre is usually painless in those with an organically based back disorder.

MOVEMENTS OF THE LUMBAR SPINE

There are three main movements of the lumbar spine. As there is minimal rotation, which mainly occurs at the thoracic spine, rotation is not so important. The movements that should be tested, and their normal ranges, are as follows:
- extension (20–30°) (Fig. 11.18a)
- lateral flexion, left and right (30°) (Fig. 11.18b)
- flexion (75–90°: average 80°) (Fig. 11.18a).

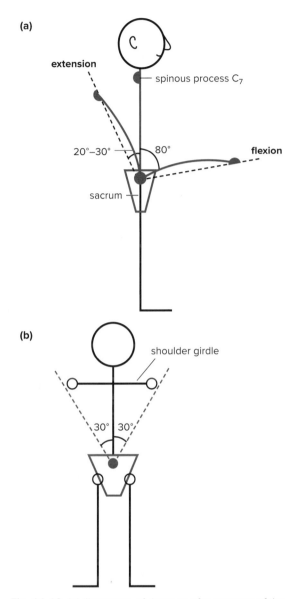

Fig. 11.18 (a) illustration of degrees of movement of the lumbar spine in flexion and extension; **(b)** illustration of the degree of lateral flexion of the lumbar spine

Reproduced from C. Kenna & J. Murtagh, *Back Pain and Spinal Manipulation*, Butterworths, Sydney, 1989, with permission.[1]

Table 11.2 Typical lumbosacral disc causes of various clinical problems

Problem	Usual causative disc prolapse
L_3 nerve root lesion	$L_2–L_3$
L_4 nerve root lesion	$L_3–L_4$
L_5 nerve root lesion	$L_4–L_5$
S_1 nerve root lesion	$L_5–S_1$
Severe low back pain, no leg pain	$L_4–L_5$
Severe sciatica, minimal low back pain	$L_5–S_1$
Low back pain with scoliosis involving lateral abnormal curvature	$L_4–L_5$

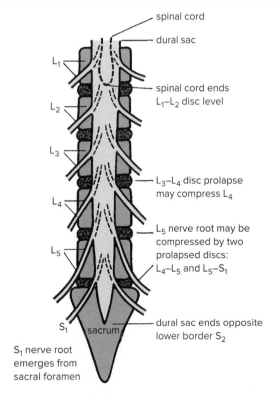

Fig. 11.19 Posterior 'window' view of lumbosacral spine, illustrating the relationships of the nerve root to the intervertebral discs

Reproduced from C. Kenna & J. Murtagh, *Back Pain and Spinal Manipulation*, Butterworths, Sydney, 1989, with permission.[1]

Measurement of the angle of movement can be made by using a line drawn between the sacrum and the large prominence of the C_7 spinous process, compared to a vertical line.

NERVE ROOTS OF LEG AND LEVEL OF PROLAPSED DISC

Pain in the leg from discogenic lesions in the lumbosacral spine is commonly due to pressure on the L_5 or S_1 nerve roots. Unlike discogenic lesions in the cervical spine, more than one nerve root can be involved with prolapses of the $L_4–L_5$ or $L_5–S_1$ discs, but this is uncommon.

Working guidelines are given in Table 11.2 and Figure 11.19. It is worthwhile to know and refer to

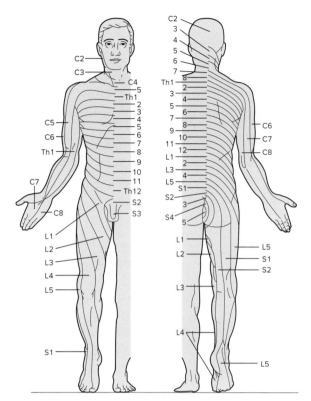

Fig. 11.20 Dermatome chart

Reproduced from J. Murtagh, *GP Companion Handbook* (7th Edn), McGraw-Hill, Sydney, 2019.[3]

the dermatome chart, especially for the lower limb (Fig. 11.20).

THE SLUMP TEST

The slump test is an excellent provocation test for lumbosacral pain and more sensitive than the straight leg raising test. It is a screening test for a disc lesion and dural tethering. It should be performed on patients who have low back pain with pain extending into the leg, and especially for posterior thigh pain.

A positive result is reproduction of the patient's pain; this may appear at an early stage of the test (at which point the test is ceased).

Method

1. The patient sits on the couch in a relaxed manner.
2. The patient then slumps forward (without excessive trunk flexion), then places the chin on the chest.
3. The unaffected leg is straightened.
4. The affected leg only is then straightened (Fig. 11.21).
5. Both legs are straightened together.
6. The foot of the affected straightened leg is dorsiflexed.

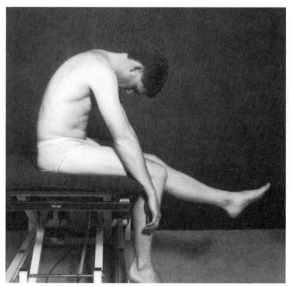

Fig. 11.21 The slump test: illustrating one of the stages

Note: Take care to distinguish from hamstring pain. Deflexing the neck relieves the pain of spinal origin, not hamstring pain.

Significance of the slump test

- It is positive if the back or leg pain is reproduced.
- If positive, it suggests disc disruption.
- If negative, it may indicate lack of serious disc pathology.
- If positive, one should approach manual therapy with caution.

ROTATION MOBILISATION FOR LUMBAR SPINE

This technique is very useful for acute low back pain of the spine, especially where manipulation is contraindicated or of doubtful value. Patients tend to prefer gentler mobilisation to spinal manipulation. There are several grades of this technique.

Method

1. The patient lies on the pain-free side, with the head supported by a pillow.
2. The lower shoulder is pulled forwards by grasping the arm at the elbow and gently rotating the spine. The uppermost arm rests on the lateral wall of the chest.
3. The uppermost leg is flexed at the hip (30–90°) and the knee flexed to a right angle. The patient places the palm of the lowermost hand under the head.
4. You stand behind the patient, opposite the pelvis.
5. Place both hands over the pelvis and apply a gentle, small-amplitude oscillatory movement (Fig. 11.22).

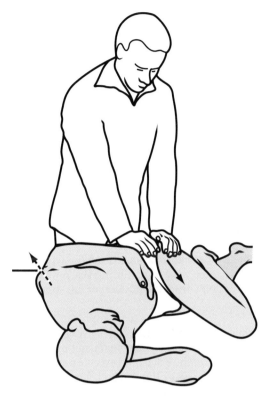

Fig. 11.22 Lumbar mobilisation in rotation (for left-sided pain)

Reproduced from C. Kenna & J. Murtagh, *Back Pain and Spinal Manipulation*, Butterworths, Sydney, 1989, with permission.[1]

6. This is a gentle 'push and pull' method, with emphasis on the push.
7. The rocking movement occupies 30 to 60 seconds. It can be repeated 2 or 3 times on any one treatment visit.

LUMBAR STRETCHING AND MANIPULATION TECHNIQUE 1

This is a traditional method used for a thrusting manipulative movement but steady stretching is simpler and safer.

Method

1. The patient lies on the pain-free side, reasonably squarely on the lower shoulder. The body should be in a straight line with the lower leg extended. The upper leg (on the painful side) can be either falling freely over the side of the couch or flexed with the foot tucked into the popliteal fossa of the lower leg. The lower arm should lie comfortably in front of the trunk. Alternatively, the hand of the lower arm can be placed under the head.

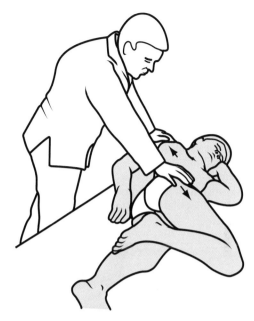

Fig. 11.23 Lumbar stretching technique 1: illustrating the direction of the applied stretching forces

Reproduced from C. Kenna & J. Murtagh, *Back Pain and Spinal Manipulation*, Butterworths, Sydney, 1989, with permission.[1]

2. Stand behind the patient at the level of the patient's waist.
3. Ask the patient to take a deep breath and breathe out.
4. When the patient has exhaled and relaxed, use one hand to push the trochanteric area of the hip forwards, and the other to gently force the front of the shoulder downwards (Fig. 11.23). It is best to keep hands in contact with the skin (avoid grasping clothing).
5. Apply steady rotational movement until a full stretch is applied to both shoulder and hip. Do not force the shoulder down too hard—take care to keep it firm and steady during the stretch.
6. Maintain sustained pressure for about 7 seconds at the end range.
7. Repeat this stretch twice.

Manipulation: If desired, this position can be used to apply a sharp rotational thrust to the hip with the force along the axis of the femur.

LUMBAR STRETCHING AND MANIPULATION TECHNIQUE 2

This is the ideal stretching or manipulative technique for the lumbar spine and is the procedure of first choice for lumbar problems. It is designed to mobilise the lower lumbosacral segments, which are responsible for most of the problems in the lower back.

The stretch

Method

1. The patient lies on the pain-free side in a relaxed position with the head on a pillow facing the therapist. The uppermost leg is flexed at the hip and the knee, both to about 45°, with the foot tucked into the popliteal fossa of the lower leg.
2. Position yourself at the level of the patient's waist.
3. Ask the patient to turn his or her head and look up at the ceiling.
4. Carefully rotate the trunk by grasping the patient's lowermost arm just above or around the elbow and gently pulling the arm outwards.

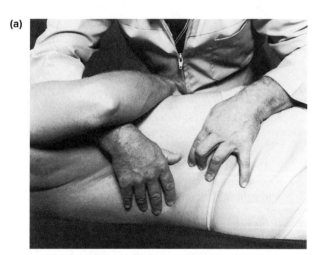

(a)

Fig. 11.24a Lumbar stretching technique 2: the method

5. Maintain smooth slow rotation of the trunk until you sense it is taut down to the upper lumbar spine.
6. Fix the trunk by asking the patient to place the hand of this arm under the head.
7. Rest the fleshy part of your upper forearm against the patient's shoulder and upper chest via the axilla, and your other forearm over the ischium, just below the iliac crest.
8. Ensure that you are properly balanced.
9. Apply a distracting force for several seconds, gently rocking back and forth with the forearms as you move towards maximal rotating stretch. This stretching is usually sufficient to achieve the desired therapeutic effect (Fig. 11.24a, b).

The manipulation

If desired, especially for a 'locked' lumbosacral level, this position can be used to perform a sharp manipulative thrust—but only from the position of full stretch.

Method

1. When all the slack is taken up by your forearms, ask the patient to take a deep breath and exhale.
2. At the end of the exhalation execute a sharp increase of rotatory pressure through both forearms, especially through the short lever to the pelvis.

Note: It is important not to dig the elbow of the proximal arm into the patient's body, since this can be painful. Likewise it is important to find a position for the distal forearm that is comfortable for the patient, and to avoid using the point of the elbow for thrusting, as the buttock area is very sensitive to sharp pressure.

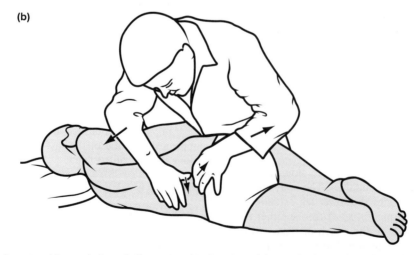

(b)

Fig. 11.24b Lumbar stretching technique 2: illustrating the direction of the applied stretching forces for left-sided problem

Reproduced from C. Kenna & J. Murtagh, *Back Pain and Spinal Manipulation,* Butterworths, Sydney, 1989, with permission.[1]

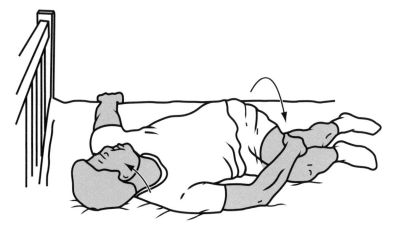

Fig. 11.25 An ideal exercise for the lower back (left-side problem illustrated)

EXERCISE FOR THE LOWER BACK

The following yoga-like exercise is highly recommended for patients with pain in the lumbosacral spine, usually after any muscle spasm has resolved.

Guidelines

It is preferable to perform the exercise on a couch or very firm bed, but it can be done on the floor. It can be performed repeatedly throughout the day but should be repeated at least twice a day for about 3 to 5 minutes at a time.

Method

1. Lie on your back.
2. Bend the leg on the painful side and stretch it across the body while turning the head to the opposite side.
3. If possible, hang onto the side of the bed or couch with your free hand (the hand that is on the same side as the leg which is crossed over).
4. Use the other hand to grasp the bent leg at the level of the knee and increase the stretch as far as possible (Fig. 11.25).
5. Relax and return to the resting position.
6. Repeat on the opposite side, especially if that side also hurts.
7. Repeat several times, concentrating on stretching the painful joints.

Note: If someone pins your shoulders to the floor or bed while you are performing this exercise, the stretch is better.

Shoulder

DISLOCATED SHOULDER

Types of dislocation

- Anterior (forward and downward)—95% of dislocations
- Posterior (backward)—difficult to diagnose
- Recurrent anterior dislocation

Anterior dislocation of the shoulder

Management

Use X-ray to check the position and exclude an associated fracture. Reduction can be achieved under general anaesthesia (easier and more comfortable) or with intravenous pethidine ± diazepam. The following methods can be used for anterior dislocation.

Kocher method (Figure 11.26)[2]

1. The patient's elbow should be flexed to 90° and held close to the body.
2. Slowly rotate the arm laterally (externally) as you apply traction.
3. Adduct the humerus across the body by carrying the point of the elbow.
4. Rotate the arm medially (internally).

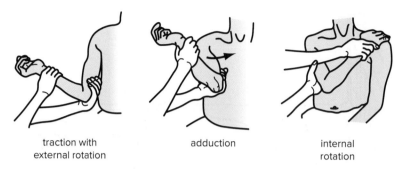

traction with external rotation

adduction

internal rotation

Fig. 11.26 Kocher method for a dislocated shoulder

Hippocratic method

Apply traction to the outstretched arm by a hold on the hand with countertraction from a stockinged foot in the medial wall of the axilla. This levers the head of the humerus back. It is a good method if there is an associated avulsion fracture of the greater tuberosity.[4]

Milch method[5] (does not require anaesthesia or sedation)

1. The patient reclines at 30° and with guidance slowly bends the elbow to 90° (Fig. 11.27a).
2. The patient is asked to lift the arm up slowly with the elbow bent so that they can pat the back of their head (requires considerable reassurance and encouragement).
3. At this position, traction along the line of the humerus (with countertraction) achieves reduction (Fig. 11.27b).

Variation of Milch method

This relies more on intervention by the therapist, who supports the shoulder with the thumb held firmly against the dislocated humeral head while the other hand facilitates adduction of the arm to the overhead position. At this position, the humeral head is pushed by the thumb into its normal socket.

Scapula pressure method

1. The patient lies prone with the dislocated arm hanging freely over the table.
2. Steady traction is applied to the arm by an assistant.
3. Firm pressure is then applied by the 'butt' of the hand to the inferolateral border of the scapula. The pressure is directed towards the glenohumeral joint.

Free-hanging method[6]

The free-hanging method is relatively painless, yet simple. It is gentler than traditional methods, without rotational

(a)

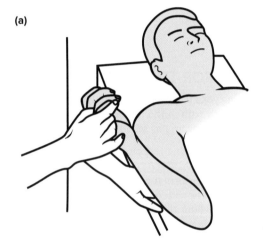

(b)

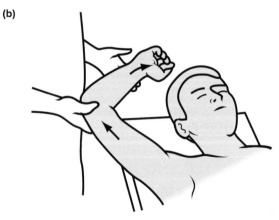

Fig. 11.27 Milch method for reduction of dislocated shoulder: **(a)** starting position with elbow bent to 90°; **(b)** patient bringing hand up to touch back of head

forces or direct pressure to the glenohumeral joint. It can be used with or without an intravenous analgesic or relaxant, which is not usually required for recurrent dislocation or in the elderly patient.

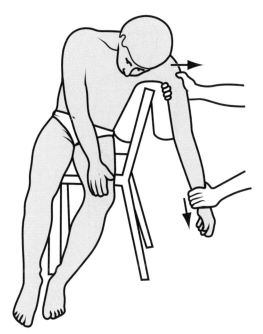

Fig. 11.28 Reduction of the dislocated shoulder: free-hanging method

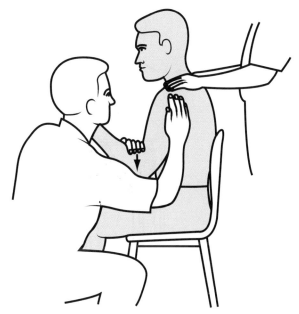

Fig. 11.29 Reduction of dislocated shoulder by gentle steady traction (as shown) in seated position

Preparation

1. Insert a 'butterfly' needle into a vein on the dorsum of the non-involved hand.
2. Prepare two solutions: (a) 10 mg of diazepam diluted to 5 mL with isotonic saline; (b) 10 mg of morphine diluted to 10 mL with isotonic saline.
3. The patient sits at right angles to the chair with only half the buttock on the seat. The affected arm hangs freely over a pillow placed on the back of the chair and tucked into the axilla. The hand with the intravenous needle rests on the opposite knee (for easy access to the practitioner).
4. You sit on a very low stool, facing the back of the chair.

Method

1. With both hands working simultaneously on the dislocated limb, grasp the patient's wrist with one hand and exert a steady, downward pressure.
2. Place the other hand in the axilla, with the palm exerting a direct outward pressure against the upper part of the shaft of the humerus (Fig. 11.28).
3. When appropriate muscle relaxation is achieved, the head of the humerus slips up and over the glenoid rim.

Analgesia and relaxation (if necessary)

Steady traction should be maintained during administration of analgesic; 3 mL morphine (3 mg) is given intravenously over 60 seconds (and may be repeated), then 1 mL diazepam (2 mg) a minute, until reduction is achieved.

Note: Carefully monitor the patient's vital signs.

THE MT BEAUTY ANALGESIA-FREE METHOD

This technique, described by Zagorski,[7] aims to reduce anterior shoulder dislocation without the need for any sedating or narcotic analgesics. It is very helpful in more remote situations and is ideal for recurrent dislocation. Fractures must be excluded.

Method (e.g. left-sided dislocation)

1. Explain the procedure to the patient, emphasising its gentleness.
2. The patient sits upright in a straight-backed chair (no arm rests).
3. An assistant stands behind the patient with a hand on each shoulder to prevent tilting of the shoulder girdle. Alternatively, the assistant can prevent the patient tipping sideways to the affected side by supporting them with a towel passing under the injured axilla across to the opposite (normal) shoulder.
4. The doctor kneels facing the patient with the left knee beside the patient's knees.
5. The patient rests his or her left hand on the doctor's left shoulder.
6. The doctor places his or her left hand on the patient's forearm just distal to the elbow (Fig. 11.29).

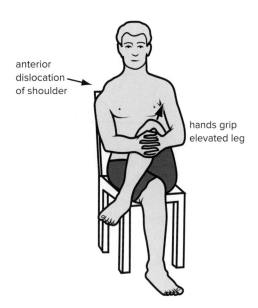
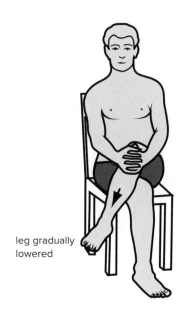

anterior
dislocation
of shoulder

hands grip
elevated leg

leg gradually
lowered

Fig. 11.30 Simple method for recurrent dislocation of shoulder

7. Very gentle downward traction is applied and gradually increased as the patient, distracted somewhat by conversation, is encouraged to relax (there should be minimal pain).
8. The doctor's right hand feels for relaxation of the shoulder and the position of the humeral head as downward traction is maintained (it usually reduces after 1 to 2 minutes).
9. If not reduced by now, very gentle external rotation is applied by leaning around the outside of the patient away from the affected side. Reduction is heralded by a gentle click. Sometimes it feels that nothing has happened so traction should be relaxed, the shoulder reassessed and, if still dislocated, traction applied. Often the release of traction leads to relocation of the joint.

Rules

- Patient must be relaxed and distracted.
- Patient must not tilt to one side.
- Gentle steady traction to avoid spasm and pain.

RECURRENT DISLOCATION OF SHOULDER

For this condition, there is a way of effecting reduction without the use of force.

Method

1. The patient sits comfortably on a chair with legs crossed.
2. The patient then interlocks hands and elevates the upper knee so that the hands grip the knee (Fig. 11.30).
3. The knee is allowed to lower gradually so that its full weight is taken by the hands. At the same time the patient has to concentrate on relaxing the muscles of the shoulder girdle.

Recurrent dislocation requires definitive surgery; the development of arthritis increases with the number of dislocations.

Elbow

PULLED ELBOW

This typically occurs in children under 8 years of age, usually at 2 to 3 years, when an adult applies sudden traction to the child's extended and pronated arm: the head of the radius can be pulled distally through the annular radioulnar ligament (Fig. 11.31a).

Symptoms and signs

- The crying child refuses to use the arm.
- The arm is limp by the side or supported in the child's lap.
- The elbow is flexed slightly.
- The forearm is pronated or held in mid-position.

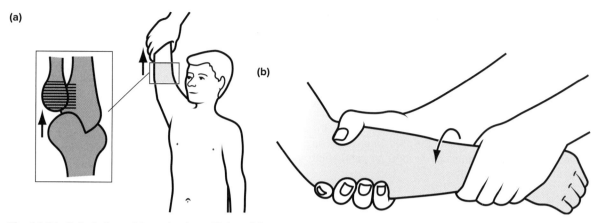

Fig. 11.31 Pulled elbow: **(a)** mechanism of injury; **(b)** supination reduction technique

Note: If atypical history, including significant pain or swelling or failed reduction, ensure that a fracture has not been overlooked.

The following methods have proven effectiveness.[8]

Supination flexion treatment method

1. Sit the child on the parent's lap. Gain the child's confidence. Ask the parent to hold the unaffected arm as the child faces you.
2. Hold the child's wrist or hand (on the affected side) as if to shake it.
3. Place one hand around the child's elbow to give support, pressing the thumb over the head of the radius.
4. Using gentle traction, firmly and smoothly twist the forearm into full supination (Fig. 11.31b) as you fully flex the forearm. A popping sound indicates relocation of the radial head. Alternatively, supinate the forearm first, then flex the elbow.

Hyperpronation flexion manoeuvre (as per RCH)

Follow steps 1–3 (above).
4. Fully pronate the forearm and then flex the elbow.

Combined manoeuvre

An alternative and preferred method to the traditional method is to very gently alternate pronation and supination through a small arc as you flex the elbow.

If you cannot get the child's cooperation apply a 'high' sling and send them home with a follow-up appointment. It may reduce spontaneously within a few days.

ELBOW FRACTURES AND DISLOCATIONS IN CHILDREN

These injuries can be very serious in children and require special care. Fractures and avulsion injuries around the elbow joint can lead to potentially severe deforming injuries. These include supracondylar fractures, fractures

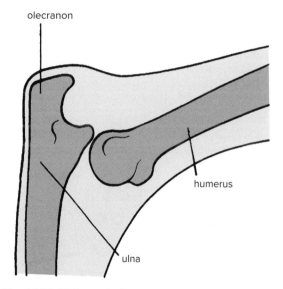

Fig. 11.32 Dislocated elbow: uncomplicated posterior dislocation

of the lateral or medial humeral condyles, and fractures of the neck of the radius. Such fractures require referral to consultants experienced in fracture management.

DISLOCATED ELBOW

A dislocated elbow is caused by a fall on the outstretched hand, forcing the forearm backwards to result in posterior and lateral displacement (Fig. 11.32). The peripheral pulses and sensation in the hand must be assessed carefully. Check the function of the ulnar nerve before and after reduction.

Usual treatment

Attempt reduction with the patient fully relaxed under anaesthesia. It is important to apply traction to the flexed elbow but allow it to extend approximately 20–30° to enable correction of the lateral displacement with the hand pushing from the side, and then the posterior displacement by pushing the olecranon forward with the thumbs.

A simple method of reduction

This method reduces an uncomplicated posterior dislocation of the elbow without the need for anaesthesia or an assistant. The manipulation must be gentle and without sudden movement.

Method

1. The patient lies prone on a stretcher or couch, with the forearm dangling towards the floor.
2. Grasp the wrist and slowly apply traction in the direction of the long axis of the forearm (Fig. 11.33).
3. When the muscles feel relaxed (this might take several minutes), use the thumb and index finger of the other hand to grasp the olecranon and guide it to a reduced position, correcting for any lateral shift.
4. After reduction the arm is held in a collar-and-cuff sling, with the elbow flexed above 90°, for 1 to 3 weeks.

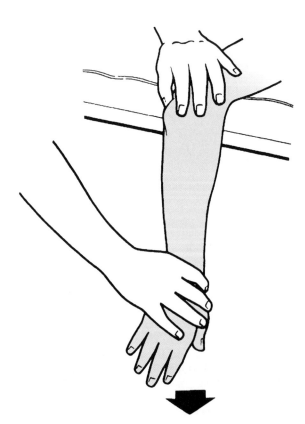

Fig. 11.33 Dislocated elbow: method of reduction by traction on the dependent arm

TENNIS ELBOW

A simple cure—the wringing exercise

Chronic tennis elbow (lateral epicondylitis) can be alleviated by a simple wringing exercise using a small hand towel.

Method

1. Roll up the hand towel.
2. With the arms extended, grasp the towel with the wrist of the affected side placed in slight flexion.
3. Then exert maximum wring pressure (Fig. 11.34):
   • first fully flexing the wrist for 10 seconds
   • then fully extending the wrist for 10 seconds
   • alternate flexion and extension between hands.

This is an isometric 'hold' contraction.

Frequency

This exercise should be performed only twice a day, initially for 10 seconds in each direction. After each week, increase the time by 5 seconds in each twisting direction until 60 seconds is reached (week 11). This level is maintained indefinitely. Apply ice for 10 minutes after completion, especially last thing at night.

Note: Despite severe initial pain, the patient must persist, using as much force as possible.

Review at 6 weeks (there is usually some relief by 4 to 6 weeks), to ensure that the patient is doing the exercise exactly as instructed.

Exercises

Stretching and strengthening exercises for the forearm muscles represent the best management for tennis elbow.[9,10] The muscles are strengthened by the use of hand-held weights or dumbbells. A suitable starting weight is 0.5 kg, building up gradually (increasing by 0.5 kg) to 5 kg, depending on the patient.

Method

1. To perform this exercise the patient sits in a chair beside a table.

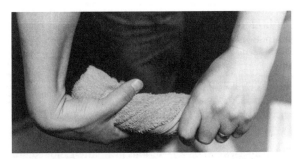

Fig. 11.34 Grip for 'wringing exercise' at the end point of the isometric hold (right wrist in full flexion and the left in extension)

2. The arm is rested on the table so that the wrist extends over the edge.
3. The weight is grasped with the palm facing downwards (Fig. 11.35a).
4. The weight is slowly raised and lowered by flexing and extending the wrist.
5. The flexion/extension wrist movement is repeated 10 times, with a rest for 1 minute and the program repeated twice.

This exercise should be performed every day until the patient can play tennis, work or use the arm without pain.

For medial epicondylitis (forearm tennis elbow, golfer's elbow), perform the same exercises but with the palm of the hand facing upward (Fig. 11.35b).

Tip: In colder conditions, keep the elbow warm with a woollen sleeve around it such as two or three modified old socks.

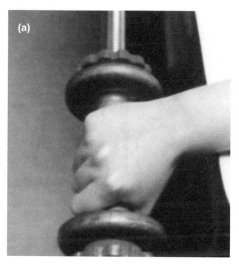
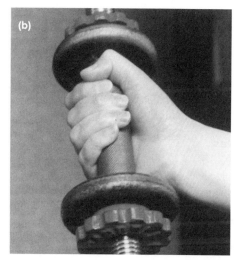

Fig. 11.35 Tennis elbow: **(a)** dumbbell exercise for classical case (palm facing down); **(b)** dumbbell exercise for medial epicondylitis—forearm tennis elbow, golfer's elbow (palm facing up)

Wrist and hand

DE QUERVAIN TENOSYNOVITIS AND FINKELSTEIN TEST

De Quervain disease is a stenosing tenosynovitis of the abductor pollicus longus or extensor pollicus brevis tendons over the radial styloid of the wrist, or both. It results from repetitive activity, such as that engaged in by staple gun operators on assembly lines, or from direct trauma.

Symptoms

The major symptoms are:
• pain during pinch grasping
• pain on thumb and wrist movement.

Tetrad of diagnostic signs

Four key diagnostic signs are:
• tenderness to palpation over and just proximal to the radial styloid
• localised swelling in the area of the radial styloid
• positive Finkelstein's sign
• pain on active extension of thumb against resistance.

Finkelstein test

Method

1. The patient folds the thumb into the palm with the fingers of the involved hand folded over the thumb.
2. Deviate the wrist in an ulnar direction (medially) to stretch the involved tendons (Fig. 11.36).
3. A positive test is indicated by reproduction of or increased pain.

SIMPLE TESTS FOR CARPAL TUNNEL SYNDROME

The carpal tunnel syndrome, caused by compression of the median nerve, is a common disorder that is usually easily diagnosed from the history. The most common and easily recognised symptoms are early-morning numbness and tingling or burning in the distribution of the median nerve in the hand. In the physical examination for the suspected carpal tunnel syndrome, a couple of simple tests can assist with confirming the diagnosis. These are

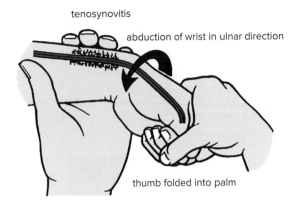

Fig. 11.36 Finkelstein test

the Tinel test and the Phalen test. The definitive test is neuromuscular conduction studies.

The Tinel test

1. Hold the wrist in a neutral or flexed position, and tap over the median nerve at the flexor surface of the wrist. This should be over the retinaculum just lateral to the palmaris longus tendon (if present) and the tendons of flexor digitorum superficialis (Fig. 11.37a).
2. A positive Tinel sign produces a tingling sensation (usually without pain) in the distribution of the median nerve.

The Phalen test

1. The patient approximates the dorsum of both hands, one to the other, with wrists maximally flexed and fingers pointed downward (Fig. 11.37b).
2. This position is held for 60 seconds.
3. A positive test reproduces tingling and numbness along the distribution of the median nerve.

SIMPLE REDUCTION OF DISLOCATED FINGER

This method employs the principle of using the patient's body weight as the distracting force to achieve reduction of the dislocation. It is relatively painless and very effective. Getting a good grip is very important, so wrap a small strip of zinc oxide adhesive plaster around the finger.

Remember to consider an associated fracture.

Method

1. Face the patient, both in standing positions.
2. Firmly grasp the distal part of the dislocated finger.
3. Request the patient to lean backwards, while maintaining the finger in a fixed position (Fig. 11.38).
4. As the patient leans back, sudden, painless reduction should spontaneously occur.

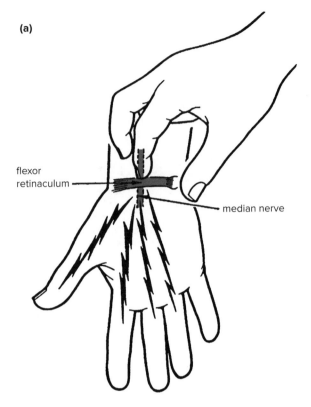

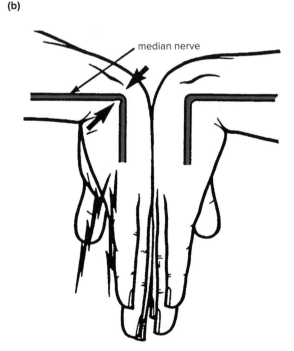

Fig. 11.37 Carpal tunnel syndrome: **(a)** Tinel test for diagnosis; **(b)** Phalen test to reproduce symptoms

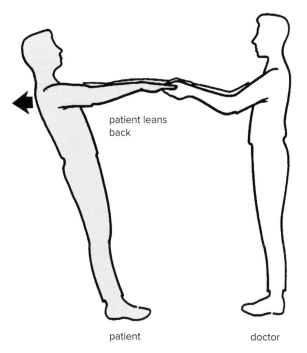

Fig. 11.38 Reduction of dislocated finger

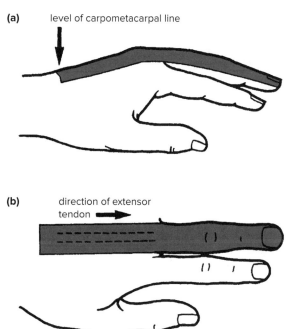

Fig. 11.39 Strapping a finger

STRAPPING A FINGER

Method

1. Instead of strapping an injured finger circumferentially, it is more comfortable and more effective to place a single strip of adhesive tape 2.5 cm or less in width on the dorsum of the finger from the tip of the nail to the carpometacarpal line (Fig. 11.39a).
2. The direction of the tape should follow the line of the extensor tendon (Fig. 11.39b). The effect is the use of the skin traction as a suspensory sling for the finger. The flexor and extensor tendons are allowed to relax with a decrease in position maintenance strain and pain. At the same time the finger is free to flex with recovery, and frozen finger is unlikely.
3. The degree of mobility of the finger is adjusted by altering the tension along the line of the tape.

MALLET FINGER

A forced hyperflexion injury to the distal phalanx can rupture or avulse the extensor insertion into its dorsal base. The characteristic swan neck deformity is due to retraction of the lateral bands and hyperextension of the proximal interphalangeal joint.

The 45° guideline

Without treatment, the eventual disability will be minimal if the extensor lag at the distal joint is less than 45°; a greater lag will result in functional difficulty and cosmetic deformity.

Treatment

Maintain hyperextension of the distal interphalangeal joint for 6 weeks, leaving the proximal interphalangeal joint free to flex. Even with treatment the failure rate is high—only about 50–60% recover.

Equipment

- Friar's Balsam (will permit greater adhesion of tape).
- Non-stretch adhesive tape, 1 cm wide: two strips approximately 10 cm in length.

Method

1. Paint the finger with Friar's Balsam (compound benzoin tincture).
2. Apply the first strip of tape in a figure-of-eight conformation. The centre of the tape must engage and support the pulp of the finger. The tapes must cross dorsally at the level of the distal interphalangeal joint and extend to the volar aspect of the proximal interphalangeal joint without inhibiting its movement (Fig. 11.40a).
3. Apply the second piece of tape as a 'stay' around the midshaft of the middle phalanx (Fig. 11.40b).

Reapply the tape whenever extension of the distal interphalangeal joint drops below the neutral position (usually daily, depending on the patient's occupation). Maintain extension for 6 weeks.

(a)

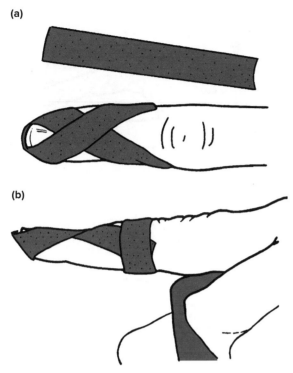

(b)

Fig. 11.40 'Mallet finger': **(a)** application of first tape; **(b)** application of 'stay' tape

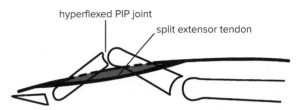

Fig. 11.41 Illustration of the mechanism of a boutonnière deformity

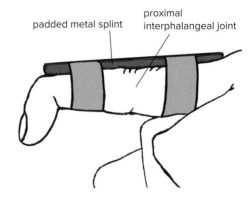

Fig. 11.42 Method of splinting for a boutonnière deformity

Other splints

There are a variety of splints. A popular one is a simple plastic mallet finger splint. One can improvise by cutting the handle of a large plastic milk carton or other similar household container.

Surgery

Open reduction and internal fixation are reserved for those cases where the avulsed bony fragment is large enough to cause instability leading to volar subluxation of the distal interphalangeal joint.

BOUTONNIÈRE DEFORMITY

The 'button hole' deformity is a closed rupture of the extensor tendon apparatus over the PIP joint, which is permanently flexed towards the palm (Fig. 11.41).

Treatment of uncomplicated deformity

1. Splint the PIP joint in full extension for 8 to 10 weeks.
2. Leave the DIP joint free for movement (Fig. 11.42).

TENPIN BOWLER'S THUMB

Tenpin bowler's thumb is a common stress syndrome in players. It usually presents as a soft-tissue swelling at the base of the thumb web (Fig. 11.43), with associated pain and stiffness of the digits used for bowling.

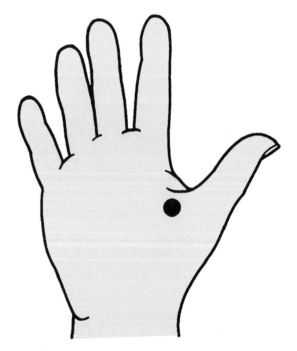

Fig. 11.43 Site of tender 'mass' at base of thumb web

Management

The patient will need:
- rest
- massage

- to bevel the bowling ball holes to reduce friction
- an intralesional injection of 0.25 mL of long-acting corticosteroid mixed with local anaesthetic (resistant cases).

SKIER'S THUMB (GAMEKEEPER'S THUMB)

A special injury is skier's thumb (also known as gamekeeper's thumb) in which there is ligamentous disruption of the metacarpophalangeal joint with or without an avulsion fracture of the base of the proximal phalanx at the point of ligamentous attachment (Fig. 11.44). This injury is caused by the thumb being forced into abduction and hyperextension by the ski pole as the skier pitches into the snow.

Diagnosis is made by X-ray with stress views of the thumb. Incomplete tears are immobilised in a scaphoid type of plaster for 3 weeks, while complete tears and avulsion fractures should be referred for surgical repair.

COLLES FRACTURE

Features

- A supination fracture of distal 3 cm of radius.
- Commonly caused by a fall onto an outstretched hand.
- The fracture features (Fig. 11.45):
  - impaction
  - posterior displacement and angulation
  - lateral (radial) displacement and angulation.

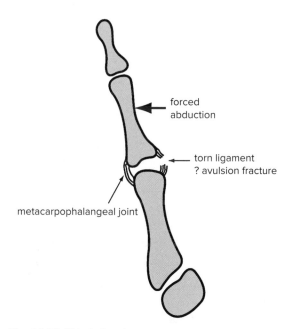

Fig. 11.44 Skier's thumb

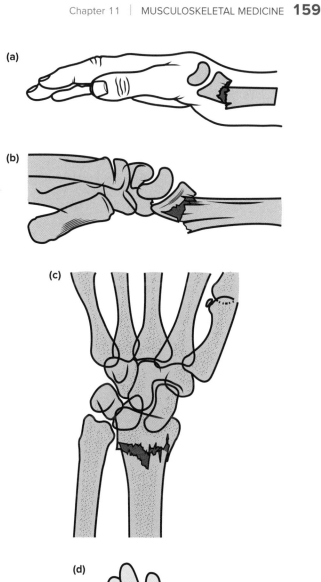

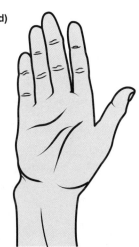

Fig. 11.45 Colles fracture: **(a)** dinner-fork deformity; **(b)** lateral X-ray view; **(c)** anteroposterior X-ray view; **(d)** radial (lateral) tilt of distal segment

Method of reduction

Under appropriate anaesthesia:
- traction on hand (to disimpact)
- an assistant maintains countertraction
- pronate
- ulnar deviation for 10° (to correct radial displacement)
- flexion (10–15°).

Immobilise the wrist and forearm in a well-padded, below-elbow plaster for 4 to 6 weeks—forearm in full pronation, wrist in corrected position (ulnar deviation, slight flexion) described above (Fig. 11.46).

SCAPHOID FRACTURE

A scaphoid fracture (Fig. 11.47) is caused typically by a fall on the outstretched hand with the wrist bent backwards (dorsiflexed). The pain may settle after the injury, so presentation may be later. One has to be careful not to treat it as a simple sprain. The signs are:

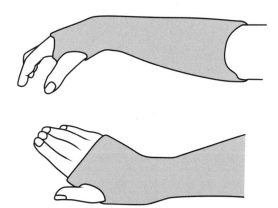

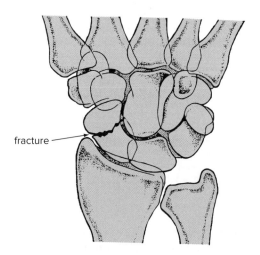

Fig. 11.46 Ideal position of the forearm in a Colles plaster. *Note:* ulnar deviation, slight flexion and pronation

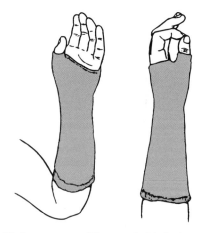

- tenderness in anatomical 'snuffbox' (the key sign)
- loss of grip strength with pain
- swelling in and around the 'snuffbox'
- pain on axial compression of thumb towards radius.

If a fracture is suspected clinically but the plain X-ray is normal, a fracture cannot be ruled out. An MRI scan is helpful (or isotope bone scan from 24 hours post injury). If scans are not available, immobilise the wrist in a scaphoid plaster for 10 days, remove it and then re-X-ray.

For an undisplaced stable fracture, immobilise for 6 weeks in a below-elbow plaster cast (Fig. 11.48). Displaced fractures require reduction (either open or closed) and, if unstable, internal fixation. All fractures require a later X-ray to check for non-union.

METACARPAL FRACTURES

Metacarpal fractures can be stable or unstable, intra-articular or extra-articular, and closed or open. They include the 'knuckle' injuries resulting from a punch, which is prone to cause a fracture of the neck of the fifth metacarpal. As a general rule, most metacarpal (shaft and neck) fractures are treated by correcting marked displacements with manipulation (under anaesthesia) and splinting with a below-elbow, padded posterior plaster slab that extends up to the dorsum of the proximal phalanx, and holds the metacarpophalangeal (MCP) joints in a position of function (Fig. 11.49).

Fig. 11.48 Appearance of the scaphoid plaster

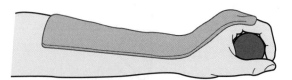

Fig. 11.49 Fracture of the metacarpal: showing position of function with posterior plaster slab and the hand gripping a roll of felt padding

fracture

Fig. 11.47 Typical appearance of a fractured scaphoid

There is often a tendency for metacarpal fractures to rotate and this must be prevented. This is best achieved by splinting the MCP joints at 90°, which corrects any tendency to malrotation. If there is gross displacement, shortening or rotation then surgical intervention is indicated. A felt pad acts as a suitable grip. The patient should exercise three fingers vigorously. Remove the splint after 3 weeks and start active mobilisation.

Hip

AGE RELATIONSHIP OF HIP DISORDERS

Hip disorders have a significant age relationship (Fig. 11.50).
- Children can suffer from a variety of serious disorders of the hip, e.g. developmental dysplasia (DDH), Perthes' disorder, tuberculosis, septic arthritis and slipped capital femoral epiphysis (SCFE), all of which demand early recognition and management.
- SCFE typically presents in the obese adolescent (10 to 15 years) with knee pain and a slight limp.
- Every newborn infant should be tested for DDH, which is diagnosed early by the Ortolani and Barlow tests (abnormal thud or clunk on abduction or adduction). However, ultrasound examination is the investigation of choice and is more sensitive than the clinical examination, especially after 8 weeks.

THE ORTOLANI AND BARLOW SCREENING TESTS[11]

Hold the leg in the hand with the knee flexed—thumb over groin (lesser trochanter) and middle finger over greater trochanter (Fig. 11.51). Steady the pelvis with the other hand.

Ortolani test (IN test)

Flex hip to about 90°, gently abduct to 45°, and then note any click or jerk as the hip reduces, allowing the hip to abduct fully (Fig. 11.51a).

Barlow (OUT test)

Flex the hip to 90°, abduct to 10-20°, and then adduct and note any click or jerk as the hip 'goes out' of the acetabulum (Fig. 11.51b).

PAIN REFERRED TO THE KNEE

Referred pain from the hip to the knee is one of the time-honoured traps in medicine. The hip joint is mainly

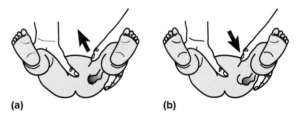

(a) (b)

Fig. 11.51 Screening for developmental dysplasia of the hip (left side): **(a)** Ortolani sign; **(b)** Barlow sign

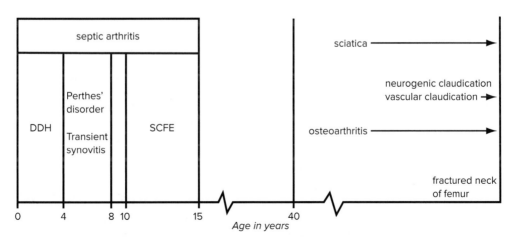

Fig. 11.50 Typical ages of presentation of hip disorders

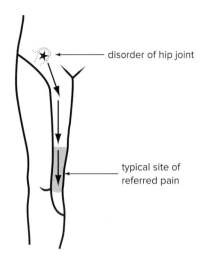

Fig. 11.52 Possible area of referred pain from disorders of the hip joint

innervated by L$_3$, hence pain is referred from the groin down the front and medial aspects of the thigh to the knee (Fig. 11.52). Sometimes the pain can be experienced on the anteromedial aspect of the knee only. It is not uncommon that children with an SCFE present with a limp and knee pain.

DIAGNOSIS OF EARLY OSTEOARTHRITIS OF HIP JOINT

The four-step stress test

Degeneration of the hip joint is a common problem in general practice, and may present with pain around the hip or at the knee. Early diagnosis is very useful, and certain tests may detect the problem. It is worth remembering that, of the six main movements of the hip joint, the earliest to be affected are internal rotation, abduction and extension. A special stress test is described here that is sensitive to diagnosing disease in the hip.

Method

1. Lay the patient in the supine position.
2. Flex the hip to about 120°.
3. Adduct to about 20–30° (Fig. 11.53).
4. Internally rotate.
5. Compress the joint through pressure down the axis of the femur.

Dysfunction of the joint may be evident when internal rotation is attempted. Any internal rotation may be virtually impossible because of stiffness or pain.

BUTTOCK PAIN

Causes to consider are: spinal dysfunction, especially lumbosacral disc radiculopathy (sciatica) and spinal

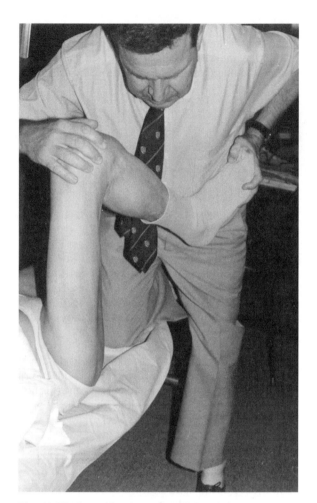

Fig. 11.53 Stress test for osteoarthritis of the hip

canal stenosis with gluteal claudication, sacroiliitis, ischial bursitis and piriformis tendinopathy.

Piriformis tendinopathy

This is caused by pressure on the sciatic nerve due to its aberrant course through piriformis muscle (Fig. 11.54). Symptoms include the gradual onset of deep-seated buttock pain, pain on and just after sitting, difficulty climbing stairs and sciatica-like symptoms centred on the buttocks. There is buttock point tenderness and pain on resisted external rotation of the flexed hip. Treatment is based on isometric stretching exercises under physiotherapist supervision.

THE 'HIP POCKET NERVE' SYNDROME

If a man presents with 'sciatica', especially confined to the buttock and upper posterior thigh (without local back pain), consider the possibility of pressure on the sciatic

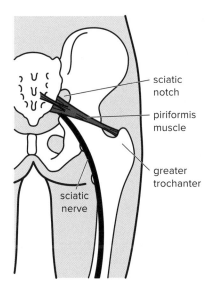

Fig. 11.54 Posterior view demonstrating the anatomy of piriformis muscle in relation to the sciatic nerve. It arises from the anterior of the sacrum, passes through the sciatic notch to insert into the upper border of the greater trochanter.

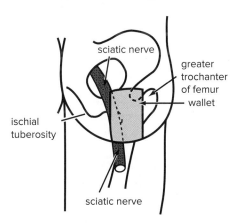

Fig. 11.55 'Hip pocket nerve' syndrome: location and relations of sciatic nerve in the buttock

nerve from a wallet in the hip pocket. This problem is occasionally encountered in people sitting for long periods in cars (e.g. taxi drivers). It appears to be related to the increased presence of plastic credit cards in wallets.

Surface anatomy

The sciatic nerve leaves the pelvis through the greater sciatic foramen and emerges from beneath the piriformis muscle at a position just medial to the midpoint of a line between the medial surface of the ischial tuberosity and the tip of the greater trochanter (Fig. 11.55). The lateral border of the nerve usually lies at this midpoint. It lies deep to the gluteus medius in the buttock.

ISCHIAL BURSITIS

'Tailor's bottom' or 'weaver's bottom', which is occasionally seen, involves a bursa overlying the ischial tuberosity. Irritation of the sciatic nerve may coexist and the patient may appear to have sciatica.

Features

- Severe pain when sitting, especially on a hard chair.
- Tenderness at or just above the ischial tuberosity.

Treatment

- Infiltration into the tender spot of a mixture of 4 mL of 1% lidocaine and 1 mL of LA corticosteroid (avoid the sciatic nerve).
- Foam rubber cushion with two holes cut out for ischial prominences.

PATRICK OR FABERE TEST

To test hip and sacroiliac joint disorders.

Fabere is an acronym for Flexion, Abduction, External Rotation and Extension of the hip.

Method

1. The patient lies supine on the table and the foot of the involved side is placed on the opposite knee.
2. Now flex, externally rotate and abduct the hip joint. This position stresses the hip joint, so that inguinal pain on that side is a pointer to a defect in the hip joint or surrounding soft tissue.
3. The range of motion for the hip joint in this position can be taken to the endpoint (thus fixing the femur in relation to the pelvis), by pressing the knee downward and simultaneously pressing on the region of the anterior superior iliac spine of the opposite side (Fig. 11.56). This stresses the hip joint as well as the sacroiliac joint on that side.

Thus, if low back pain is reproduced, the cause is likely to be a disorder of the sacroiliac joint. Such a lesion is uncommon, but is seen in nursing mothers and in those with inflammatory disorders of the joint (e.g. ankylosing spondylitis and reactive arthritis) and with infection (e.g. tuberculosis).

SNAPPING OR CLICKING HIP

Some patients complain of a clunking, clicking or snapping hip. This represents a painless, annoying problem.

Causes

One or more of the following:

- a taut iliotibial band (tendon of tensor fascia femoris) slipping backwards and forwards over the prominence of the greater trochanter

- the iliopsoas tendon snapping across the iliopectineal eminence
- the gluteus maximus sliding across the greater trochanter
- joint laxity.

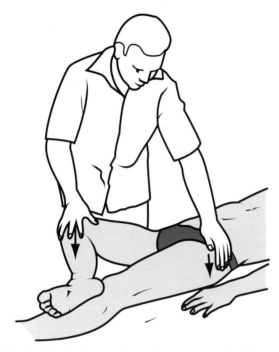

Fig. 11.56 The Patrick (Fabere) test for right-sided hip or sacroiliac joint regions, illustrating directions of pressure from the examiner

Treatment method

There are two major components of the treatment:

  a. explanation and reassurance
  b. exercises to stretch the iliotibial band.

1. The patient lies on the 'normal' side, and flexes the affected hip (with the leg straight and a weight around the ankle; Fig. 11.57) to a degree that produces a stretching sensation along the lateral aspect of the thigh.
2. This iliotibial stretch should be performed for 1 to 2 minutes, twice daily.

DISLOCATED HIP

Posterior dislocation of the hip is usually caused by a direct blow to the knee of the flexed leg (knee and hip flexed, as in a motor vehicle).

The painful shortened leg is held in:

- internal rotation
- adduction
- slight flexion (Fig. 11.58a).

With anterior dislocation, the shortened leg is held in abduction, external rotation and flexion.

Principles of management

- Adequate analgesia, e.g. IM morphine for pain.
- X-rays to confirm diagnosis and exclude associated fracture.
- Reduction of the dislocated hip under relaxant anaesthesia with some urgency since devascularisation of the femoral head is a concern.

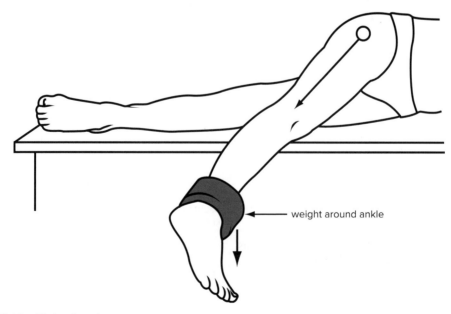

weight around ankle

Fig. 11.57 Clicking hip treatment

(a)

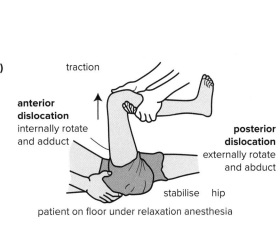

Fig. 11.58 (a) Posterior dislocation of hip with internal rotation; **(b)** dislocated hip: classic reduction method

- Follow-up X-ray to confirm reduction and exclude any fractures not visible on the first X-ray.

Method of reduction A

Standard method for posterior dislocation

With the patient under relaxant anaesthesia and lying on the floor and with an assistant steadying or fixing the pelvis by downward pressure:[4]
- Apply traction as the hip is flexed to 90°.
- Then apply gentle external rotation and abduction (maintaining traction) with hand pressure over the femoral head (Figs. 11.58 a, b).

For anterior dislocation, the leg is internally rotated and adducted under traction.

Method of reduction B

Dependent reduction method

This is especially useful if there is an associated fracture of the femur on the same side (Fig. 11.59).

The anaesthetised patient lies prone on the table:
- drop the leg and flex the dislocated hip over the edge of the table
- apply steady downward traction on the flexed hip

- gently rotate externally with hand pressure on femoral head (from gluteal region).

FRACTURED FEMUR

Emergency pain relief can be provided by a femoral nerve block with local anaesthesia (see pp. 31–32).

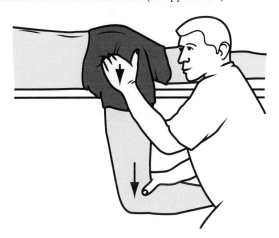

Fig. 11.59 Dependent method of reduction of the dislocated hip

Knee

COMMON CAUSES OF KNEE PAIN

A UK study has highlighted the fact that the most common cause of knee pain is simple ligamentous strains and bruises due to overstress of the knee or other minor trauma. Traumatic synovitis may accompany some of these injuries. Some of these so-called strains may include a variety of recently described syndromes such as the synovial plica syndrome, patellar tendinopathy and infrapatellar fat-pad inflammation (Fig. 11.60).

Low-grade trauma of repeated overuse such as frequent kneeling may cause prepatellar bursitis, known variously as 'housemaid's knee' or 'carpet layer's knee'. Infrapatellar bursitis is referred to as 'clergyman's knee'.

Osteoarthritis of the knee, especially in the elderly, is a very common problem. It may arise spontaneously or be secondary to previous trauma with associated internal derangement and instability.

The most common overuse problem of the knee is the patellofemoral joint pain syndrome (often previously referred to as chondromalacia patellae).

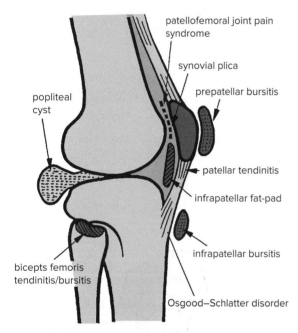

Fig. 11.60 Lateral view of knee showing typical sites of various causes of knee pain

DIAGNOSIS OF MENISCAL INJURIES OF THE KNEE

Injuries to the medial and lateral menisci of the knee are common in contact sports, and are often associated with ligamentous injuries.

Table 11.3 is a useful aid in the diagnosis of these injuries. There is a similarity in the clinical signs between the opposite menisci, but the localisation of pain in the medial or lateral joint lines helps to differentiate between the medial and lateral menisci (Fig. 11.61).

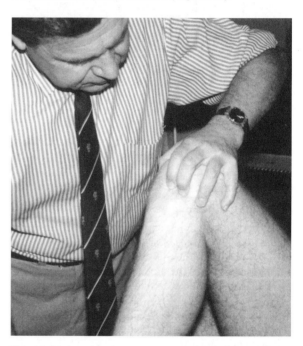

Fig. 11.61 Localised tenderness over the outer joint line with injury to the lateral meniscus

Table 11.3 Typical symptoms and signs of meniscal injuries

	Medial meniscus tear	Lateral meniscus tear
Mechanism	• Abduction (valgus) force • Internal rotation of femur on tibia	• Adduction (varus) force • External rotation of femur on tibia
Symptoms 1. Knee pain during and after activity 2. Locking 3. Effusion	Medial side of knee Yes + or −	Lateral side of knee Yes + or −
Signs 1. Localised tenderness over joint line (with bucket handle tear) 2. Pain on hyperextension of knee 3. Pain on hyperflexion of knee joint 4. Pain on rotation of lower leg (knee at 90°) 5. Weakened or atrophied quadriceps	Medial joint line Medial joint line Medial joint line On external rotation May be present	Lateral joint line (may be cyst) Lateral joint line Lateral joint line On internal rotation May be present

Note: The diagnosis of a meniscal injury is made if three or more of the five examination findings ('signs' in Table 11.3) are present.

LACHMAN TEST

The Lachman test is a sensitive and reliable test for the integrity of the anterior cruciate ligament. It is an anterior draw test with the knee at 20° of flexion. At 90° of flexion, the draw may be negative but the anterior cruciate torn.

Method

1. Position yourself on the same side of the examination couch as the knee to be tested.
2. Hold the knee at 20° of flexion by placing a hand under the distal thigh and lifting the knee into 20° of flexion. The patient's heel rests on the couch.
3. Ask the patient to relax, allowing the knee to 'fall back' into your steadying hand and roll slightly into external rotation.
4. Perform the anterior draw with your second hand grasping the proximal tibia from the medial side (Fig. 11.62) while holding the thigh steady with your other hand.
5. Carefully note the feel of the endpoint of the draw. Normally there is an obvious jar felt as the anterior cruciate tightens. In an anterior cruciate deficient knee there is excess movement and no firm endpoint. Compare the amount of draw to the opposite knee. Movement greater than 5 mm is usually considered abnormal.

Note: Functional instability due to anterior cruciate deficiency is best elicited with the pivot shift test. This is more difficult to perform than the Lachman test.

OVERUSE SYNDROMES

The knee is very prone to overuse disorders. The pain develops gradually without swelling, is aggravated by activity and relieved with rest. It can usually be traced back to a change in the sportsperson's training schedule, footwear, technique or related factors. It may be related also to biomechanical abnormalities ranging from hip disorders to feet disorders.

Overuse injuries include:
- patellofemoral joint pain syndrome ('jogger's knee', 'runner's knee')
- patellar tendinopathy ('jumper's knee')
- synovial plica syndrome
- infrapatellar fat-pad inflammation
- anserinus bursitis/tendinopathy
- biceps femoris tendinopathy
- semimembranous bursitis/tendinopathy
- quadriceps tendinopathy/rupture
- popliteus tendinopathy

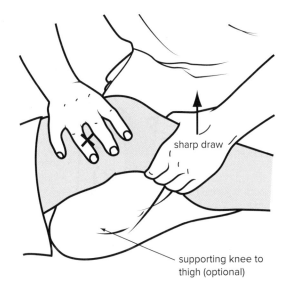

Fig. 11.62 Lachman test

- iliotibial band friction syndrome ('runner's knee')
- the hamstrung knee.

It is amazing how often palpation identifies localised areas of inflammation (tendinopathy or bursitis) around the knee, especially from overuse in athletes and in the obese elderly (Fig. 11.63a, b).

PATELLAR TENDINOPATHY ('JUMPER'S KNEE')

'Jumper's knee' or patellar tendinopathy (Fig. 11.64a) is a common disorder of athletes involved in repetitive jumping sports, such as high jumping, basketball, netball, volleyball and soccer. The diagnosis is often missed because of the difficulty localising the signs.

The condition is best diagnosed by eliciting localised tenderness at the inferior pole of the patella with the patella tilted.

Method

1. Lay the patient supine in a relaxed manner with head on a pillow, arms by the side and quadriceps relaxed (a must).
2. The knee should be fully extended.
3. Tilt the patella by exerting pressure over its superior pole. This lifts the inferior pole.
4. Now palpate the surface under the inferior pole. This allows palpation of the deeper fibres of the patellar tendon (Fig. 11.64b).
5. Compare with the normal side.

Very sharp pain is usually produced in the patient with patellar tendinopathy.

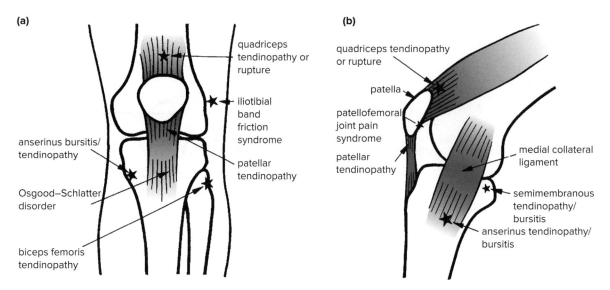

Fig. 11.63 Typical painful areas around the knee for overuse syndromes: **(a)** anterior aspect; **(b)** medial aspect

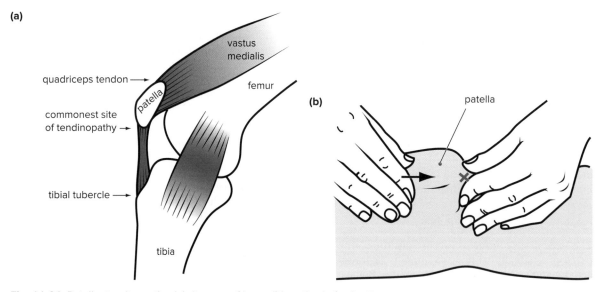

Fig. 11.64 Patellar tendinopathy: **(a)** diagram of knee; **(b)** method of palpation

Treatment

Explanation and conservative management including activity modification, stretching exercises and a strengthening program are the first-line treatment. However, the problem can be stubborn, and surgery has an important place in the management.

ANTERIOR KNEE PAIN

Pain felt in the anterior part of the knee is very common and is most commonly caused by the patellofemoral joint pain syndrome. It needs to be distinguished from arthritis of the knee joint. It is common in sports medicine and is referred to sometimes as 'jogger's knee', 'runner's knee' or 'cyclist's knee'.

DIAGNOSIS AND TREATMENT OF PATELLOFEMORAL JOINT PAIN SYNDROME

This syndrome, also known as chondromalacia patellae, is characterised by pain and crepitus around the patella during activities that require flexion of the knee under loading (e.g. climbing stairs).

Signs

Patellofemoral crepitation during knee flexion and extension is often palpable, and pain may be reproduced by compression of the patella onto the femur as it is pushed from side to side with the knee straight or flexed (Perkins test).

One method for the patella apprehension test (Fig. 11.65)

1. Have the patient supine with the knee extended.
2. Grasp the superior pole of the patella and displace it inferiorly.
3. Maintain this position and apply patellofemoral compression.
4. Ask the patient to contract the quadriceps (a good idea is to get the patient to practise quadriceps contraction before applying the test).
5. A positive sign is reproduction of pain under the patella and hesitancy in contracting the muscle.

Treatment

Figure 11.66 illustrates a simple quadriceps exercise. A series of isometric contractions are each held for about 4 seconds and alternated with relaxation of the leg. This exercise can be repeated many times in one period and throughout the day.

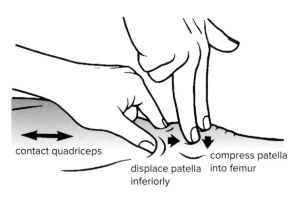

Fig. 11.65 Patellar apprehension test for patellofemoral joint pain syndrome

DISLOCATED PATELLA

Typical features

- An injury of children and young adults (especially females). Also common in sport.
- Caused by contraction of quadriceps with a flexed knee.
- There is always lateral displacement.
- Knee may be stuck in flexion.

Method of immediate reduction

The following can be attempted without anaesthesia (preferably immediately after the injury) or by using morphine and IV diazepam as a relaxant.

1. Place your thumb under the lateral edge of the patella.
2. Push it medially as you extend the knee.

Important points

- Exclude an osteochondral fracture with X-rays.
- Post-reduction rest with knee splinted in extension and crutches for 4 to 6 weeks.
- Arthroscopic inspection and repair may be advisable.
- Recurrent dislocation in young females (14 to 18 years) requires surgery.

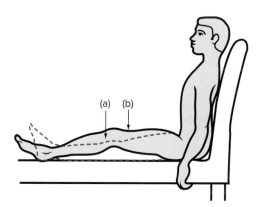

Fig. 11.66 Quadriceps exercise: tighten muscle by straightening the knee to position **(a)** from the relaxed position **(b)**

Leg

OVERUSE SYNDROMES IN ATHLETES

Athletes, especially runners and joggers, are prone to painful problems in the lower legs (Fig. 11.67). Diagnosis of the various syndromes can be difficult, but Table 11.4 will be a useful guide. The precise anatomical site of the painful problem is the best pointer to a diagnosis.

TORN 'MONKEY MUSCLE'

The so-called torn 'monkey muscle', or 'tennis leg', is actually a rupture of the medial head of gastrocnemius at

Table 11.4 Clinical comparisons of overuse syndromes

Syndrome	Symptoms	Common cause	Treatment
Anterior compartment syndrome	Pain in the anterolateral muscular compartment of the leg, increasing with activity. Difficult dorsiflexion of foot, which may feel floppy.	Persistent fast running (e.g. squash, football, middle-distance running).	Modify activities. Surgical fasciotomy is the only effective treatment.
Iliotibial band tendinopathy	Deep aching along lateral aspect of knee or lateral thigh. Worse running downhill, eased by rest. Pain appears after 3–4 km running.	Running up hills by long-distance runners and increasing distance too quickly.	Rest from running for 6 weeks. Special stretching exercises. Correct training faults and footwear. Consider injection of LA and corticosteroids deep into tender areas.
Tibial stress syndrome or shin splints	Pain and localised tenderness over the distal posteromedial border of the tibia. Bone scan for diagnosis.	Running or jumping on hard surfaces.	Relative rest for 6 weeks. Ice massage. Calf (soleus stretching). NSAIDs. Correct training faults and footwear.
Tibial stress fracture	Pain, in a similar site to shin splints, noted after running. Usually relieved by rest. Bone scan for diagnosis.	Overtraining on hard (often bitumen) surfaces. Faulty footwear.	Rest for 6–10 weeks. Casting not recommended. Graduated training after healing.
Tibialis anterior tenosynovitis	Pain over anterior distal third of leg and ankle. Pain at beginning and after exercise ± swelling, crepitus. Pain on active or resisted ankle dorsiflexion.	Overuse—excessive downhill running.	Rest, even from walking. Injection of LA and corticosteroid within tendon sheath.
Achilles tendinopathy	Pain in the Achilles tendon aggravated by walking on the toes. Stiff and sore in the morning after rising but improving after activity.	Repeated toe running in sprinters or running uphill in distance runners.	Relative rest. Ice at first and then heat. 10 mm heel wedge. Correct training faults and footwear. NSAIDs. Consider steroid injection.
Plantar fasciitis	Pain in medial or central aspect of base of the heel, worse with weight bearing. Sharp pain upon getting up to walk after sitting.	Running on uneven surfaces with feet pronated.	Relative rest. Orthotics in shoes. Injection of LA and corticosteroid.

the musculoskeletal junction where the Achilles tendon merges with the muscle (Fig. 11.68). This painful injury is common in middle-aged tennis and squash players who play infrequently and are unfit.

Clinical features

- A sudden sharp pain in the calf (the person thinks he or she has been struck from behind, e.g. by a thrown stone).
- Unable to put heel to ground.
- Walks on tip toes.
- Localised tenderness and hardness.
- Dorsiflexion of ankle painful.
- Bruising over site of rupture.

Management

- RICE treatment for 48 hours.

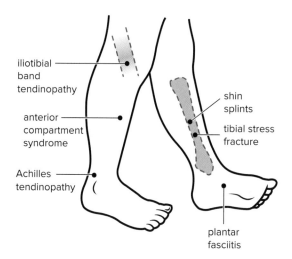

Fig. 11.67 Common sites of lower leg problems

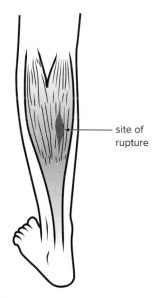

Fig. 11.68 'Tennis leg' or 'monkey muscle'—illustrating typical site of rupture of the medial head of gastrocnemius at the junction of muscle and tendon (left leg)

- Ice packs immediately for 20 minutes and then every 2 hours when awake (can be placed over the bandage).
- A firm elastic bandage from toes to below the knee.
- Crutches can be used if severe.
- A raised heel on the shoe (preferably both sides) aids mobility.
- Commence mobilisation after 48 hours rest, with active exercises.
- Physiotherapist supervision for gentle stretching massage and then restricted exercise.

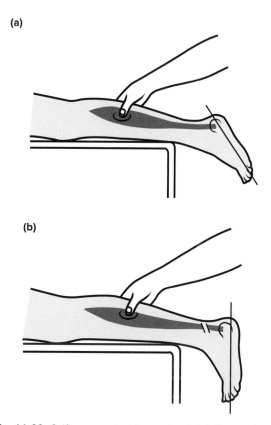

Fig. 11.69 Calf squeeze test for ruptured Achilles tendon: **(a)** intact tendon, normal plantar flexion; **(b)** ruptured tendon, foot remains stationary

COMPLETE RUPTURE OF ACHILLES TENDON

A complete rupture of the Achilles tendon can be misdiagnosed because the patient remains able to plantar flex the foot by virtue of the deep long flexors. Two tests should be performed to confirm the diagnosis.

Palpation of tendon

Palpate for a defect in the Achilles tendon. This defect could be masked by haematoma if the examination is performed more than a couple of hours after the injury.

The 'calf' squeeze test

With the patient prone and both feet over the edge of the couch (or kneeling on a chair facing the back), squeeze the gastrocnemius soleus complex of both legs. Plantar flexion of the foot indicates an intact Achilles tendon (Fig. 11.69a); failure of plantar flexion indicates total rupture (Fig. 11.69b).

TREATMENT OF SPRAINED ANKLE

Most of the ankle 'sprains' or tears involve the lateral ligaments (up to 90%), while the stronger tauter medial (deltoid) ligament is less prone to injury.

The treatment of ankle ligament sprains depends on the severity of the sprain. Most grade I (mild) and II (moderate) sprains respond well to standard conservative measures and regain full, pain-free movement in 1 to 6 weeks, but controversy surrounds the most appropriate management of grade III (complete tear) sprains.

Grades I & II sprains

R rest the injured part for 48 hours, depending on disability
I ice pack for 20 minutes every 3 to 4 hours when awake for the first 48 hours
C compression bandage, e.g. crepe bandage
E elevate to hip level to minimise swelling
A analgesics, e.g. paracetamol
R review in 48 hours, then 7 days
S special strapping

Use partial weight bearing with crutches for the first 48 hours or until standing is no longer painful, then encourage early full weight bearing and a full range of movement with isometric exercises. Use warm soaks, dispense with ice packs after 48 hours. Walking in sand, e.g. along the beach, is excellent rehabilitation. Aim towards full activity by 2 weeks.

Strapping of the ankle

Method

1. Maintain the foot in a neutral position (right angles to leg) by getting the patient to hold the foot in that position by a long strap or sling.
2. Apply small protective pads over pressure points.
3. Apply one or two stirrups of adhesive low-stretch 6–8 cm strapping from halfway up the medial side, around the heel and then halfway up the lateral side to hold the foot in slight eversion (Figs. 11.70a, b, c).
4. Apply an adhesive bandage, e.g. Acrylastic (6–8 cm), which can be rerolled and reused.
5. Reapply in 3 to 4 days.
6. After 7 days, remove and use a non-adhesive tubular elasticised support until full pain-free movement is achieved. An alternative is to use an ankle brace such as a Velcro brace (Fig. 11.71) to allow activity and comfort.

Hiking (bushwalking) tip for rolled sprained ankle

Some experienced leaders carry Voltaren (or similar) gel and plastic wrap when taking a walking group. If

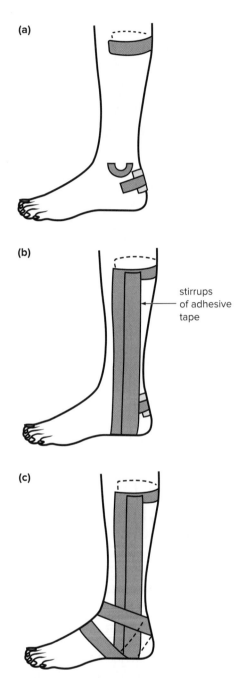

(a)

(b)

stirrups of adhesive tape

(c)

Fig. 11.70 Supportive strapping for a sprained ankle: **(a)** Step 1 apply protective pads and stay tape; **(b)** Step 2 apply stirrups to hold foot in slight eversion; **(c)** Step 3 apply an ankle lock tape

the ankle is injured (sprain is a common problem) and ICE treatment is unavailable, apply the gel or ointment to the injured ankle, cover with plastic wrap and then bandage.

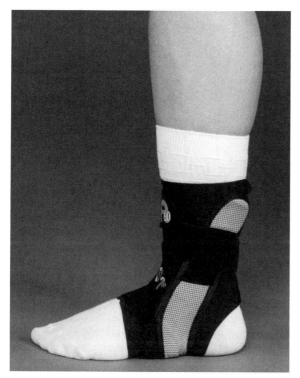

Fig. 11.71 Ankle braces—a variety of braces are available

Source: P. Brukner & K. Khan, *Brukner & Khan's Clinical Sports Medicine, Volume 1: Injuries* (5th Edn), McGraw-Hill, Sydney, 2017.

MOBILISATION OF THE SUBTALAR JOINT

The medial-lateral gliding mobilisation of the subtalar joint is indicated where there is a loss of function of the subtalar ankle joint, commonly with chronic post-traumatic ankle stiffness, with or without pain. The most common cause is the classic 'sprained' ankle.

The objective of therapy is to increase the range of inversion and eversion.

Method

1. The patient lies on the side (preferably the problematic side), with the affected leg resting on the table. The foot hangs over the end of the table with the lower leg supported by a flexible support, such as a rolled-up towel, small pillow, sandbag or lumbar roll. The foot is maintained in dorsiflexion by support against the therapist's thigh.
2. Stand at the foot of the table facing the patient's leg.
3. Grasp the patient's leg with the stabilising hand just above the level of the malleolus.
4. The mobilising hand firmly grasps the calcaneum.
5. Apply a firm force to the foot at right angles to the long axis of the foot, so that an even up and down

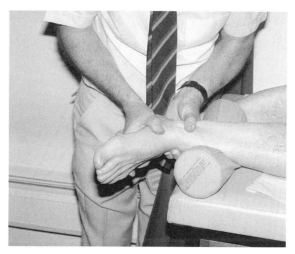

Fig. 11.72 Position of foot for mobilisation of the subtalar joint

(medial-lateral) rocking movement is achieved. The movement should be smooth (not too forceful or jerky) and of consistent amplitude (Fig. 11.72).

WOBBLE BOARD (AEROPLANE) TECHNIQUE FOR ANKLE DYSFUNCTION

Proprioception exercises

Strengthening of the leg muscles and the ligaments of the ankle can be improved by the use of a wobble board. The patient stands on the board and shifts his or her weight from side to side in neutral, forward or extended body positions to improve proprioception and balance.

An improvised wobble board

Patients can construct a simple wobble board by attaching a small piece of wood (10 cm × 10 cm × 5 cm (deep)) to the centre of a 30 cm square piece of plywood or similar wood about 2 cm thick. (Suitable for patients with good balance.)

Alternative

Patients can simply place their slab of wood on a dome-shaped mound of earth.

The Bosu-Ball

This is a fitness training device for yoga gym exercises. It is ideal for ankle exercises since it is a half sphere with a round bottom half and a flat surface on top.

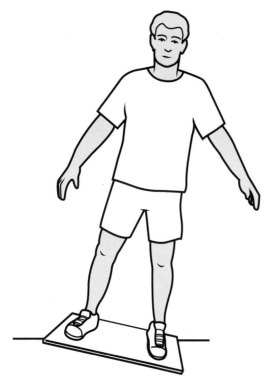

Fig. 11.73 Wobble board technique for ankle dysfunction

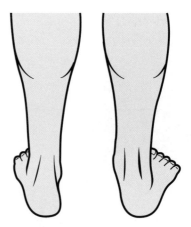

Fig. 11.74 Tibialis posterior rupture (right foot): the 'too many toes' posterior view

The 'aeroplane' exercise

1. Instruct the patient to stand in a neutral position and shift his or her weight from side to side to improve balance and proprioception.
2. After 2 or 3 days, perform the balancing exercises by leaning forwards in addition to using the neutral position (Fig. 11.73).
3. After a further 2 or 3 days, practise the exercise by leaning backwards—thus adding to the difficulty of the exercise.

TIBIALIS POSTERIOR TENDON RUPTURE

Rupture of the tibialis posterior tendon after inflammation, degeneration or trauma is a relatively common and misdiagnosed disorder. It causes collapse of the longitudinal arch of the foot, leading to a flat foot. It is uncommon for patients to feel obvious discomfort at the moment of rupture. Most cases in middle age can be treated conservatively. Severe problems respond well to surgical repair, which is usually indicated in athletes.

Features

- Middle-aged females and athletes.
- Usually presents with 'abnormal' flat foot.
- Pain in the region of the navicular to the medial malleolus.
- Gross eversion of the foot.
- 'Too many toes' test (Fig. 11.74).
- Single heel raise test (unable to raise heel).
- On palpation, thickening or absence of tibialis posterior tendon.

'Too many toes' test

More toes are seen on the affected side when the feet are viewed from about 3 m behind the patient (Fig. 11.74).

Useful investigations

- Ultrasound—the most economical.
- MRI and CT scan—gives the clearest image.

Plastering tips

PLASTER OF PARIS

The bucket of water

- Line the bucket with a plastic bag for easy cleaning.
- The water should be deep enough to allow complete vertical immersion.
- Use cold water for slow setting.
- Use tepid water for faster setting.

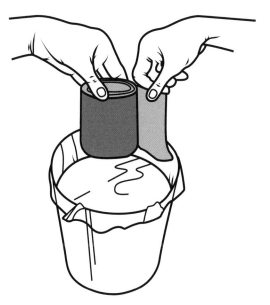

Fig. 11.75 Holding the plaster roll

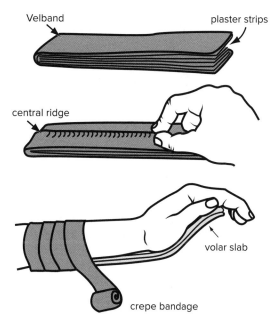

Fig. 11.76 Preparation of volar arm plaster splint; apply with the wrist dorsiflexed 30°

- Do not use hot water: it produces rapid setting and a brittle plaster.

The plaster rolls

- Do not use plaster rolls if water has been splashed on them.
- Hold the roll loosely but with the free end firm and secure (Fig. 11.75).
- Immerse in water until bubbles have ceased coming from the plaster surface. Ensure that the centre of the plaster is fully wet.
- Drain surface water after removal from the bucket.
- Gently squeeze the roll in the middle: do not indent.
- Use about 2 × 10 cm and 1 × 8 cm rolls for below elbow and upper limb plasters.
- Use 4 × 15 cm rolls for below knee leg plaster.

Padding

- Use Velband or stockinet under the plaster.
- With Velband, moisten the end of the roll in water to allow it to adhere to the limb.
- For legs, make extra padding around pressure areas such as the ankle and heel.
- Use two layers of padding but avoid multiple layers.

Method

1. Use an assistant to support the limb where possible (e.g. hold the arm up with fingers of stockinet).

2. Lay the bandage on firmly but do not pull tight.
3. Lay it on quickly. Avoid dents.
4. Overlap the bandage by about 25% of its width.
5. Use only the flat of the hand so as to achieve a smooth cast.

PREPARING A VOLAR ARM PLASTER SPLINT (FRONT SLAB)

A plaster splint can be prepared with minimal mess and maximal effectiveness by following this procedure.

Procedure

1. Measure the length of the required plaster splint.
2. Select Velband of the same width as the plaster and measure a length slightly more than twice the length of the splint.
3. On a flat bench top, lay out the length of the Velband on a piece of newspaper or undercloth.
4. Fold the plaster (10 cm roll for adults) according to the number of strips required (usually eight) and after immersing it in cool or lukewarm water and draining off excess water, place it on the Velband as shown in Figure 11.76.
5. Fold the Velband over the plaster to produce a 'sandwich' effect.
6. Using the fingers through the upper layer of Velband, mould two to three ridges along the length of the plaster on the outer surface of the slab. This provides reinforced strength for the splint.

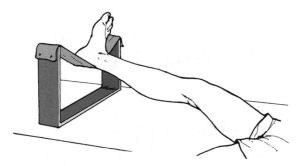

Fig. 11.77 Supportive device for application of leg plaster

7. Take a crepe bandage and apply the splint to the arm with appropriate moulding to hold the wrist in about 30° of extension.
8. This method can be adapted for plaster slabs for other areas.

LEG SUPPORT FOR PLASTER APPLICATION

The awkward task of applying a leg plaster including a plaster cylinder can be aided by the use of a simple supportive device (Fig. 11.77).

The support, which should be at least 30 cm high, can be made by pinning a broad leather strap across a U-shaped frame.

WATERPROOFING YOUR PLASTER CAST

A suitable plastic protective cover for a plaster cast, especially for one on the arm, is a veterinary plastic

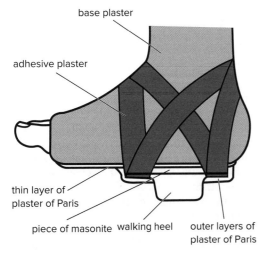

base plaster
adhesive plaster
thin layer of plaster of Paris
piece of masonite   walking heel   outer layers of plaster of Paris

Fig. 11.78 Plaster walking heel

glove, which is ideally long and fits on the arm like a mega 'glove'. These are the gloves used in rural practice!

A LONG-LASTING PLASTER WALKING HEEL

To avoid the plaster underlying the walking heel (incorporated into a leg plaster) becoming soft and therefore uncomfortable for walking (thus requiring repair), the following method can be used (Fig. 11.78).

It involves incorporating a small piece of masonite (or similar wooden material) into the plaster cast at the time of affixing the heel. This is performed 24 hours after application of the original base plaster cast.

Method

1. Apply a thin layer of plaster of Paris to the underside of the base of the cast.
2. Place the piece of masonite (or wood) against the plaster.
3. Place the heel over the wood.
4. Wrap adhesive plaster (such as Elastoplast) around the wood and heel to 'fix' the unit.
5. Apply the final coating of plaster of Paris to fix the heel.
6. Weight bearing can commence 24 hours later.

SUPPORTING SHOE FOR A WALKING PLASTER

Method A

An economical method is to get the patient to bring an old pair of rubber sneakers and cut out the front half (including the tongue) but leave the laces intact. On review (day 2), the plaster cast is fitted into the sneaker and tied over with the laces.

Method B

A better alternative to the walking heel is the 'open-toe cast shoe', with its open heel and toe areas that can accommodate a wide variety of foot and cast types. The rocker sole, which is manufactured from EVA (a synthetic rubber), has three layers and minimises microtrauma to joints. The upper is made from reinforced canvas with Presto-flex adhesive straps.

The shoes come in at least three sizes and fit neatly onto the plaster. They can be washed and will last throughout the life of a normal walking plaster. The shoes are available from various surgical suppliers.

USE OF SILICONE FILLER

An economical walking plaster can be improvised by obtaining silicone filler (preferably resin type) from a

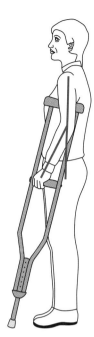

Fig. 11.79 Correct fitting for crutches

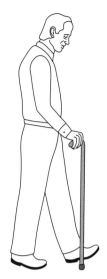

Fig. 11.80 Correct cane height

hardware store and layering it over the base of the plaster with extra thickness over pressure areas.

PRESCRIBING CRUTCHES

Patients with leg injuries are often given crutches without ensuring they are the correct height. The following guidelines are useful:
- Wear the shoes that are usually worn.
- Stand erect and look straight ahead, shoulders relaxed.
- For fitting, the end of each crutch should be placed about 5 cm from the side of the shoe and about 15 cm in front of the toe.

- The top of the crutch should be about 2–3 finger breadths (about 5 cm) below the apex of the axilla.
- The hand grip should be adjusted with the elbow bent 20–30° (Fig. 11.79).
- The patient should have a trial walking practice under supervision before discharge.

WALKING STICK ADVICE

The walking stick has been proved to be beneficial for osteoarthritis of the knee.[12] It should be held in the hand on the opposite side to the 'bad leg'. When prescribing a walking stick (cane) instruct the person to place the tip of the cane on the ground at the same time as the affected side (knee) is placed on the ground. Advise the correct height so that the patient's elbow will be bent at slightly less than 30° when maximum force is applied (Fig. 11.80).

References

1. Kenna C, Murtagh JE. *Back pain and spinal manipulation* (2nd edn). Oxford: Butterworths Heinemann, 1997.
2. Chakraverty R, Pynsent P & Isaacs K. Which spinal levels are identified by palpation of the iliac crests and the posterior superior iliac spines? *J Anat,* 2007; 210(2): 232–6.
3. Murtagh J, *General Practice Companion Handbook* (7th Edn), McGraw-Hill, Sydney, 2019.
4. Huckstep RL. *A simple guide to trauma.* Edinburgh: E&S Livingstone, 1970: 101, 141.
5. Milch H. Treatment of dislocation of the shoulder. Surgery, 1938; 3: 732–8.
6. White AD. Dislocated shoulder—a simple method of reduction. Med J Aust, 1976; 2: 726–27.
7. Zagorski M. Analgesia-free reduction of anterior dislocation of the shoulder joint. Aust J Rural Health, 1995; 3: 53–5.
8. Krul M, van der Wouden JC, van Suijlekom-Smit LWA, Koes BW. Manipulative interventions for reducing pulled elbow in young children (Review). Cochrane database of systematic reviews, 2012; 1.

9. Sims S, Miller K, Elfar J, Hammert W. Non-surgical treatment of lateral epicondylitis: a systematic review of randomized controlled trials. Hand, 2014; 9: 419–46.

10. Cullinane F, Boocock M, Trevelyan F. Is eccentric exercise an effective treatment for lateral epicondylitis? A systematic review. Clin Rehab, 2014; 28(1): 3–19.

11. Gwee A, Rimer R, Marks M (Eds.). *Paediatric handbook: RCH* (9th edn). West Sussex: Wiley Blackwell, 2015: 220–21.

12. Jones A, Silva PG, Colucci M, Tuffanin A, Jardim JR, Natour J. Impact of cane use on pain, function, general health and energy expenditure during gait in patients with knee osteoarthritis: a randomised controlled trial. Ann Rheum Dis, 2012; 71: 172–9.

Chapter 12

ORODENTAL PROBLEMS

EMERGENCY DENTAL KIT

The dental emergency basic kit is useful for practitioners working where no dentist is readily available, particularly in rural and remote locations. The kit should have the material requirements for temporary relief of:

- a broken or lost piece of tooth
- a broken or lost filling
- irritated gums, tongue or cheek from a broken tooth or sharp braces.

KNOCKED-OUT TOOTH

If a permanent (second) tooth is knocked out (e.g. in an accident or fight) but is intact, it can be saved by the following, immediate procedure. The tooth should not be out of the mouth for longer than 20 to 30 minutes from the time of injury.

Method

1. Using a glove hold the tooth by its crown and replace it in its original position, preferably immediately (Fig. 12.1); if dirty, put it in milk before replacement or, better still, place it under the tongue and 'wash' it in saliva. Alternatively, it can be placed in contact lens saline or the solution in the 'Dentist in a Box' kit (www.dentistinabox.com.au). *Note:* Do not use water, and do not rub or wipe (it removes dentine) or touch the root.
2. Fix the tooth by moulding strong aluminium foil over it and the adjacent teeth. If none is available, substitute with a large wad of Blu Tack. Moulding foil can be difficult: an alternative is to suture with

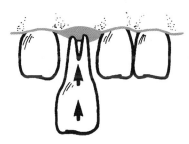

Fig. 12.1 Replacement of a knocked-out tooth

a figure-of-eight silk suture to encompass the tooth. It can also be secured to the two adjoining teeth with a strip of tape cut from a disc in the 'Dentist in a Box' kit.

3. Refer the patient to his or her dentist or dental hospital as soon as possible. Tell the patient to avoid exerting any direct biting force on the tooth.

Note: If a blood clot is present, remove it after a nerve block. Teeth replaced within 20 to 30 minutes have a 90% chance of successful reimplantation.

LOOSE OR PARTIALLY DISLODGED TOOTH

Loosening is excessive movement of a permanent tooth with no displacement.

Splint the mobile tooth to a neighbouring tooth with the splinting material from the kit (see above). Alternatively, use chewing gum or Blu Tack. Refer the patient to a dentist.

CHIPPED TOOTH

Rinse the mouth with warm water. Cover the exposed area, which is usually painful, with dental tape. Recover and store the tooth fragment for use by the dentist. If possible, secure the broken fragment with splinting material from the kit. Refer the patient to a dentist.

LOST FILLING

A temporary measure is to stick a piece of chewed sugarless gum into the filling or use an OTC dental cement. Refer to the dentist ASAP.

LOST CROWN

Make appointment to visit dentist ASAP.

If area is sensitive, apply a little clove oil. Slip crown back over the tooth after coating the inner surface with OTC dental cement (or from Box kit). Do not use 'superglue'.

CHILD WITH A BLEEDING MOUTH

A bleeding lip or tongue in a crying child is quickly settled with half a teaspoon of sugar, which acts not only as a distraction, but also as a styptic.

To palpate the teeth, wear gloves and further protect yourself from a bite injury by inserting a wooden tongue depressor sideways in between the teeth.

IMPACTED WISDOM TOOTH

This may present as an impacted tooth in the molar region, with pain and swelling, possible local infection and 'frozen' jaw. Rinse with warm salt water, applying an ice pack, and organise a dental appointment ASAP. Prescribe antibiotics if dental care is delayed.

INFECTIONS—TOOTH ABSCESS, WISDOM TOOTH OR ROOT CANAL INFECTION

Localise the affected tooth by percussing firmly along the chewing surface of each tooth with the tip of a tongue depressor—a yelp will indicate you have reached your destination.

Dental attention—if severe:
- amoxicillin.

If unresponsive:
- amoxicillin/clavulanate and metronidazole.

BLEEDING TOOTH SOCKET

First aid treatment method

Enquire about blood-thinning medication. Wipe away the blood on top of the socket. Instruct the patient to bite very firmly on a gauze swab moistened with saline or water or a rolled-up moistened clean cotton handkerchief over the bleeding socket. Bite hard for up to 30 minutes. This simple measure is sufficient to achieve haemostasis in most instances. Biting on a recently used moist tea bag is a readily available alternative.

Surgical treatment for persistent bleeding

1. Remove excess blood clot, using a piece of sterile gauze.
2. Bite on a firm gauze pack (as above).
3. If still bleeding, infiltrate LA with adrenaline, insert an absorbable suture.
4. Using a reverse suture, approximate the anterior and posterior mucosal remnants (Fig. 12.2). The idea is not to close the socket but to tense the mucoperiosteum against the bone.

If a vessel in soft tissue is bleeding, either ligate or cauterise it.

Avoid aspirin, rinsing and alcohol.

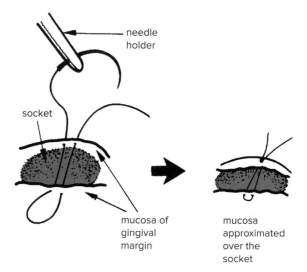

Fig. 12.2 Treatment for persistent bleeding of tooth socket

DRY TOOTH SOCKET

Clinical features

- Tooth extraction 1 to 3 days earlier especially a wisdom tooth.
- Very severe pain, unrelieved by analgesics.
- Continuous pain on the side of the face.
- Foetid odour.
- Mainly in the lower molars, especially the third (wisdom teeth).

Examination shows a socket with few or no blood clots, and sensitive bone surfaces covered by a greyish-yellow layer of necrotic tissue.

Treatment method

1. Self-limiting healing 10 to 14 days.
2. Refer to the dentist for special toilet and dressing (palliative).

If you have to treat:
- irrigate with warm saline in a syringe
- pack socket with 1 cm ribbon gauze in iodiform paste or pack a mixture of a paste of zinc oxide and oil of cloves or (usual dental formulation) zinc oxide and eugenol dressing. Leave 10 days.
- analgesics
- mouth wash.

Note: Antibiotics are of no proven value unless infection supervenes.

The differential diagnosis for the dry tooth socket is descending infection.

A SIMPLE WAY OF NUMBERING TEETH

Dentists utilise codes in which the teeth are numbered 1 to 8 from the midline.

International notation

Each of the four quadrants is numbered, starting at the upper right:

Permanent teeth (n = 32; Fig. 12.3)

$$\text{R.} \quad \frac{^{1}87654321}{_{4}87654321} \bigg| \frac{12345678^{2}}{12345678_{3}} \quad \text{L.}$$

Deciduous teeth (n = 20)

There are five teeth in each quadrant, and the four quadrants are notated 5 to 8.

$$\text{R.} \quad \frac{^{5}54321}{_{8}54321} \bigg| \frac{12345^{6}}{12345_{7}} \quad \text{L.}$$

Examples:
- 1.6 = upper right first molar
- 3.2 = lower left lateral incisor
- 6.3 = upper left deciduous canine.

Palmer notation

In this notation a cross is drawn to represent quadrants, but the numerals are used as above for permanent teeth. Deciduous teeth are represented by the letters A–E.

The quadrants are noted by four right angles:

R ⫢ L

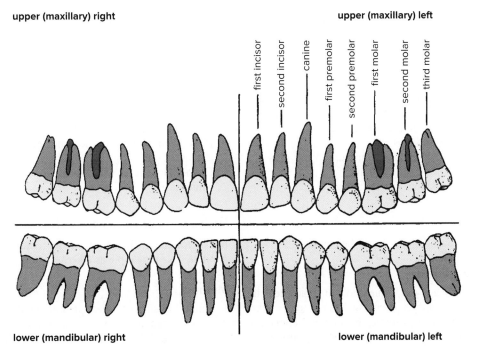

upper (maxillary) right   **upper (maxillary) left**

first incisor — second incisor — canine — first premolar — second premolar — first molar — second molar — third molar

lower (mandibular) right   **lower (mandibular) left**

Fig. 12.3 Permanent teeth

Examples:
- └ 5 = upper left second premolar
- ┐ C = lower right deciduous cuspid.

Wisdom teeth

These are the third molars. They are usually normal teeth, but are prone to troublesome eruption usually in the late teens and difficult extraction when impacted.

APHTHOUS ULCERS (CANKER SORES)

These acutely painful ulcers on the mobile oral mucosa are a common problem in general practice and puzzling in their cause and response to treatment. Their cause is unknown, but several factors indicate a localised abnormal immune reaction.
Minor ulcers: < 5 mm in diameter—last 5 to 10 days.
Major ulcers: > 8 mm in diameter—last weeks and heal with scarring.

Associations to consider

Blood dyscrasias, denture pressure, Crohn disease, pernicious anaemia, iron deficiency.

Precipitating factors

Stress and local trauma.

Treatment methods

These treatments should be used early when the ulcer is most painful. Several optional healing methods are presented.

Symptomatic relief

Apply topical lidocaine gel or paint, e.g. SM-33 adult paint formula or SM-33 gel (children) every 3 hours. If applied before meals, eating is facilitated.
Alternatively, use a mixture of:
- diphenhydramine (Benadryl mixture) 5 mL plus
- Mylanta (or Gaviscon) 5–10 mL.
Gargle well and swallow 4 times a day.

Healing

One of the following methods can be chosen.

The teabag method

Consider applying a wet, squeezed out, black teabag directly to the ulcer regularly, such as 3 to 4 times daily. The tannic acid promotes healing and alleviates pain. Another method is to prepare a strong cup of tea (concentrated), cool and dip in a cotton bud or ball and hold it against the ulcer for 3 minutes.

Topical corticosteroid paste

Triamcinolone 0.1% (Kenalog in Orobase®) paste. Apply 8 hourly and at night.

Topical corticosteroid spray

Spray beclomethasone onto the ulcer 3 times daily.

Topical chloramphenicol

Use 10% chloramphenicol in propylene glycol. Apply with a cotton bud for 1 minute (after drying the ulcer) 6 hourly for 3 to 4 days.

Tetracycline suspension rinse for multiple ulcers

1. Empty the contents of a 250 mg tetracycline capsule into 20–30 mL of warm water and shake it.
2. Swirl this solution in the mouth for 5 minutes every 3 hours.
An alternative method is to apply the solution soaked in cotton wool wads to the ulcers for 5 to 10 minutes.
Note: This has a terrible taste but reportedly shortens the life of the ulcers considerably.[1] We recommend spitting out the rinse, although some authorities suggest swallowing the suspension.

Topical sucralfate

Dissolve 1 g sucralfate in 20–30 mL of warm water. Use this as a mouth wash.

GEOGRAPHIC TONGUE (ERYTHEMA MIGRANS)

Treatment

Explanation and reassurance.
- No treatment if asymptomatic.
- Cepacaine gargles, 10 mL tds, if tender.
- If persistent and troublesome, low-dose spray of glucocorticoid (e.g. beclomethasone 50 mcg tds). Do not rinse after use. Warn about the risk of oral candidiasis.

BLACK, GREEN OR HAIRY TONGUE

Brush tongue with a toothbrush to remove stained papillae. Use pineapple as a keratolytic agent.

Method

1. Cut a thin slice of pineapple into eight segments.
2. Suck a segment on the back of the tongue for 40 seconds and then slowly chew it.

3. Repeat until all segments are completed.
4. Do this twice a day for 7 to 10 days. Repeat if symptoms recur.
   Alternate: sodium bicarbonate mouthwash.

CALCULUS IN WHARTON DUCT

The most common site for a salivary calculus is in the duct of the submandibular gland (Wharton duct). Obstruction to the gland by the calculus causes the classic presentation of intermittent swelling of the gland whenever the patient attempts to eat. The following method applies if the clinician can easily palpate the calculus with the finger under the tongue.

Method

1. Localise the calculus in the duct by finger palpation.
2. Anaesthetise the area with a small bleb of LA or surface anaesthetic (preferable if available), e.g. 5% cocaine placed under the tongue.
3. Insert a stay suture around the duct immediately behind the calculus (Fig. 12.4), and use this to steady the stone by elevation.
4. Make an incision over the long axis of the duct (the calculus easily slips out).
5. Remove the stay suture and leave the wound unsutured.

A 'NATURAL' METHOD OF SNARING A CALCULUS

1. Fast for about 6 hours.
2. Squeeze an unripe lemon and drink the juice.
3. Place a slice of lemon on the tongue. The calculus usually appears at the opening—it may then be possible to extract it using the preceding or following methods.

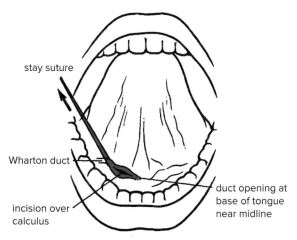

stay suture

Wharton duct

incision over calculus

duct opening at base of tongue near midline

Fig. 12.4 Excision of calculus in Wharton duct

SIMPLE REMOVAL OF CALCULUS FROM WHARTON DUCT

If the calculus is visible at the opening of the duct it can be removed using the round end of a Jacob–Horne probe.

The round end of the probe is placed over the meatus and firmly pressed inwards.

Digital pressure is then applied from the opposite side of the frenulum. The calculus may 'pop out' quite readily.

RELEASE OF TONGUE TIE (FRENULOTOMY)

The ideal time to release a tongue tie (ankyloglossia) is in infancy, when it may cause maternal nipple pain. Although a 2017 Cochrane review found no benefit for breastfeeding after frenulotomy, evidence was scant and the review also found no serious complications from the procedure.[2]

Early signs

- Tongue may appear as heart-shaped.
- Infants should be able to lift the tongue halfway to the roof when the mouth is open.
- Infants should be able to protrude the tongue over the lower lip.

Tongue tie has been postulated to cause symptoms later in childhood, including speech defects (e.g. a lisp), dental problems with the lower teeth, and accumulation of food in the floor of the mouth. However, a 2011 literature review done at The Royal Children's Hospital Melbourne found insufficient evidence to implicate tongue tie in these symptoms.[3]

Treatment in infants (usually under 4 months, best at 3 to 4 months)

Note: The frenulum is thin and avascular and there is minimal or no bleeding.
1. Ideally, a frenulum spatula should be used.
2. When the spatula is in place the tongue is stretched upwards.
3. Use a scalpel blade or sterile iris scissors to slit the frenulum just above the floor of the mouth.

Alternative to frenulum spatula

The infant is held by an assistant on the examination table with arms positioned either side of the head. The operator holds the frenulum between the index finger and thumb of the non-dominant hand and stretches it firmly (Fig. 12.5). The frenulum is then snipped with sterile scissors, taking care not to damage structures in the floor of the mouth and under the tongue. Another method, requiring referral, is to use laser excision, which is very effective for those with the acquired skills.

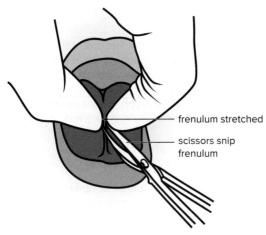

frenulum stretched

scissors snip frenulum

Fig. 12.5 Tongue tie release

Treatment in adults or older children

1. Perform the procedure under local or general anaesthesia.
2. When the tongue is elevated, use a no. 15 scalpel blade to incise the frenulum horizontally, taking care to avoid the Wharton ducts.
3. Tongue traction will then convert the horizontal incision into a vertical one, which can be closed in a vertical plane with interrupted plain catgut sutures.

References

1. Henriesson V, Axial T, *Treatment of recurrent aphthous ulcers with aureomycin mouth rinse or zedium dentifrice,* Acta odontol Scand, 1985, 43: 47–52.
2. O'Shea J et al, *Frenotomy for tongue-tie in newborn infants,* Cochrane Database Syst Rev, 2017, 11: 3.
3. Royal Children's Hospital, Change to 'tongue tie' outpatient speech pathology service. Melbourne: 2011, https://www.rch.org.au/uploadedfiles/main/content/speech/changes_to_tongue_tie_service.pdf.

Chapter 13
EAR, NOSE AND THROAT

URTIs and sinus problems

DIAGNOSING SINUS TENDERNESS

Eliciting sinus tenderness is important in the diagnosis and follow-up of sinusitis.

Firm pressure over any facial bone, particularly in the patient with an upper respiratory infection, may cause pain. It is important to differentiate sinus tenderness from non-sinus bone tenderness.

Method

1. This is best done by palpating a non-sinus area first and last (Fig. 13.1), systematically exerting pressure over the temporal bones (T), then the frontal (F), ethmoid (E) and maxillary (M) sinuses, and finally zygomas (Z), or vice versa.
2. Differential tenderness both identifies and localises the main sites of infection.

DIAGNOSIS OF UNILATERAL SINUSITIS

A simple way to assess the presence or absence of fluid in the frontal sinus, and in the maxillary sinus (in particular), is the use of transillumination. It works best when one symptomatic side can be compared with an asymptomatic side.

It is necessary to have the patient in a darkened room and to use a small, narrow-beam torch.

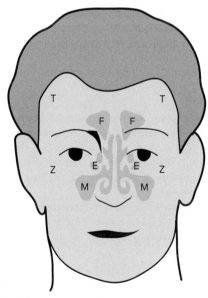

Fig. 13.1 T (temporal) and Z (zygoma) represent no sinus bony tenderness, for purposes of comparison (F = frontal sinuses; E = ethmoid sinuses; M = maxillary sinuses)

Frontal sinuses

Shine the torch above the eye in the roof of the orbit (touching the skin under the eyebrow) and also directly over the frontal sinuses, and compare the illuminations.

Maxillary sinuses

Remove dentures (if any). Shine the light inside the mouth (touching the mucosa), on either side of the hard palate, pointed at the base of the orbit. A dull glow seen below the orbit indicates that the antrum is air-filled. Diminished illumination on the symptomatic side indicates sinusitis.

Unblocking maxillary sinuses

Particularly in light of recommendations against antibiotics in most cases of sinusitis, a 'hydrate and vibrate' approach to clearing the mucus is worth trying.

Squirt 8 sprays of saline into the nostril on the affected side (bilaterally if indicated). Position an electric toothbrush against the upper molars and vibrate for up to five minutes. Blow and clear the nose, using further saline sprays as necessary.

INHALATIONS FOR URTIS

Simple inhalations for upper respiratory tract infections (including upper airways obstruction from the oedema and secretions of rhinitis and sinusitis) can promote symptomatic relief and early resolution of the problem. The positive effect of making the patient responsible for active participation in management often helps to counterbalance the occasional disappointment when no antibiotic is prescribed.

The old method of towel over the head and inhalation bowl can be used, but it is better to direct the vapour at the nose.

Equipment

- Container. This can be an old disposable bowl, a wide-mouthed bottle or tin, or a plastic container.
- The inhalant. Several household over-the-counter preparations are suitable: e.g. Friar's Balsam (5 mL), Vicks VapoRub (one teaspoon), Euky Bear, eucalyptus oil or menthol (5 mL).
- Cover. A paper bag (with its base cut out), a cone of paper (Fig. 13.2a) or a small cardboard carton (with the corner cut away; Fig.13.2b).

Method

1. Add 5 mL or one teaspoon of the inhalant to 0.5 L of boiled water (allow to cool for 5 to 10 minutes) in the container.
2. Place the paper or carton over the container.
3. Get the patient to apply nose and mouth to the opening to breathe the vapour in deeply and slowly through the nose, and then out slowly through the mouth.
4. This should be performed for 5 to 10 minutes, 3 times a day, especially before retiring.

After inhalation, upper airway congestion can be relieved by autoinsufflation.

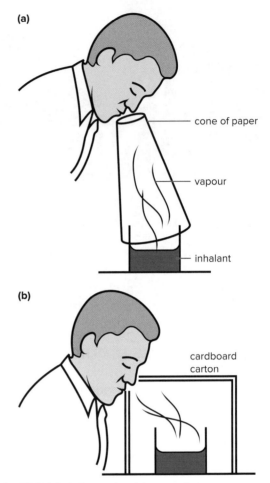

Fig. 13.2 Inhalations using: **(a)** cone of paper; **(b)** cardboard carton

Hot water bottle method

A relatively safe and convenient way is to use a hot water bottle for inhalations. The top fits neatly over the mouth and nose.

Vacuum flask method

An old vacuum flask (thermos) is an ideal container to fill with very hot/boiling water and the inhalant. It is also portable.

Warning: Avoid using these hot water methods in children.

A practical inhalation method for busy workers

Some practitioners claim great success using a coffee cup for inhalations. By placing the inhalant, e.g. Vicks, on a teaspoon then adding boiling water, an inhalation bowl is made by placing the hands over the cup to suit the nose and mouth. People find this easy to use during meal/coffee breaks.

NASAL POLYPS

Nasal polyps are small 'bags' of fluid and mucus following engorgement of the mucosa of the sinuses, usually due to allergic rhinitis. They pop out through the sinus openings into the nasal cavity (Fig. 13.3). They are best treated by medical polypectomy using topical corticosteroid sprays for small polyps and oral corticosteroids for extensive polyps, e.g. prednisolone 50 mg per day for 5 to 7 days (avoid aspirin). Antibiotics are occasionally needed for infection.

Surgery is usually reserved for failed medical treatment. Polyps can be simply removed under local anaesthetic by snaring the base or stalk with a loop of cutting wire. More severe cases may require sophisticated surgery.

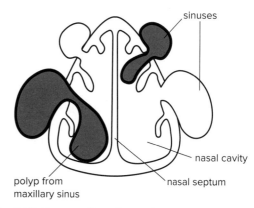

Fig. 13.3 Cross-section of nose demonstrating origin of nasal polyps

The ear and hearing

A RAPID TEST FOR SIGNIFICANT HEARING LOSS

The age of the digital watch has meant a decline in the use of the 'ticking watch' test as a rough screening procedure for hearing loss.

In children and in adults with a reasonable amount of hair, an alternative method can be used.

Method

1. Grasp several scalp hairs close to the external auditory canal lightly between the thumb and index finger.
2. Rub lightly together (Fig. 13.4) to produce a relatively high-pitched 'crackling' sound.

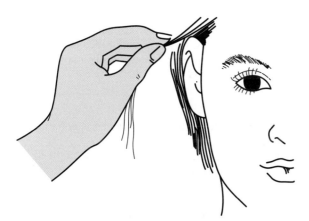

Fig. 13.4 Test for hearing loss in a child

If this sound cannot be heard, a moderate hearing loss is likely (usually about 40 dB or greater). If a hearing loss is detected, tuning fork assessment and other investigations will then be required.

The whispered voice test

The whispered voice test has been proved as an accurate screening test for hearing impairment. It is less accurate in children than in adults.

It is important to exhale quietly before whispering.

Method

1. Stand 60 cm behind the patient.
2. Mask the non-test ear by gently occluding the auditory canal and rubbing the tragus in a circular motion.
3. Exhale quietly before whispering a combination of numbers and letters (e.g. '5, M, 2, A').
4. If the patient responds correctly (i.e. repeats at least 3 out of 6 numbers and letters correctly), hearing is considered normal.
5. If the patient responds incorrectly, repeat the test using a different number-and-letter combination.
6. Test each ear individually, beginning with the better ear. Use a different number–letter combination each time.

Crumpled paper test

Another simple rapid test for adults and older children is to use the sound of paper. Gently rub two pieces of paper together about 1 cm from the ear and request the patient to indicate if they hear the sound. The sound is approximately equivalent to 30 dB. For infants over 3 months of age, crush a piece of paper behind the ear and note their response, including observing for eye movement towards the sound. Infants over 6 months should turn their whole head.

The chewing apple screening test

Get the patient to chew an apple or other crunchy morsel and note if the sound is louder in one ear to differentiate between conductive and nerve deafness.

Mobile phone apps

Free audiological screening apps can be downloaded onto a mobile phone. (See p247)

WATER- AND SOUNDPROOFING EARS

Waterproofing ears with Blu Tack

An excellent earplug can be made with Blu Tack, which can be gently moulded to the external auditory canal. It is ideal for children if they need to keep an ear dry when swimming or showering, for example those with perforations, ventilating grommets and recurrent otitis externa ('swimmer's ear'). Ideally, a swimming cap should also cover the ear and diving should be advised against.

The Blu Tack provides excellent waterproofing, stays in place and is reusable. Do not use in hot saunas, where it softens easily.

Children should be instructed not to keep poking the 'tack' into their ears with their fingers.

Be prepared to remove retained bits of Blu Tack sometimes. Surfers should probably invest in a more custom-designed plug.

Cotton ball and petroleum jelly plugs

Melt some petroleum jelly (e.g. Vaseline) on low heat on the stove, add a pack of cotton balls to the saucepan and mix with a potato masher. When cool, store these ear plugs in a jam jar.

New type of ear plug

A new form of ear protection is the expanding ear plug. The plugs can be used during exposure to excessive noise and for middle ear protection while swimming, especially for children with ventilating tubes inserted in their ears.

Made of compressible foam, when cut in half the plug can be rolled into a cylindrical shape that fits neatly in a child's ear. Keeping a finger on the outer part of the ear canal allows the plug to expand and fill the canal. A small coating of petroleum jelly and a standard rubber bathing cap make them waterproof, but the child should not dive under water.

Parents who have tried to use a full-sized ear plug for a child have sometimes found that the bathing cap rubbed on the end of it, pulling it out of the ear—hence the reason for cutting them in half. (E.A.R. Plugs are available from most acoustic services for approximately $1.00 a pair. They are washed easily in warm, soapy water, and a pair will last between 6 and 12 months.)

USE OF TISSUE 'SPEARS' FOR OTITIS EXTERNA AND MEDIA

The debris from otitis externa and the discharge from otitis externa or media can be mopped out with 'spears' fashioned from toilet paper or other tissue. They are widely recommended in Indigenous children prior to inserting ear drops. In otitis externa this toileting can be followed by acetic acid 0.25% washout—then topical steroid and antibiotic drops or ointment if necessary.

PREVENTING SWIMMER'S OTITIS EXTERNA

Get patients to rinse ears out with fresh water (possibly using a 5 mL syringe) and then dry with a hair dryer on the lowest warming setting. Avoid poking with cotton buds or similar objects.

Treatment and prevention of swimmer's ear

Use a drying topical medication, e.g. Aquaear or Ear Clear (acetic acid and isopropyl alcohol). An alternative less expensive preparation is a 'homebrew' mixture of acetic acid (vinegar) and methyl alcohol (methylated spirits), 3 parts to 7. Instil 2 to 3 drops daily during the swimming season.

CHRONIC SUPPURATIVE OTITIS MEDIA AND EXTERNA

Wash the canal with dilute povidone-iodine (Betadine) 5% solution using a 20 mL syringe with plastic tubing 1, 2 or 3 times daily. Dry mop with rolled tissue paper 'spears'. Teach this method to family members. If available, suction kits are useful.

TROPICAL EAR

For severe painful otitis externa, which is common in tropical areas:
- prednisolone (orally) 15 mg statim, then 10 mg 8 hourly for six doses, followed by
- compressed-sponge ear wick (e.g. Merocel) or ichthammol and glycerine wick
- topical Locacorten Vioform or Sofradex drops for 10 days.

Getting ointment into ear canals

Filling an ear canal with ointment has a longer lasting effect on otitis externa than ear drops. Use corticosteroid/antibacterial combination ointments that already contain an antifungal (e.g. Kenacomb Otic) or combine equal parts of the ointment (e.g. Celestone VG) with an antifungal cream (e.g. clotrimazole).

- Generously coat an ear wick in ointment and insert, or
- Remove the plunger from a 3 mL syringe, squirt 1.5 mL of ointment into the barrel and replace the plunger. Attach a butterfly needle to the nozzle and cut off the needle, leaving 3 cm of tubing. Slowly and gently insert the tubing deep into the canal, then fill from near the tympanic membrane outwards.

Assist temporary retention with a plug of cotton wool or gauze.

EAR PIERCING

This simple method of ear piercing (for the insertion of 'sleepers') requires only an 18- or 19-gauge sterile needle. Local anaesthesia is optional. A freezing spray can be used.

Method

1. Carefully place marks on the ear lobe (this is better done by the patient or patient's parents).
2. Introduce the needle through the selected site (Fig. 13.5a). One can use a cork or piece of potato on the exit side to avoid stabbing the patient's neck or your hand.
3. Insert the pointed end of the sleeper into the bore of the needle, ensuring that it fits tightly, and withdraw the needle (Fig. 13.5b).

EAR WAX AND SYRINGING

Ear syringing is a simple and common procedure, but it should be performed with caution and by an experienced professional. *Cautionary advice*: Medical negligence claims related to complications of ear syringing are common.[1]

Contraindications

Important contraindications include:
- perforation of the tympanic membrane
- the ear is the sole hearing ear
- the presence of a grommet
- previous ear surgery to the ear.

Syringing should not be performed in the acute stages of otitis media or when perforation of the tympanic membrane cannot be excluded. In these instances, wax should be cleared with a hook or curette under direct vision (Fig. 13.6a).

In otitis externa, syringing may be performed to remove debris from the canal. Meticulous drying after the procedure is mandatory.

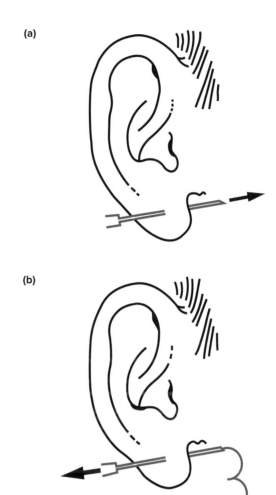

(a)

(b)

Fig. 13.5 Ear piercing method

Wax softeners

The average wax production is 2.8 mg/week. Most ear wax clears spontaneously without treatment. Proprietary preparations may be used as an alternative to syringing or to assist removal. These include hydrogen peroxide, carbamide peroxide (Ear Clear) and docusate sodium (Waxsol), but these should not be used if perforation is suspected. Sodium bicarbonate (available on prescription) or olive oil drops may also be used. Culinary vegetable oil can be used by the patient prior to visiting the office, preferably warming the dropper container slightly under a hot tap.

A study by Kamien led to the conclusion 'that the most effective, cheapest and least messy cerumenolytic is a 15% solution of sodium bicarbonate'.[2] It can be readily made by dissolving ¼ teaspoon of sodium bicarbonate in 10 mL of water. Apply it with a dropper.

Another simple method is to fill the ear with liquid soap. Ask the patient to 'pump' their tragus for a couple of minutes then attempt syringing.

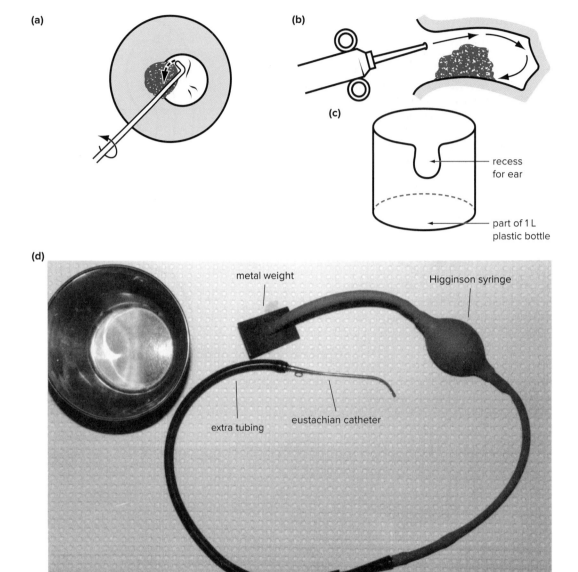

Fig. 13.6 Removal of wax: **(a)** a hook is rotated behind the wax to remove it; **(b)** syringing technique, in which water is directed around (not at) wax; **(c)** ear 'cup' to collect water; **(d)** the Higginson syringe with special attachments

For the procedure, the patient should be seated in a comfortable chair with a towel over the shoulder on the same side as the ear to be syringed. The patient holds the kidney dish just under the ear.

Ear syringing

Method 1

The syringe should have a properly fitting nozzle and an airtight plunger. Friction in a metal syringe can be reduced by coating the inner plunger with petroleum jelly; it can also be primed with liquid soap. Water at body temperature (37°C), as judged by your finger, is a satisfactory solution (vertigo, nausea and vomiting may be precipitated by excessively hot or cold fluid coming in contact with the tympanic membrane).

Rest the nozzle of the syringe just inside the auditory meatus and angle the syringe slightly upwards (Fig. 13.6b). Water directed along the roof of the external auditory canal cascades around and behind the plug of wax. Pull the pinna upward and slightly backward to straighten the canal, and assist partial separation of the wax plug. The stream of water is syringed firmly but not too rapidly. Stop syringing immediately if there is any pain.

While a kidney dish is the traditional collecting vessel for the syringed fluid, an empty plastic ice cream 'bucket' is a practical alternative: the pliable sides mould easily into the shape of the neck. Another improvised ear 'cup' can be cut out from a suitably sized 1–1.5 L plastic bottle. A small recess can be made for the ear (Fig. 13.6c).

Method 2

This is a very effective system that provides a constant flow of water, maximum safety and a free hand when syringing the ear.

The apparatus consists of:
- a Higginson syringe (a one-way bulb pump)
- a heavy metal washer (acts as a weight)
- a metal eustachian catheter
- additional tubing.

The washer maintains the rubber syringe in the basin of water during the ear syringing. The metal eustachian catheter provides an accurate jet of water, which is aimed superiorly above the wax in the usual, recommended manner (Fig. 13.6b).

Post-syringing

If the patient complains of deafness due to water retention, instil acetic acid-alcohol drops (Aquaear or Ear Clear). This gives instant hearing. Some doctors routinely use these drops after syringing out the wax.

A 'gentle' ear syringe

A simple ear syringe can be improvised from a 20 mL or 50 mL syringe and a plastic 'butterfly' intravenous cannula.

Method

Firmly attach the 'butterfly' cannula to the syringe and cut off the tubing, leaving it about 3–4 cm long (Fig. 13.7).

Use

This 'ear syringe' is flexible, safe and easy to use, especially for children. The curve at the end of the tubing permits good positioning in the ear canal.

Note: Some doctors testify to the value of adding a small quantity of povidone-iodine solution to the water, especially if otitis externa is present. Others prefer hydrogen peroxide (100 mL bottles of 30 mg/mL are available in supermarkets) for ear toilet, especially with low-grade otitis externa.

Hair spray and hard wax

People who use hair sprays are prone to developing hard wax if the spray finds its way into the ear canal. Advise these people to cover their ears when they use the spray.

Keratosis obturans—a pearly white plug of keratin—can develop.

RECOGNISING THE 'UNSAFE' EAR

Examination of an infected ear should include inspection of the attic region, the small area of drum between the lateral process of the malleus, and the roof of the external auditory canal immediately above it. A perforation here renders the ear 'unsafe' (Fig. 13.8a); other perforations, not involving the drum margin (Fig. 13.8b), are regarded as 'safe'.

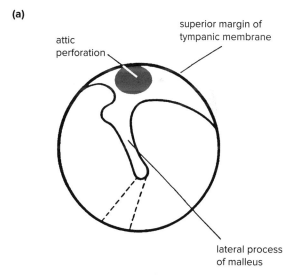

(a)

attic perforation

superior margin of tympanic membrane

lateral process of malleus

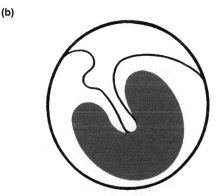

(b)

Fig. 13.8 Infected left ear: **(a)** unsafe perforation; **(b)** safe perforation

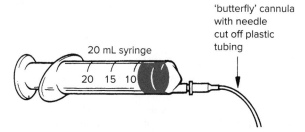

20 mL syringe

20 15 10

'butterfly' cannula with needle cut off plastic tubing

Fig. 13.7 A 'gentle' ear syringe

The status of a perforation depends on the presence of accumulated squamous epithelium (termed cholesteatoma) in the middle ear, because this erodes bone. An attic perforation contains such material; safe perforations do not.

Cholesteatoma is visible through the hole as white flakes, unless it is obscured by discharge or a persistent overlying scab. Either type of perforation can lead to a chronic infective discharge, the nature of which varies with its origin. Mucus admixture is recognised by its stretch and recoil when this discharge is being cleaned from the external auditory canal. The types of discharge are compared in Table 13.1.

Table 13.1 Comparison of types of discharge

	Unsafe	**Safe**
Source	Cholesteatoma	Mucosa
Odour	Foul	Inoffensive
Amount	Usually scant, never profuse	Can be profuse
Nature	Purulent	Mucopurulent

Management

If an attic perforation is recognised or suspected, specialist referral is essential. Cholesteatoma cannot be eradicated by medical means: surgical removal is necessary to prevent a serious intratemporal or intracranial complication.

AIR PRESSURE PAIN WHEN FLYING

Ear pain during descent can be helped by instilling a nasal decongestant such as oxymetazoline (Drixine) 1 hour beforehand, and also by chewing gum during descent.

EXCISION OF EAR LOBE CYSTS

Small ear lobe cysts can be removed by simple excision with the aid of ring forceps (meibomian clamps). Such forceps are especially useful when they can be applied over accessible areas, such as eyelids, lips, webbing, scrotum and ear lobes. They enable a firm hold over a small cyst and help to control haemostasis.

Method

1. For a small ear lobe cyst apply the forceps over the ear, and clamp so that the surface chosen for excision occupies the open ring.

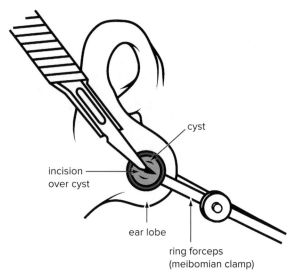

Fig. 13.9 Excision of ear lobe cysts

2. Make an incision over the cyst with a small scalpel blade and dissect the cyst gently away from adherent tissue (Fig. 13.9).
3. Once it is relatively free, it may be possible to squeeze out the entire cyst by digital pressure on either side.

INFECTED EAR LOBE

The cause is most likely a contact allergy to nickel in the jewellery, complicated by a *Staphylococcus* infection.

Management method

1. Discard the earrings.
2. Clean the site to eliminate residual traces of nickel.
3. Swab the site, then commence antibiotics (broad-spectrum antistaphylococcus).
4. Get the patient to clean the site daily, then apply the appropriate ointment.
5. Use a 'noble metal' stud to keep the tract patent.
6. Advise the use of only gold, silver or platinum studs in future. *Note:* Cheaper silver-plated studs may eventually wear down to expose underlying nickel.

EMBEDDED EARRING STUD

The embedded earring stud can be difficult to remove, but a simple technique using curved mosquito artery forceps can disimpact the stud easily. The typical stud consists of a post that slots into a butterfly clip.

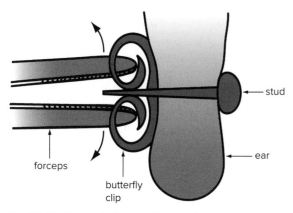

Fig. 13.10 Removal of embedded earring stud

The nose

TREATMENTS FOR EPISTAXIS

Remember to use protective eyewear if there is significant bleeding.

Simple tamponade

In most instances, haemostasis can be obtained by pinching the 'soft' part of the nose between a finger and thumb for 5 minutes and applying ice packs to the bridge of the nose (Fig. 13.11).

Other simple office methods

- Remove any clots—blow nose and then apply 5-6 sprays of a decongestant nasal spray (e.g. Drixine).
- A cotton wool ball soaked in lignocaine with adrenaline or a decongestant is also a useful method.

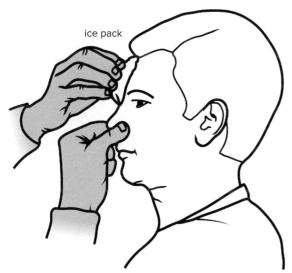

Fig. 13.11 Simple tamponade method for epistaxis

Method

1. Insert the tips of the mosquito artery forceps into the two openings of the butterfly clip.
2. Open the forceps, thus gently springing apart the butterfly clip (Fig. 13.10). This manoeuvre removes the pressure on the post, and the stud can then be separated.

PROBLEMS WITH COTTON BUDS

Avoid cotton buds to instil ointment and other material in the ear. Advise against the use of cotton buds to clean the ear. They tend to impact wax and other debris.

Matchstick tamponade

Several practitioners claim excellent results using a matchstick (¾ of its length) jammed up in a horizontal position under the upper lip to the roof of the gum reflection on the teeth. Leave it in place for several minutes. It compresses the superior labial arteries that also supply the nasal septum.

Note: Dental packing (hard cotton wool roll) is ideal and preferable to a matchstick.

Simple cautery of Little's area

Local anaesthetic

CoPhenylcaine Forte Spray—leave 5 minutes;
or
an equal mixture of 10% cocaine HCl and adrenaline 1:1000 (0.5 mL of each) soaked in a small piece of cotton wool about the size of a 5 cent piece. This pledget is gently compressed against the area and left for 2 minutes.

Cautery methods

The three common methods of cautery are:
- electrocautery
- trichloroacetic acid (pure)
- silver nitrate stick (preferred).

Fashion cotton wool onto the end of the silver nitrate stick to dry the treated site. Put the silver nitrate directly onto the small vessels. Beware of silver nitrate stains. Apply petroleum jelly twice daily to the cauterised area.

Use of a dental broach for treatment of epistaxis

A dental broach can be modified to pick up a small but adequate amount of trichloroacetic acid (TCA) for nasal cautery.

Method

1. A small loop can be made in the broach by bending the wire around the tip of fine forceps.
2. The loop is placed in the TCA so that a small amount fits neatly in the loop.
3. The loop is then applied to the appropriate site on Little's area in the nasal septum (Fig. 13.12). The small amount of acid is delivered accurately and cauterises a specific area, without spillage to the healthy adjacent tissue.

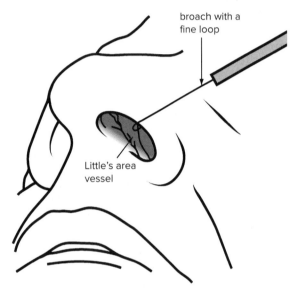

Fig. 13.12 Shows loop of broach applied to the site of bleeding

Intermittent minor nose bleeds

If not actively bleeding:
- avoid nose blowing
- avoid digital trauma
- apply petroleum jelly (e.g. Vaseline) or an antibiotic ointment twice daily for 2 to 3 weeks.

Recurrent anterior epistaxis

For patients with recurrent epistaxis from Little's area, especially in the presence of localised rhinitis, several topical options are available:
- Nasalate cream tds for 7 to 10 days, or
- Aureomycin or Bactroban ointment bd or tds for 10 days, or
- Rectinol ointment.

Rectal ointment containing local anaesthetic and a vasoconstrictor, e.g. Rectinol, is a very useful topical agent.

Persistent anterior bleed

Use a Merocel (surgical sponge) nasal tampon or a Kaltostat pack or a vaginal tampon.

Severe posterior epistaxis

Occasionally, severe posterior nasal bleeding cannot be controlled by an anterior pack. Insertion of a nasopharyngeal pack via the oropharynx is technically difficult and distressing for the patient. A simple and effective method of applying postnasal pressure uses a Foley catheter.

The traditional ribbon nasal pack with bismuth iodoform paraffin paste (BIPP) can still be used, or glycerine can be used instead of BIPP.

Method

1. Anaesthetise the nasal passage.
2. Select a small Foley catheter (no. 10, 12, 14 or 16) with a 30 mL balloon and self-sealing rubber stopper.
3. Lubricate the deflated catheter and pass it directly into the nasal passage along the floor of the nose until resistance is felt in the nasopharynx (the tip might be visible behind the soft palate).
4. Using a 20 mL syringe, partially inflate the balloon with 5–8 mL of saline or, preferably, air.
5. Gradually withdraw the catheter until resistance is felt; inject another 5 mL of saline or air.
6. Draw the catheter taut so that the balloon fits snugly in the nasopharynx against the choana (Fig. 13.13).
7. Pack the anterior chamber with ribbon gauze in the usual manner.

Note: The patient should be admitted to hospital. Administration of oxygen might be necessary for the elderly patient whose respiration is compromised.

The Epistat catheter: A special catheter called the Epistat has been developed specifically for this method. It is ideal but relatively costly. It has two inflatable balloons, one to act as a stay posteriorly and a wider 'anterior' balloon. There is a central airway in the device. This catheter can be autoclaved for further use.

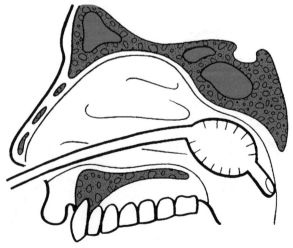

Fig. 13.13 Semi-inflated Foley catheter in nasopharynx and posterior nasal cavity

Rapid Rhino nasal packing for anterior and posterior epistaxis

This practical kit is a balloon covered in a self-lubricating hydrocolloid fabric. The sequence of steps are:
1. Soak the fabric in sterile water for at least 30 seconds.
2. Insert it horizontally into the nostril along the nasal floor until the blue indicator is past the nares.
3. Use a 20 mL syringe to inflate the balloon with air until it feels firmly wedged then tape the tag to the patient's cheek for about 24–72 hours.

INSTILLING NOSE DROPS

To achieve the best results from nasal drops instil as follows:
- to insert into the left side, tilt head slightly to the left
- for the right side, incline the head to the right.

OFFENSIVE SMELL FROM THE NOSE

Ensure no foreign body present.

Treatment

- Mupirocin 2% nasal ointment (Bactroban) instil 2 to 3 times a day (with 5th fingertip or cotton bud) or
- Kenacomb ointment instil 2 to 3 times a day

STUFFY, RUNNING NOSE

Treatment

- Blow nose hard into disposable paper tissue or handkerchief until clear.
- Nasal decongestant for 2 to 3 days only.
- Steam inhalations with Friar's Balsam or menthol.
- Oral antihistamines (e.g. Phenergan 25 mg nocte) do have an effect, but 'too small to be relevant', according to a Cochrane review.[3]

NASAL IRRIGATION

This is used to flush out excess mucus and other 'debris' with hypertonic sterile saline. A suitable solution can be prepared with two cups of warm water (distilled water or previously boiled water) with ¼ to ½ teaspoon of non-iodised salt and a pinch of baking soda.

Method

Lean to one side over a basin and forwards about 30°–40°. Introduce the wash on one side of the nose with a squeeze bottle, large plastic syringe or bulb spray with the tip just inside the nose. Some of the fluid drains out through the other nostril. Gently blow the nose. Perform about 3 times a week.

Follow-up: corticosteroid nebuliser or nasal inhaler twice daily.
Note: Tissue spears classically used for ear toileting can also be gently introduced along the nasal airways to mop up purulent discharge.

SENILE RHINORRHOEA

This is a common, distressing problem in the elderly, caused by failure of the vasomotor control of the mucosa. It may be associated with a deviated septum and dryness of the mucosa. The treatment is to keep the nasal passages lubricated with an oil-based preparation e.g. insufflation with an oily mixture (a commercial preparation is Nozoil, which is sesame oil based). Topical decongestants can cause serious side effects in the elderly.

Conditions suitable for Nozoil (sesame oil preparation)

This can be used when temporary relief of dry and crusting nasal tissue is required. This can be caused by:
- dry air
- CPAP and oxygen
- drugs such as isotretinoin
- age-related dryness ± rhinorrhoea
- post-surgery including cautery for epistaxis
- nasal steroid use
- nasal crusting from colds and influenza.

NASAL FACTURES

Fractures of the nose can occur in isolation or combined with fractures of the maxilla or zygomatic arch. They may result in nasal bridge bruising, swelling, non-alignment and epistaxis. Always check for a compound fracture or head injury and, if present, leave alone and refer. If the patient is seen immediately (such as on a sports field) with a straightforward lateral displacement, reduction may be attempted 'on the spot' with digital manipulation before distortion from soft tissue swelling. This involves simply using the fingers to push laterally on the outside of the nose towards the injured side to realign the nose.

Tips

- X-rays are generally unhelpful unless excluding other facial skeletal injuries.
- If a deformity is present, refer the patient to be seen within 7 days, ideally days 3 to 5.
- Skin lacerations (i.e. a compound fracture) usually require early repair.
- The optimal time to reduce a fractured nose is about 10 days after injury. There is a window period of 2 to 3 weeks before the fracture unites.

- Closed reduction under local or general anaesthetic is the preferred treatment.
- Open reduction is more suitable for bilateral fractures with significant septal deviation, bilateral fractures with major dislocations or fractures of the cartilaginous pyramid.

Refer

- Uncontrolled epistaxis
- Recurrent epistaxis
- Concern about cosmetic alignment

Miscellaneous ENT pearls

HANDS-FREE HEADLIGHT

Ideal hands-free lights to examine the ears, nose and throat include the Vorotek headlight kit or the Welch Allyn portable binocular microscope, the LumiView—a headband flat surface magnifier.

A considerably less expensive alternative is an LED caving headlamp. See Chapter 18.

SELF-PROPELLED ANTRAL AND NASAL WASHOUT

This method works well for patients with persistent catarrh and sinus problems.

Equipment

The patient will need:
- a drinking straw
- a tea cup
- warm water with 1 teaspoon of salt and 1 teaspoon of sodium bicarbonate.

Method

1. Place the straw in the water and the other end in the nostril.
2. Holding the other nostril closed with a finger, inhale the fluid rapidly into the nostril and then expectorate.

USE OF FLO SINUS CARE

This preparation is a sinus douche of physiological 'extracellular fluid' (salt–sugar). It can be delivered as a nasal metered pump, which limits the distribution to the nose only, or as a 200 mL douche bottle to thoroughly wash nasal and sinus cavities.

HICCOUGHS (HICCUPS)

Hiccoughs (singultus) are due to involuntary repetitive diaphragmatic spasms, which if prolonged can have serious consequences especially in infants.

For simple brief episodes, try any of the following.
- Rebreathe air in a paper bag (as for hyperventilation).
- Hold the breath.
- Suck ice/swallow iced water.
- Plug both ears and drink a glass of cold water without pause.

- Swallow a teaspoon of granulated table sugar. An old study quotes a 19/20 success rate, postulating an irritation of the vagus nerve fibres via the pharynx.[4]
- Swallow a teaspoon of malt vinegar.
- More pleasurably, swallow 20 mL of spirits (37% or more alcohol) e.g. whisky, gin, Benedictine or sambuca.
- Apply pressure on the eyeballs.
  When persistent (assuming exclusion of the organic diseases):
- chlorpromazine orally or IV, or
- sodium valproate.
  Consider acupuncture, hypnosis or phrenic nerve block.

Newborn

Tend to occur during feeding, especially with a bottle. Advise the parent to take a break and facilitate burping to expel air.

Toddlers

Lie the child prone and apply natural pressure to the epigastrium. Apply quick downward (gentle) pressure movements and try and coincide it with the hiccoughs (not evidence based).

Nasal catheter for hiccoughs

Persistent hiccoughs can be arrested quickly by irritation of the nose with a soft rubber or plastic nasal catheter. The method is particularly useful for the post-operative patient.

A catheter is introduced into one of the nasal passages and withdrawn as soon as the patient shows irritation.

Worth a try?

Ask the patient what they ate for breakfast 2 days ago. The thoughtful pause that 'freezes' the diaphragm may work!

SNORING

Important strategies to prevent snoring include:
- avoid sleeping on the back: try wearing a tennis ball in a sock pinned to back of clothing, or in the pocket of a pyjama top worn back-to-front
- weight reduction to ideal weight
- no alcohol in the evening.

Otherwise refer to a medical consultant in sleep disorders. Continuous positive airway pressure (CPAP) delivered through a special face mask may be prescribed if apnoea is present.

Nasal device

If the snoring originates from the anterior nose, a device suitable to prevent 'collapsing' of the front of the nose is Nozovent, which is a simple medical-grade plastic device that fits into the nostrils. The device, invented by a Swedish ENT surgeon, increases the diameter of the nostrils and prevents them from collapsing on inhalation. An Australian version is the Breathing Wonder, which is inexpensive and widely available.

TINNITUS

Precautions

- Exclude drugs (including marijuana), vascular disease, depression, aneurysm and vascular tumours.
- Be mindful of lonely elderly people living alone (suicide risk).

Management

- Educate and reassure the patient.
- Encourage the patient to use relaxation techniques.
- Encourage background 'noise', e.g. music playing during night.
- Tinnitus maskers.
- Hearing aids.

Drug trials to consider (limited efficacy)

- Betahistine (Serc) 8–16 mg daily (max 32 mg)
- Carbamazepine (Tegretol)
- Antidepressants
- Sodium valproate (Epilim, Valpro, Valprease)

Acute severe tinnitus

Slow IV injection of 1% lidocaine (as for migraine—see p. 239). Up to about 5 mL is very effective.

SWALLOWING WITH A SORE THROAT

Rather than painful sipping of fluids, advise the patient to fill the mouth with as much fluid as possible and then swallow.

Beware of the sneeze

A BMJ case report warns against holding the nose and closing the mouth when sneezing. Cases have been reported of a ruptured/perforated posterior pharynx, neck injury, perforated tympanic membrane, pneumomediastinum and ruptured cerebral aneurysm.[5] Children (and adults) should be encouraged to sneeze into their sleeve rather than their hands, if no tissue is available, to reduce the spread of fomites.

EUSTACHIAN TUBE DYSFUNCTION AND GLUE EAR

This common condition, particularly in children, causes discomfort in the affected ear or ears. Symptoms include muffled or dull hearing, ear 'fullness', buzzing, ringing or 'popping' noises. One consequence, particularly in younger children, is glue ear.

Treatment strategy

Physical

If the problem is mild, as often follows an URTI, no treatment apart from clearing the snuffly nose is required. All cases can be helped by inhalations of steam with menthol (or similar) added to the water.

Auto-sufflation (auto-inflation) can be used with good effect. This involves Valsalva manoeuvres in which you breathe out slowly with your mouth closed several times and then, while pinching your nose, blow out hard against the back of your hand. This may unblock mucus in the tube.[6]

Proprietary devices

These include the balloon-based device Otovent and an air-pump device such as Ear Popper.

Otovent consists of a balloon attached to a nosepiece. The child with a glue ear holds the nosepiece to the nostril and inflates the balloon to the size of a grapefruit while keeping the other nostril compressed with a finger and the mouth firmly closed. It acts as a Valsalva manoeuvre to open up the Eustachian tube. The balloon is then allowed to deflate while the child swallows. It is performed 2 to 3 times a day for 2 to 3 weeks.[7]

Decongestants: These agents such as pseudoephedrine and phenylephrine taken by mouth or as a spray or drops (5 to 7 days) can be effective.

Antihistamines: These taken orally or used as a nasal spray are effective for allergic causes such as hay fever.

Corticosteroids: Nasal steroids are commonly used particularly if there is an allergic basis to the problem. Steroids taken orally for short periods, especially if the symptoms are severe with considerable congestion and swelling, can be effective.

AURISCOPE AS AN ALTERNATIVE TO NASAL SPECULA

An auriscope with the widest possible attachment will allow an excellent view of the nasal cavity. The patient should mouth breathe during the inspection. If the auriscope has an opening for a pneumatic bulb, occlude the opening with your finger to prevent lens condensation.

CHRONIC ANOSMIA FOLLOWING URTI

For patients complaining of loss of the sense of smell following an upper respiratory infection, prescribe a nasal decongestant such as Spray-Tish Menthol for 5 to 7 days (maximum).

TICKLISH THROAT

For an irritated persistent ticklish throat, instruct the patient to make a trilling musical sound like an opera singer for 2 to 3 minutes.

DOCTOR-ASSISTED TREATMENT FOR BENIGN PAROXYSMAL POSITIONAL VERTIGO

Theory[8]

This condition is considered to be caused by displacement of floating crystalline calcium carbonate deposits (otoconia) in the posterior semicircular canal. This creates the illusion of motion. The Brandt–Daroff exercises can be performed by the patient at home. The particle repositioning manoeuvres of Semont and Epley can be performed as office procedures by the therapist.

The Epley manoeuvre[9]

This exercise should be tried first. The basic manoeuvres are (Fig. 13.14):
- move the patient's head into four different positions
- hold the head in each postural position for 1 minute
- after doing this sit still for 10 minutes to allow the crystals to settle.

Method (right-sided ear problem shown)

1. The patient sits on the bed with the head slightly extended and turned 45° in the direction that precipitated the vertigo (Fig. 13.14a).

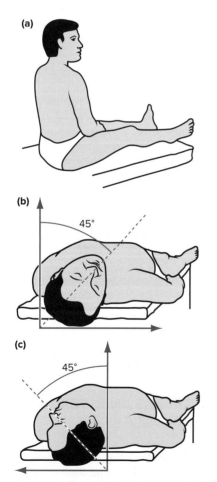

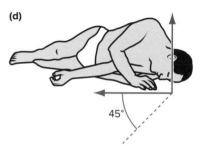

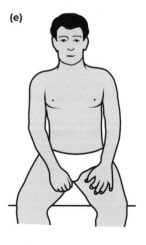

Fig. 13.14 **(a)** to **(e)** The Epley manoeuvre for treatment of right-sided disease (reverse head position for left-sided disease)
Reproduced from *Therapeutic Guidelines: Neurology,* 2011, with permission.[10]

2. Lie the patient on their back with the head hanging over a pillow placed at the shoulder level (this is the basic Hallpike test). Wait 1 minute (Fig. 13.14b).
3. Once the provoked vertigo and nystagmus settles, from this position turn the head through 90° to the opposite side and wait 1 minute (Fig. 13.14c).
4. Turn the head through a further 90° and roll onto that side so that the ear is parallel to the floor. Wait another minute (Fig. 13.14d).
5. Slowly sit the patient upright and still for 10 minutes (Fig. 13.14e).

Follow-up: Get the patient to sleep in a semi-upright position. Repeat until the attacks abate.

The Semont manoeuvre (Fig. 13.15)

1. Sit the patient upright in the middle and on the edge of the bed or couch. Turn the head 45° to the side opposite to that which precipitated the vertigo (the unaffected ear).
2. While maintaining the head position, tip the patient to the affected side so that they are lying on the affected side (with nose up) and wait 1 minute.
3. Move the patient quickly 180° through the upright position (maintaining the original head position) and lower to the other side (nose now pointing down). Wait 1 minute.
4. Slowly return the patient to the upright position and then rotate the head to the normal position. Sit still in this position for 10 minutes.

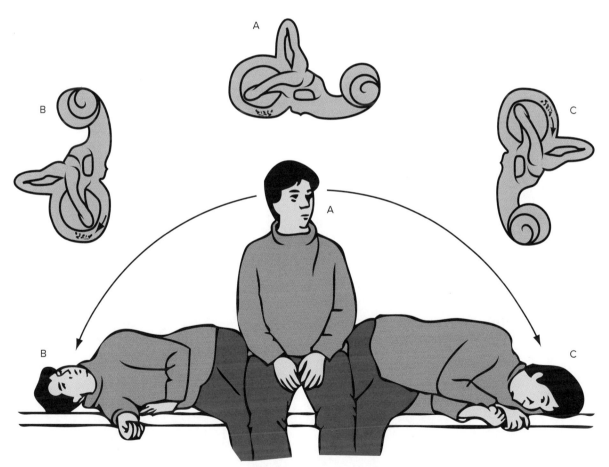

Fig. 13.15 (A) to (C) The Semont manoeuvre. For right-sided problems, the labelled boxes show the orientation of the vestibular labyrinth in each head position with the corresponding positions of the free-floating deposits that eventually fall into the utricular cavity on completion of a successful particle repositioning manoeuvre

Reproduced from *Therapeutic Guidelines: Neurology,* 2003, with permission.[11]

References

1. Watson A. Are you playing Russian roulette with your patients? In: Murtagh J. *Cautionary tales* (2nd edn). Sydney: McGraw-Hill Australia, 2011: 111–13.

2. Kamien M. *Which cerumanolytic?* Aust Fam Physician, 1999; 28: 817.

3. De Sutter AIM, Saraswat A, van Driel ML. *Antihistamines for the common cold.* Cochrane Database Syst Rev, 2015, 11, Art no: CD009345.

4. Engleman EG, Lankton J, Lankton B. *Granulated sugar as treatment for hiccups in conscious patients.* N Eng J Med, 1971, 285: 1489.

5. Yang W, Sahota RS, Das S. *Snap, crackle, and pop: when sneezing leads to crackling in the neck: Case report.* BMJ, 2018; doi:10.1136/bcr-2016-218906

6. Perera R, Glasziou PP, Heneghan CJ, McLellan J, Williamson I. *Autoinflation for hearing loss associated with otitis media with effusion (glue ear).* Cochrane Database Syst Rev, 2013; Issue 5: Art no: CD006285.

7. Willamson I, Vennik J, Harnden A et al. *Effect of nasal balloon autoinflation in children with otitis media with effusion in primary care: an open randomized controlled trial.* CMAJ, 2015; DOI: 10.1503/cmaj.141608.

8. Neurology Expert Group. Therapeutic Guidelines: Neurology. Melbourne: Therapeutic Guidelines Ltd, 2011.

9. Hilton MP, Pinder DK. The Epley (canalith repositioning) manoeuvre for benign paroxysmal positional vertigo. Cochrane Database Syst Rev, 2014; Issue 12: Art no: CD003162.

10. Neurology Expert Group. Therapeutic Guidelines: Neurology. Melbourne: Therapeutic Guidelines Ltd, 2011.

11. Neurology Expert Group. Therapeutic Guidelines: Neurology. Melbourne: Therapeutic Guidelines Ltd, 2003.

Chapter 14
THE EYES

BASIC KIT FOR EYE EXAMINATION

As recommended by the Royal Victorian Eye and Ear Hospital, an eye kit should include equipment for removal of corneal foreign bodies, and eye-testing charts at 18 inches (46 cm) and 10 feet (305 cm):

- multiple pin holes
- fluorescein sterile paper strips, e.g. Flourets
- torch
- eyelid speculum
- magnification (necessary to examine cornea)
- sterile isotonic saline solution to irrigate eyes
- local anaesthetic (oxybuprocaine 0.4% e.g. Minims unidose)
- sterile cotton buds
- glass rod to double-evert eyelids in chemical burns
- non-allergenic tape (e.g. Micropore).

Eye tip: The eye holds only one drop of liquid, which usually remains in the eye for only a few seconds. The action can be prolonged by pinching on either side of the nose to occlude the lacrimal duct for 60 seconds.

EVERSION OF THE EYELID

Paperclip method

No eye examination is complete without eversion of the upper eyelid to exclude hidden pathology, particularly a foreign body.

The method generally taught is to evert the lid over a matchstick, but this can be difficult. The use of a paperclip can simplify this examination.

1. By bending the long arm of the paperclip to make a right angle, you can create an instrument with a fine diameter, which is easy to withdraw and has a handle that keeps fingers out of the field of inspection (Fig. 14.1).
2. Care must be taken not to slide the end of the clip over the lid but to place it gently and precisely along the appropriate line (about 15 mm from the edge of the lid and parallel to it).
3. You must also make sure not to slide the end of the clip across the lid and scratch it on removal.

Care must also be taken with uncooperative children.

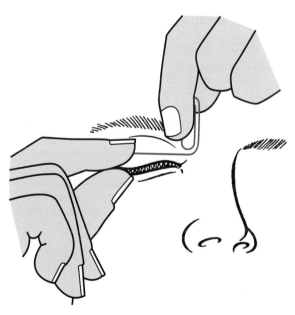

Fig. 14.1 Paperclip method for eyelid eversion

Cotton bud method

The use of a cotton bud is recommended for eyelid eversion. Its effectiveness depends on correct placement.
1. Ask the patient to put the chin up and to look down.
2. Gently grasp the eyelashes of the upper lid between the index finger and thumb of the non-dominant hand and pull gently downwards.
3. Apply the cotton bud 15 mm above the upper eyelid margin.
4. With gentle pressure, push the bud back while lifting the lashes upward.
5. Eversion of the lid can be maintained even after removal of the cotton bud.

BLEPHARITIS

Blepharitis is inflammation of the lid margins and is commonly associated with secondary ocular effects such as styes, chalazia and conjunctival or corneal ulceration. There are two main causes or types:
- anterior blepharitis—staphylococcal
- posterior blepharitis—seborrhoeic and rosacea: associated with facial seborrhoea.

Precautions

Corneal ulceration, recurrent staphylococcal infections.

Management

- Eyelid hygiene is the mainstay of therapy. The crusts and other debris should be gently cleaned with a cotton wool bud dipped in clean, warm water or a 1:10 dilution of baby shampoo or a solution of sodium bicarbonate, once or twice daily.

  An alternative is to apply a warm water or saline soak with gauze for 20 minutes followed by a rest for 60 minutes. Proprietary lid solutions or wipes can also be used.
- If not controlled, treat infection with an antibiotic ointment smeared on the lid margin (e.g. tetracycline 1% or chloromycetin 1% ointment to lid margins once or twice daily). This may be necessary for four weeks, then review.
- For chronic blepharitis, short-term use of a corticosteroid ointment, e.g. hydrocortisone 0.5%, can be very effective.
- Ocular lubricants such as artificial tear preparations may greatly relieve symptoms of keratoconjunctivitis sicca (dry eyes), e.g. hypromellose 1%.
- Control scalp seborrhoea with regular medicated shampoos, e.g. ketoconazole.
- Systemic antibiotics may be required for lid abscess.
- Discontinue wearing contact lenses until the problem has cleared.

FLASH BURNS

A common problem usually presenting at night is bilateral painful eyes from keratitis caused by ultraviolet 'flash burns' to both corneas some 5 to 10 hours previously.

Sources of UV light such as sunlamps and snow reflection can also cause a reaction.

Management

- Local anaesthetic (long-acting) drops, e.g. amethocaine 1% eye drops: once only application (do not allow the patient to take home more drops).
- Instil homatropine 2% drops statim.
- Analgesics, e.g. paracetamol, for 24 hours.
- Broad spectrum antibiotic eye ointment in lower fornix (to prevent infection).
- Firm eye padding for 24 hours, when eyes reviewed (avoid light).
- A cold compress applied to the lid can be soothing.

  The eye usually heals completely in 48 hours. If not, check for a foreign body. Use fluorescein if in doubt.

  Note: Contact lens 'overwear syndrome' gives similar symptoms.

WOOD'S LIGHT AND FLUORESCEIN

After fluorescein is instilled into the eye, look for a dendritic ulcer with a Wood's light. Cheap ultraviolet LED lights can replace traditional fluorescent tubes.

SIMPLE TOPICAL ANTISEPTICS FOR MILD CONJUNCTIVITIS

- Saline: prepare a saline solution by dissolving a dessertspoon of salt in 500 mL of boiled water, then bathe the eye regularly (1 to 2 hourly) with cotton wool or gauze.
- Dilute povidone-iodine solution: dilute Betadine solution 1 in 10 parts water and use this to clean the eye.

REMOVING 'GLITTER' FROM THE EYE

Make-up glitter can adhere to the conjunctiva and cornea. Its removal can be aided by ointment such as chloromycetin or hydrocortisone, which binds it and 'flushes' it to the inner canthus where it can be removed by wiping with a tissue or gauze.

DRY EYES

Dry eyes can cause burning or stinging, itching, a gritty sensation, redness and a feeling of 'something in the eye'.

Simple test

Hold the eyelids wide apart for about 20 seconds—it will reproduce symptoms such as burning, stinging or dryness.

Treatment

For uncomplicated dry eyes it is usual to use artificial tear preparations, which relieve the symptoms. In some people these may be needed for life.

There are three main types of artificial tears:
- Lubricating drops: these are instilled during the day, usually 1 to 2 drops about 4 times a day or as often as required.
  Examples: Liquifilm, Teardrops, Murine Tears, Isopto Tears, Tears Naturale, Methopt.
- Lubricating gels or ointments: these are instilled at bed time.
  Examples: Poly Visc, Duratears, Lacri-Lube.
- Stimulant drops: these are given in the same ways as lubricating drops and are very effective.
  Examples: TheraTears, Cellufresh.

Remember that bathing the eyes with clean water will help relieve dry eyes. Room humidifiers also help in rooms where there is dry heating.

EYELASH DISORDERS

Irritation of the eye by lashes rubbing on it is usually caused by either entropion or ingrowing lashes.

Entropion

With entropion, the eyelashes of the lower lid are pushed to the side by the regular inturning. The condition can be demonstrated by asking the patient to close the eyes tightly and then open the eyes. The danger is ulcerative scarring of the cornea by the eyelashes, so it should be examined by staining with fluorescein.

Entropion in the frail elderly can be corrected by the use of a strip of hypoallergenic, non-woven surgical tape (1 cm × 3 cm). Attach one end to the lower lid just below the lashes, with tension sufficient to hold the lid everted, and the remainder to the face (Fig. 14.2). It should be changed as often as necessary and may be done by a relative, the doctor or a district nurse.

Ingrowing eyelashes (trichiasis)

In this condition the lid is in a normal position but the eyelashes may grow inward. Magnification may be necessary.

For only a few ingrowing lashes, epilation is the best method. Use fine-artery forceps, jeweller's forceps or, better still, eyebrow tweezers (available from chemists) to pluck out the offending eyelashes. The lashes tend to regrow, and regular epilation may be necessary.

If there are many ingrowing eyelashes, the best options are electrolysis of the hair roots or cryotherapy.

REMOVAL OF CORNEAL FOREIGN BODY

Use adequate magnification with a magnifying loupe, ideally one with an inbuilt light source. Use local anaesthetic (e.g. oxybuprocaine 0.4%). Test visual acuity. Examination—inspect conjunctivae, cornea, upper and

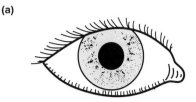

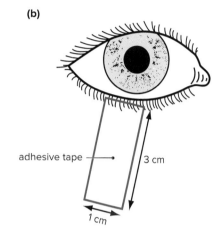

adhesive tape — 3 cm — 1 cm

Fig. 14.2 Treatment of entropion: **(a)** before; **(b)** after

lower lids (evert), pupils and cornea. Fluorescein detects an epithelial defect. Slit light examination is optional. If there is a concern about an ocular foreign body, a plain X-ray or CT scan can be revealing.

Recent and superficial

Attempt removal of the foreign body (FB) by using a sterile cotton bud, lightly moistened with a drop of local anaesthetic or saline to gently lift it off.

Embedded

Use a sterile, disposable needle (25- or 23-gauge) with a small syringe or a tightly wedged cotton bud attached to steady the needle. It is best to bend the end of the needle (bevel) so that it forms a scoop.

Hold the unit with a pen grip and keep the needle tangential away from the eye with bevel upwards. Introduce the needle horizontally so that the tip lifts the edge of the FB (Fig. 14.3a). Finally, irrigate the ocular surface and upper and lower fornices with sterile saline to flush out residual tissue.

The rust ring

The needle can lift loosely bound rust.

A sterile dental burr can be used but best avoided. The burr, which is applied vertically, should be rotated gently once and then the cornea inspected after each

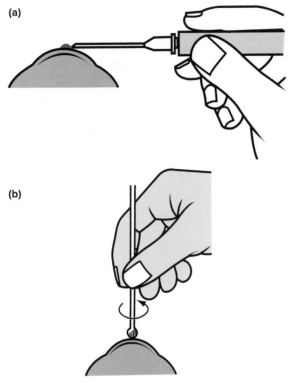

Fig. 14.3 Removal of foreign body: **(a)** disposable needle steadied with syringe using a horizontal approach; **(b)** dental burr rotated once, using a direct vertical approach

rotation (Fig. 14.3b). This should not be attempted on deep rust or central FBs.

An 'automatic' safety burr can be used. The flat part of a no. 15 scalpel blade can be useful to remove the ring.

Assessing the depth of injury—Seidal test

This test can evaluate suspected global rupture but a slit lamp with a cobalt blue filter is ideal. Apply 2% fluorescein eye drops and observe to see if the dye is diluted by leaking aqueous fluid. The ruptured area stains weakly while bright green concentrated dye surrounds the leak site—urgent referral is required.

Follow-up

Instil antibiotic drops and pad the eye for 30 minutes only. Review at 24 hours. Inspect and stain the cornea with fluorescein. Continue to instil antibiotic drops 3 times a day for 3 days. (Drops are preferable to ointment.)

Precautions

- Do not give LA for pain relief.
- Refer deep rust stains to experts.
- Never forcibly rub the cornea.
- Do not use corticosteroids on the eye initially.

- Get patients to wait until LA wears off (about 20 minutes). They should drive home without an eye pad.

CORNEAL ABRASION AND ULCERATION

The many causes of abrasions include trauma from a foreign body, fingernails including false nails, contact lenses, UV burns and insects.

The abrasion may be associated with an ulcer, which is a defect in the epithelial cell layer of the cornea.

Symptoms

- Ocular pain
- Watering of the eye
- Foreign body sensation
- Blurred vision

Think corneal abrasion if the eye is 'watering' and painful.

Diagnosis

This is best performed with a slit lamp using a cobalt blue filter and fluorescein staining. Place a drop of LA on the end of a fluorescein strip (or two drops into the conjunctival sac). If a slit lamp is unavailable, the direct ophthalmoscope can be used to provide illumination as well as blue light for corneal examination, although this blue is considerably less effective than UV at making the dye fluoresce. Magnifying loupes can then be used for viewing the illuminated cornea. You usually see an epithelial flap of tissue on the cornea.

Management

- Stain with fluorescein and look for a foreign body.
- Treat with chloramphenicol 1% ointment ± homatropine 2% (if pain due to ciliary spasm).
- Consider double eye pad for 24 hours (max.).
- Give analgesics.
- Consider an ice pack on the eyelid (best avoided).
- Review in 24 hours.
- Consider specialist referral.

The recurrent erosive syndrome

Be aware of this syndrome especially with fingernail injuries. Pain is triggered upon opening the eye first thing in the morning because the lid pulls off epithelium. Treatment is Lacri-Lube applied at night.

EYE EXAMINATION IN INFANTS

If closed eyes preclude an examination in newborns, ask the parent to hold the infant vertically and then tilt them backwards down to horizontal. The eyes usually open in response.

Consider the diagnosis of corneal abrasion in newborn babies with sudden inconsolable crying. A linear fingernail scratch will be visible with fluorescein under UV light.

EXCISION OF MEIBOMIAN CYST

The meibomian cyst (tarsal cyst, chalazion) is simple to treat by incision of the cyst and curettage of its wall.

Equipment

You will need:
- a small syringe and needle
- a chalazion clamp
- a chalazion curette
- a scalpel handle and no. 11 blade.
  Note: Disposable kits are available.

Method

1. Instil LA drops (e.g. Minims oxybuprocaine, benoxinate HCl).
2. Inject about 1 mL of 2% lidocaine around the cyst through the skin (see Fig. 14.4a).
3. Apply the chalazion clamp, with the solid plate on the skin side.
4. Tighten the clamp just enough to stop the bleeding.
5. Evert the eyelid to expose the bulging cyst in the ring.
6. Make a vertical incision in the cyst (Fig. 14.4b) to avoid damage to other glands.
7. Vigorously scrape out cyst contents with the curette (Fig. 14.4c).
8. Apply a small quantity of chloramphenicol eye ointment.
9. Remove the clamp and then double-pad the eye, folding one pad over to ensure firm pressure.

Advise the patient to change the eye pad 24 hours later and to clean away the debris with warm water or saline. Apply the ointment daily until the conjunctiva has healed (3 to 5 days).

LOCAL ANAESTHETIC FOR THE EYELID

For minor surgical procedures of the eyelid, such as a meibomian cyst, it is advisable to infiltrate local anaesthetic just under the skin of the eyelid around the lump.

Start from the outer (lateral) aspect of the lid with the needle entry being about 10 mm below the eyelid margin for cysts of the lower lid.

Keep the needle tangential to the globe (Fig. 14.4a) and use about 1.5–2 mL of 1 or 2% lidocaine with adrenaline.

NON-SURGICAL TREATMENT FOR MEIBOMIAN CYSTS

Before proceeding to excision of a meibomian cyst (chalazion), another method is worth attempting.

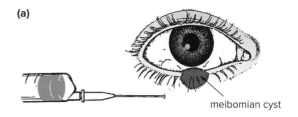

(a)

meibomian cyst

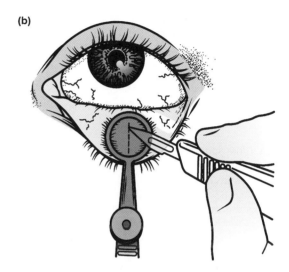

(b)

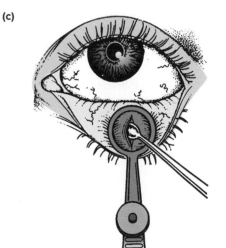

(c)

Fig. 14.4 Removal of meibomian cyst: **(a)** the cyst; **(b)** incising with clamp in place; **(c)** curetting contents

Method

- Twice daily 'hot spoon' the eye. Pad a spoon with cotton wool and a bandage, dip in hot water and gradually bring it up to the eye—similar to steaming the painful eye (Fig. 14.5). An alternative is to use a wooden spoon without padding.

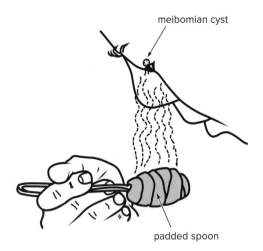

meibomian cyst

padded spoon

Fig. 14.5 Simple treatment for meibomian cyst

- After 'hot spooning' for 5 minutes, instil GoldenEye ointment (or soframycin eye ointment if use of mercury compounds is undesirable).
- Massage the ointment into the chalazion for 5 minutes.
- Using this method twice a day, it usually takes 2 to 4 weeks for the meibomian cysts to resolve.

PADDING THE EYE

The materials used are single packs of sterile gauze eye pads and 25 mm non-allergenic (Micropore) tape. A single, flat eye pad is satisfactory for protection, but for healing, especially for the cornea, more care is required.

Method

1. Two pads are required for healing.
2. Fold the first eye pad so that the folded edge rests just below the eyebrow (Fig. 14.6).

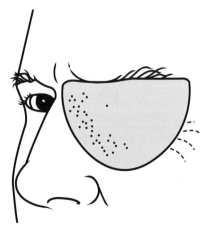

Fig. 14.6 Method of eye padding

3. The pad is then reinforced by a single, flat pad over the top.
4. Secure the pads firmly and apply 25 mm non-allergenic tape carefully to the skin.
   Precaution: Never pad a discharging infected eye.

MANAGING STYES

A stye is an acute abscess of a lash follicle or associated glands, caused usually by *Staphylococcus aureus*.

Treat as for any acute abscess, by drainage when the abscess has pointed.

Method

1. Direct steam from a thermos onto the closed eye (Fig. 14.9), or use a hot compress. This helps the stye to discharge.
2. Perform lash epilation to allow drainage of pus. (Incise with a D11 blade if epilation does not work.)
3. Use chloramphenicol ointment if the infection is spreading locally.

APPLICATION OF DROPS

The following instructions are advisable for patients:
1. Avoid contamination of the tip of the dropper bottle (fingers, eyelashes, etc.).
2. Lie down or sit with head over the back of a lounge chair.
3. Look up, spread the lower eyelid and instil the drops into the lateral conjunctival sac.
4. Close the eyes and press a finger against the lacrimal sac to stop quick drainage.

VISUAL ACUITY

A representation of a Snellen eye chart, comparing the metric and British 'feet' distances, is shown in Figure 14.7.

Choose the appropriate distance and ask the patient to cover one eye and note the eye being tested. Don't use fingers as a cover, to avoid the patient peeking through a crack. If the patient has a pair of distance glasses, ask them to read the lowest possible line left to right. Then test the other eye, reading the lines from right to left. If the acuity is reduced out of either eye, then a pinhole must be used to help compensate for an uncorrected refracture error. Up to two errors on the smaller lines is acceptable, but these should be noted (e.g. 6/12 − 2). Finally assess acuity with both eyes open and glasses on.

THE PINHOLE TEST FOR BLURRED VISION

The pinhole test (Fig. 14.8a) is a useful and under-utilised test in clinical practice.

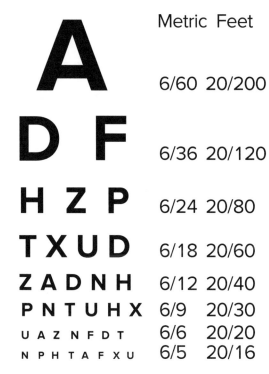

Metric Feet

	Metric	Feet
A	6/60	20/200
D F	6/36	20/120
H Z P	6/24	20/80
T X U D	6/18	20/60
Z A D N H	6/12	20/40
P N T U H X	6/9	20/30
U A Z N F D T	6/6	20/20
N P H T A F X U	6/5	20/16

Fig. 14.7 Snellen eye chart comparing the metric and 'feet' classification

It is important to use the test for any patient presenting with indistinct or blurred vision, whether it is sudden or gradual, painful or painless.

Theory

The pinhole reduces the size of the blur circle on the retina in the uncorrected eye.

A pinhole acts as a universal correcting lens and a 1 mm pinhole will improve acuity in refractive errors. If not, further investigation is mandatory as the defective vision is not due to a refractive error.

Using a multiple pinhole occluder

Multiple pinhole occluders are widely available (Fig. 14.8b). The patient is given the occluder and tests vision in one eye by covering the other eye and then examining an eye chart through any pinhole. The other eye is tested by reversing the procedure for the eyes.

If no pinhole is available, an otoscope cover (small aperture) can substitute.

If the blurred vision is normalised and no other abnormality is discovered on ophthalmic examination, the patient should be referred for a sight test. If the blurred vision is unchanged, an organic cause should be suspected and appropriate referral arranged.

(a)

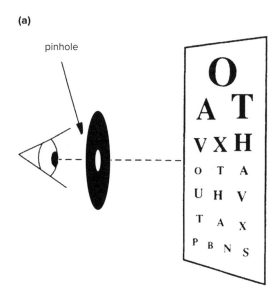

pinhole

(b)

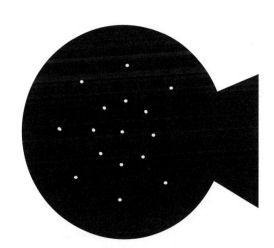

Fig. 14.8 (a) Pinhole test for blurred vision; **(b)** multiple pinhole occluder

RELIEF OF OCULAR PAIN BY HEAT

Heat, in the form of steam, applied to the closed eye is practical and very effective for the symptomatic relief of any ocular pain. Indications for the use of steam include styes, meibomian cysts and iritis.

Method

1. Using a thermos of boiled water, allow steam to rise onto the painful eye.
2. The eye must be closed for this treatment (Fig. 14.9).
3. The steaming, which should be comfortable to the sore eye, is used for about 15 minutes.

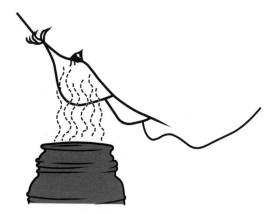

Fig. 14.9 Steaming the painful eye

CHEMICAL BURNS TO THE EYE

Acid or alkali injury to the eye may occur from domestic and industrial products, especially household cleaning products and cosmetics.

Alkali injury (e.g. oven and drain cleaners, lime, cement, plaster and fertilisers) is more common and more severe.

Alkali causes liquefactive necrosis of the surface epithelium of the eye. Acid (e.g. from toilet cleaner, pool cleaners, bleaches and battery fluid) causes coagulative necrosis of the cornea.

Equipment for treatment

1 L bag of Hartmann or normal saline solution, IV tubing, litmus paper, cotton buds, oxybuprocaine eye drops.

Treatment

- Apply immediate copious irrigation of the eye for 30 minutes. Commence with tap water irrigation followed by Hartmann or N saline solution via IV tubing until the pH is normalised.
- The pH square on a urine test strip can give a rough guide as to when the conjunctival pH reaches 7; cut off all the squares beyond the pH and apply the strip to the conjunctiva.
- Ask the patient to look in all directions during irrigation.
- Give a topical anaesthetic (oxybuprocaine drops).
- Sweep the upper and lower fornices with a moistened cotton-tipped applicator as you lift the eyelids away from the eye and remove any debris, including loose conjunctival tissue.
- Stain with fluorescein. Test and record vision and refer for specialised assessment.

PROTECTIVE INDUSTRIAL SPECTACLES

All workers at risk of eye injury should wear protective spectacles. One recommended set of economical spectacles with polycarbonate lenses is Alsafe 20-20 (made by New Zealand Safety Ltd).

Features

- One-piece wrap-around safety spectacles manufactured from high-impact-resistant polycarbonate material with scratch-resistant, coated lens.
- Available in clear, amber, green and infrared for harmful infrared and ultraviolet radiation.

EFFECTIVE TOPICAL TREATMENT OF EYE INFECTIONS

The application of eye ointment or drops for such infections as conjunctivitis can be rendered ineffective by the presence of debris, such as mucopurulent exudate.

Method

One simple method is to use a warm solution of saline to bathe away any discharge from conjunctivae, eyelashes and lids. The solution of saline is obtained by dissolving a teaspoonful of kitchen salt in 500 mL of boiled water.

HYPHAEMA

This is usually caused by injury from a fist/finger or ball, e.g. squash ball.

Management

- First, exclude a penetrating injury.
- Avoid unnecessary movement: vibration will aggravate bleeding. (For this reason, do not use a helicopter if evacuation is necessary.)
- Avoid smoking and alcohol.
- Do not give aspirin (can induce bleeding).
- Prescribe complete bed rest for 5 days and review the patient daily.
- Apply padding over the injured eye for 4 days.
- Administer sedatives as required.
- Beware of 'floaters', 'flashes' and field defects.
  Arrange follow-up ophthalmic consultation to exclude glaucoma and retinal detachment (within 1 month).

SUBCONJUNCTIVAL HAEMORRHAGE

If an orbital fracture is excluded and the haemorrhage has a definite posterior limit, the common spontaneous subconjunctival haemorrhage can be assumed. No local therapy is necessary. The blood absorbs over 2 weeks. Patient education and reassurance, including measurement of blood pressure, is appropriate management.

TIPS ON TREATING CHILDREN

MAKING FRIENDS

- A good aphorism is: never examine the child until you have made the parent laugh.
- Establish rapport in the waiting area with children—show interest, use considerable eye contact and make favourable comments.
- Ask them what they like to be called.
- Have special stickers to put on the backs of their hands, T-shirts, etc.
- Take time to converse and/or play with them.
- Have interesting toys for them to handle while listening to their parents.
- Compliment the child on, for example, a clothing item or a toy or book they are carrying.
- Ask them about their teacher or friends.
- Try to examine them on their parent's lap.

DISTRACTING CHILDREN

Children are sometimes difficult to examine but can be readily distracted, a characteristic the general practitioner can use effectively in carrying out the all-important examinations.

In the consulting room, a small duck with a rattle inside can be used for palpating the abdomen of young children. This seems more acceptable to them, as it becomes a game and you obtain the same information as if you had palpated with your hand.

Another method of examining the abdomen in an upset child is to use a soft toy to play a game on the abdomen and then slip your other hand under the toy for closer assessment.

Alternatively, use the diaphragm of your stethoscope (preferably one with a small soft toy attached) to apply pressure, starting lightly and then pressing harder while watching the child's reaction. 'Small talk' can also be employed, such as asking the child to note how cold the stethoscope feels. Rebound tenderness can also be tested.

Perhaps the best abdominal palpation method is to use the child's hand under yours to palpate.

When performing painful procedures, a recommended technique for infants (especially under 3 months) is 'the three Ss' method:
- swaddling for firm containment
- swaying (where appropriate)
- sucking using a pacifier (dummy) with a little honey.

Another way of diverting a child's attention, especially if giving an injection, is to blow up a balloon in front of them and let the air out slowly through a narrow opening to make a high-pitched 'squealing' sound—or let it go and 'shoot' around the room.

When examining the ears of young children sitting on their parent's lap, difficulty is encountered when the child follows the auroscope light and moves his or her head. A small rabbit or other animal on the desk, which, at the press of a button under the desk, will play a drum, distracts the child sitting to the right and enables you to get a good look into the left ear.

Similarly, over the examination couch, a clockwork revolving musical toy will distract the child for examination of the ear. It is also a distraction for the examination of children on the couch, and can become a most useful instrument. A decorated, ticking second hand on a clock fastened to the ceiling above the couch can be useful.

An excellent method to distract upset or uncooperative children is to blow bubbles for them. Have a bubble blowing kit on hand for this.

Another technique when giving an injection is to get the child to take a deep breath followed by a series of rapid blowing, during which the injection is given.

Then there is the 'cough trick' whereby the child is asked to perform a 'warm up' cough of moderate intensity, followed by a second cough to coincide with the vaccine needle puncture.

MANAGEMENT OF PAINFUL PROCEDURES

The treatment of painful procedures in children requires special consideration and planning because pain preventive measures reduce both short-term and long-term morbidity. Current evidence indicates that pain and distress in children is poorly managed and children continue to suffer unnecessarily. This can lead to anticipatory anxiety, needle phobia and the avoidance of health care. Obviously, it is impossible to make many basic procedures such as immunisation and other injections painless, but there are strategies to minimise the pain. Before inflicting pain on a child, always consider if the procedure is justified.

'BITE THE BULLET' STRATEGY

A novel method of achieving the cooperation of some children for an uncomfortable procedure, such injecting local anaesthetic for suturing, is to distract them by asking them to 'bite the bullet' at the appropriate time. Boys of primary school age in particular seem very attracted to this novelty, as they equate it with being brave and tough.

Rather than use a dead (gunpowder removed) .38 or .45 calibre bullet, which is too hard, a 'toy' bullet made out of a plastic or rubber compound is ideal (e.g. from a Nerf gun).

Method

1. Explain the method to the child and parents.
2. Place the 'bullet' between the child's teeth and ask a parent or assistant to hold the end of the bullet firmly.
3. Ask the child to bite the bullet as you perform the painful part of the procedure.

Biting on a chocolate with a hard coating and a soft centre is another novel tip.

USING PACIFIERS (DUMMIES) TO EASE PAIN

A study[1] reported in the 1999 BMJ recommended that all newborn babies undergoing minor procedures (e.g. veneuncture, IV injections, lumbar puncture) should be given a dummy to ease the pain. This is reinforced using a sweet substance such as honey on the pacifier (dummy).

SWEET SOLUTIONS FOR PROCEDURAL PAIN IN INFANTS

Infants up to 12 months of age may be suitable for decreasing short-term pain during minor procedures.[1,2,3,4] These solutions can be administered directly onto the tongue by a medical syringe. Suitable solutions are 24% sucrose or 30% glucose.

Examples of pre-packed products:
- TootSweet 24% sucrose solution by MedTel
- Sucrose oral solution 24% by Phebra
- Sweet-Ease Natural by Philips.[1,2]

DEEP BREATH WITH BLOWING DISTRACTION

A distraction technique for giving children injections, e.g. routine immunisations, is to get them to take a deep breath followed by a series of rapid blows (similar to childbirth exercises).

TAKING MEDICINE

There are many tricks used by parents to get their children to swallow medicine.
- Apply the mixture to a chocolate ripple (or other suitable) biscuit.
- Mix it into a small glass of a cola drink.
- Instead of a medicine cup, use a syringe—squirt the liquid well back into the oropharynx and on one side.
- Mix crushed tablet into ice cream along with 100s and 1000s or sprinkles.
- Crush tablet into fine powder and coat it over a piece of chocolate softened to room temperature.

SWALLOWING A TABLET

Ask the child to put the tablet on the tip of the tongue and then take a big suck on a straw from soft drink or other fluid.

ADMINISTRATION OF FLUIDS

Improving fluid intake in a small child

Place a child who is refusing oral fluids in a bath with a face washer in such a way that the child is encouraged to suck the wet washer. Some children will do this even when they refuse to take fluids in the conventional manner.

This method will help to reduce fever, if present.

WEIGHING A CHILD

Where no baby scales are available, or where a toddler refuses to step onto the scales, ask the parent to stand on the scales while carrying the child, then subtract the parent's own weight.

HOW TO OPEN THE MOUTH

Some children refuse to open their mouths to have an examination of their throat. Getting the spatula between clenched teeth is not easy. Hold their nose closed by gently pinching the nostrils together and they will reflexively open their mouth.

One tip is to ask the child to take a deep breath while you inspect the pharynx with your torch. Another tip is to ask them to look up at a 45° angle and yawn, or ask them to make a loud noise like a tiger. This may need to be repeated.

In younger children who are reluctant, it is often better to 'be cruel to be kind' and get in and out fast. Instead of the GP and parent unsuccessfully coaxing the child for minutes of increasing agitation, try the following:

- Leave the oral examination until last.
- The parent sits the child on their lap, facing forwards and wraps one arm in a 'hug' across the whole front of the child's body, including their arms.
- The parent's other hand holds the forehead, to stop the head turning at the crucial moment (Fig. 15.1).
- If the child snaps the teeth shut, gently wiggle the spatula between the front teeth and lever it up and down (without pushing) until the teeth open momentarily. Take that opportunity to reach the back of the tongue, ensuring your light and eyes are focused on the tonsillar area during the brief gag.

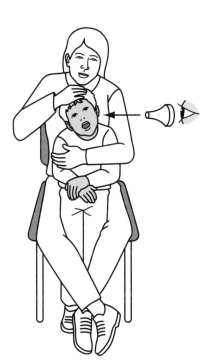

Fig. 15.1 Restraint for ear, nose and throat examination

- The whole 'upsetting' part of the manoeuvre takes just a few seconds, followed by a distracting cuddle with the parent.

SPATULA SKETCHES FOR CHILDREN

Many young patients have quickly forgotten any inspection of their throats while observing the preparation of a 'present' in the form of a drawing on the wooden spatula used in one practitioner's examination.

After the examination they are informed of their special present, and you can then proceed to draw on the unused end of the spatula. The drawings take about 15 seconds.

Figure 15.2 illustrates three sketches from one repertoire: a penguin (with optional bow tie), a caterpillar and a racing car.

Tip: Use an ink pad with special stamps, e.g. Disney characters, Bananas in Pyjamas, to stamp onto the spatulas.

Another idea is to make a human face on the spatula then make a split of about 1–2 cm at the top of the spatula. Insert wisps of cotton wool or tissue to create the impression of hair.

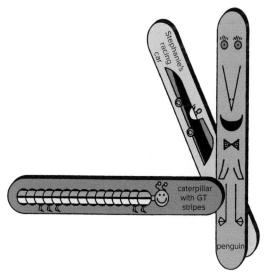

Fig. 15.2 Spatula sketches

INSTILLING NOSE DROPS

A trick to get a toddler to inhale nose drops is to instil a drop or two at the nasal openings and cover the child's mouth. The reverse of the 'pinch the nose' mouth-opening tip.

INSTILLING EYE DROPS IN CHILDREN

Method

1. Gently hold the lower lid down.
2. Get the child to look up, and instil the necessary drops.

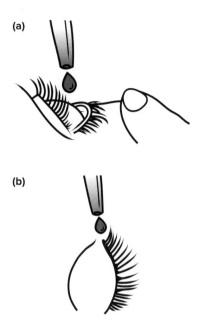

Fig. 15.3 Instilling eye drops in cooperative children

3. Ensure that the tip of the bottle does not touch the eye (Fig. 15.3a).

If the child is unable to keep the eyes open:
1. Lay the child on his or her back.
2. When the eyes are 'screwed up', instil the drops into the depression formed above the inner canthus (Fig. 15.3b).
3. When the child opens the eyes (preferably slowly), the drops soon gravitate into the eye.

Note: This is suitable for antibiotic drops, but unsuitable for drops acting through the autonomic nervous system.

INTRAVENOUS CANNULA INSERTION

The preferred site is the dorsum of the non-dominant hand. Other sites are the radial aspect of the forearm, the dorsum of the foot, great saphenous vein or cubital fossa.

Give topical local anaesthetic and consider an injection of local anaesthetic (preferable).

Keep the child as still as possible by wrapping in a sheet. Grasp the wrist and hand to facilitate insertion into the dorsum of the hand. Keep the cannula as still as possible at an angle of 10–15° and advance it gently into the vein (Fig. 4.2). Splint the arm and wrap the whole arm in a firm crepe bandage. See 'Venepuncture and intravenous cannulation' in Chapter 4.

Use of subcutaneous local anaesthetic

An intravenous cannulation can be very painful so insertion of subcutaneous local anaesthetic is recommended.

Method

Draw up 1% lidocaine into an insulin syringe. After skin preparation, the skin overlying the target vessel is pulled laterally and a small volume (about 0.2 mL) is injected into the subcutaneous tissue. When the skin returns to its former position, wait for 1 to 2 minutes and then insert the cannula.

DIFFICULT VEIN ACCESS

To raise a vein for cannulation in chubby children, consider the methods described in 'Venepuncture and intravenous cannulation' in Chapter 4, but remember that a neat vein can be raised over the fourth metacarpal on the dorsum of the hand.

EASIER ACCESS TO A CHILD'S ARM

To achieve relaxation in an arm, for example to insert an intravenous line, distract the child by getting them to squeeze a special toy (as used in children's hospitals) with the hand of the opposite arm. This muscular activity of one arm leads to relaxation of the opposite arm.

SWALLOWED FOREIGN OBJECTS

Hard objects swallowed by children are common emergencies in general practice.

A golden rule

The natural passage of most objects entering the stomach can be expected. Once the pylorus has been traversed, the foreign body usually continues. Typical presenting foreign bodies are:
- coins
- buttons
- sharp objects
- open safety pins
- glass
- drawing pins.
  Special cases are:
- very large coins (e.g. 50 cent pieces): watch carefully
- hair clips (usually cannot pass duodenum if under 7 years).
  High-risk foreign bodies:
- Large objects: > 6 cm long, > 2.5 cm wide
- Button batteries
- Magnet plus metal object
- > 1 magnet ingestion
- Lead-based objects (if impacted leads to lead toxicity)
- Abnormal GIT: previous surgery, tracheoesophageal fistulas or stenosing lesions.

Management
- Manage conservatively.
- Investigate unusual gagging, coughing and retching with X-rays of the head, neck, thorax and abdomen (check nasopharynx and respiratory tract).

- Watch for passage of the foreign body in stool (usually 3 days). Avoid giving aperients.
- If not passed, order an X-ray in 1 week.
- If a blunt foreign body has been stationary for 1 month without symptoms, remove at laparotomy.

Button and disc battery ingestion

If not in the stomach, these (and especially lithium batteries) create an emergency if in the oesophagus, because the electric current they generate destroys mucous membranes and causes perforation within 6 hours. They must be removed ASAP—within hours.

This also applies to the ear canal and nares.

Impacted foreign bodies

Obstruction of the oropharynx and tracheal opening by a larger foreign body (especially a large food bolus) can be rapidly fatal. As a rule, the obstruction can usually be removed by asking patients to cough (first line) or by giving them a sharp blow to the back. Sweeping a finger around the pharynx to hook out the bolus is another good method.

In children, a blow to the back is usually the first line method. A sternal thrust over the lower end of the sternum can be used to depress the chest by about one-third of its diameter. Yet another method is to place the child over your knees with head down, and apply blows to the back with a firmness applicable to the child's age.

WOUND REPAIR

Wherever possible it is worth using a simple painless technique without compromising good healing.

Scalp lacerations

If lacerations are small but gaping, use the child's hair as the suture. This, of course, only pertains to children with long hair. *Do not* use this method for large wounds.

Method

1. Make a twisted bunch of the child's own hair of appropriate size on each side of the wound. (The longer the hair, the better the result.)
2. Tie a reef knot and then an extra holding knot to minimise slipping (Fig. 15.4).
3. As you tie, ask an assistant to drip compound benzoin tincture solution (Friar's Balsam) or spray plastic skin or similar compound on the hair knot.
4. As this congeals, the knot is further consolidated against slipping.

Leave the hair suture long. The parents can cut the knot about 5 days later when the wound is healed.

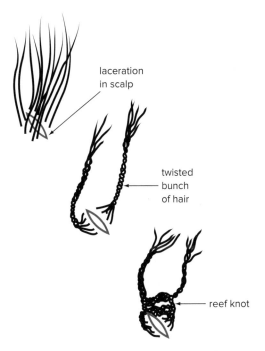

laceration in scalp

twisted bunch of hair

reef knot

Fig. 15.4 Method of using hair to repair scalp lacerations

The whole procedure is painless until tetanus toxoid is given (if indicated).

Forehead lacerations

Despite the temptation, avoid using reinforced paper adhesive strips (Steri-Strips) in children for open wounds. They will merely close the dermis and cause a thin, stretched scar. They can be used only for very superficial epidermal wounds or in conjunction with sutures.

Lacerated lip or gums

A practical method to soothe and distract an upset child with a mouth wound is to ask the child to suck on a teaspoon of sugar. The sugar acts as a 'styptic', alleviating oozing of blood.

Glue for children's wounds

A tissue adhesive glue can be used successfully to close superficial, smooth and clean skin wounds, particularly in children. It is useful for wounds less than 3 cm.

Skin glues—an alternative to sutures

Cyanoacrylate tissue adhesions are available for wound closure. These glues act by polymerising with the thin water layer on the skin's surface to form a bond. Those available include Histoacryl, Dermabond and Epiglu. Some practitioners find that a similar type, such as superglue, also serves the purpose but sterility and toxicity have to be considered and so this is not recommended.

Precautions

The glue should be used only for superficial, dry, clean and fresh skin wounds. It must not be applied for deep wounds or wounds under excessive tension. Special care is required near the eye since the glue can readily glue the eyelids together. Contact with the cornea or conjunctiva must be avoided, as this can cause adhesions. The glue must not be used on mucosal surfaces.

The protective 'window' method: If applying glue near the eye or other sensitive structure, cut a hole in a protective adherent cover such as Tegaderm in order to localise the glue application.

Method

- Ensure the wound is clean and dry and the wound edges are precisely opposed. No gaps are permissible with the glue method (Fig. 15.5).
- Clean the wound with normal saline or aqueous chlorhexidine and let dry.
- Apply a thin layer of glue directly to the tissue edges to be joined with the fine end of the tapered plastic ampoule (Fig. 15.6)—squeeze out gently.
- Press the tissue surfaces together for 30 seconds.
- Remove any excess glue immediately with a dry swab.
- Apply Steri-Strips to prevent access to the wound, e.g. 'picking' by the child.

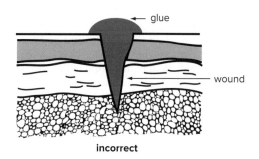

incorrect

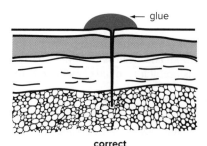

correct

Fig. 15.5 Application of glue to a wound

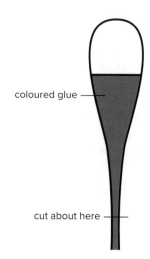

Fig. 15.6 The ampoule of Histoacryl

- Do not wash the wound for 3 to 4 days.
  Follow instructions in the product data sheet.
  Caution: The glue bonds skin and eye tissue in seconds.
If spilt on skin, remove with acetone as soon as possible.

Topical local anaesthesia for children's lacerations

Topical anaesthetic drugs that can be used for instilling in minor wounds in children are listed in Table 15.1. The preparations include a variety of drugs, so toxicity and safety factors have to be considered. Cocaine is very effective, but it is relatively toxic and as a rule should be avoided in open wounds. Adrenaline-containing preparations should be used with caution in wounds in end-artery areas, such as digits, pinnae, tip of the nose and penis, and are best avoided on mucous membranes such as inside the mouth where rapid absorption may

Table 15.1 Topical preparations for local analgesia

Topical preparation	Contents
Laceraine (previously ALA)	adrenaline 1:1000, lidocaine 4%*, tetracaine 4%
LAT	lidocaine 4%, adrenaline 1:2000, tetracaine[†] 2%
TAC	tetracaine[†] 0.5%, adrenaline 1:2000, cocaine 11.8%
AC gel	adrenaline, cocaine
AnGel	amethocaine 4%
EMLA	lidocaine, prilocaine

*lidocaine = lignocaine
[†]tetracaine = amethocaine

occur. The recommended topical combinations are Laceraine and LAT (see Table 15.1), but these may have to be prepared by a hospital or compounding pharmacy. A variation of LAT and Laceraine is the readily available preparation EMLA cream. It requires at least 60 minutes of skin contact to be effective and is not recommended for open wounds.[3]

Method

- Thoroughly clean the wound (should be less than 5 cm).
- Use LAT or Laceraine in a dose 0.1 mL/kg bodyweight.
- Apply this solution on a piece of gauze or cotton wool placed inside the wound and hold in place with an adhesive clear plastic dressing.
- Leave for 20 to 30 minutes (an area of blanching about 1 cm wide will appear around the wound).

Anaesthesia is obtained about 20 to 30 minutes after instillation. Test the adequacy of anaesthesia by washing and squeezing the wound or prodding it with forceps—if this is pain free, suturing will usually be painless.

Note: Use these solutions with caution. Death and convulsions with doses greater than 3 mL of TAC in infants have been reported.

Lignocaine 1% can be used as a topical agent whereby a few drops can be placed onto the wound. Wait a few minutes before injecting into the wound.

Improvised topical 'anaesthesia'

Some practitioners use an ice block or a wet ice-cold piece of gauze to chill the lacerated site in children. The child or parent is asked to hold the ice, then lift it while a suture is rapidly inserted or while local anaesthetic is introduced.

Liquid nitrogen topical 'anaesthesia'

A useful technique for a variety of topical anaesthesia, especially useful in older children, is to spray liquid nitrogen or other vapocoolant over the skin where a procedure such as incising an abscess is necessary.

WOUND INFILTRATION

For a larger wound requiring suturing, infiltrate lidocaine 1% into the wound edges using a small 27-gauge (or smaller) needle with a 3 mL syringe. The pain of injection can be reduced by:

- using topical anaesthesia first
- injecting slowly
- placing the needle into the wound through the lacerated surface, not through intact skin
- passing the needle through an anaesthetised area into an unanaesthetised area

- buffering the acidic solution with 8.4% sodium bicarbonate in a 9:1 ratio, that is, 9 mL lidocaine 1% with 1 mL sodium bicarbonate.

FRACTURES

Skeletal injuries in children differ from adults in many respects and fractures should be considered in children presenting with unusual loss of function such as walking or use of an arm.

Occult (hidden) fractures

These arise because of the large amount of cartilage in immature bones, especially around the epiphyses, which are radiolucent because they have not yet ossified. These include:

- epiphyseal fractures—which may masquerade as dislocations
- condylar fractures
- humerus-condylar fractures (beware of overlooking in under-3-year-olds)
- elbow-epiphyseal fractures—X-rays can appear normal
- hip-fractures—difficult to detect because of avascular changes to the femoral head
- spine—spinal cord damage may be present without radiological evidence of a fracture
- head injuries—because of the resilience of the skull there may be no evidence of a fracture in the presence of severe brain damage; this also applies to lung, heart and upper abdominal injuries without evidence of a rib fracture
- femoral shaft and tibia—deformity can result if crush injuries and minor displacement of the epiphyseal growth plate are misdiagnosed.

Significant differences

- Children's fractures differ in nature and management due to bone plasticity and other factors.
- Epiphyseal or growth plate fractures provide challenging management problems.
- As a rule, sprains do not occur in childhood.
- Greenstick fractures, which involve one cortical surface only; if undiagnosed, can cause overgrowth of the affected limb.
- Buckle fractures due to compressed metaphyseal bone.
- Child abuse must be considered as a cause of fractures in infants under 6 months.
- Meticulous X-rays are required for fractures around the elbow joint.

Specific fractures

- The 'toddler's fracture', *spiral fracture of tibia*—often no history of injury; requires immobilisation in an above knee plaster.

- *Clavicle*—requires a simple sling for 2 weeks.
- *Shaft fracture of humerus*—treat conservatively with collar and cuff sling ± supportive plaster slab holding arm against chest.
- *Supracondylar fracture of humerus*—a potentially complex and serious injury usually requiring referral for specialised treatment. Circulation and major nerve injuries are a concern.
- *Condylar fractures of humerus*—also 'tiger country' if epiphyseal plates and metaphyses involved. Requires orthopaedic referral.
- *Forearm fractures*—often are areas for greenstick fractures but beware of the *Monteggia fracture* with associated dislocation of the radius. Include the elbow and wrist joints in X-rays.

Rule: If a pre-school child presents holding an apparently painful arm, consider a 'greenstick' fracture (foremost) or a **pulled elbow** (see Chapter 11). The pulled elbow is common in children and reduction is important.

SPLINTS FOR MINOR GREENSTICK FRACTURES

Non-displaced fractures of the arm can be splinted using one or two plastic tongue depressors under the bandage as an alternative to a plaster backslab.

REMOVING PLASTER CASTS FROM CHILDREN

To facilitate removal of plaster, especially a plaster cylinder from a child, request that the patient soaks the plaster in warm water prior to seeing you, ideally for about 15 minutes or longer on the evening or morning prior to the visit. Alternatively, the plaster can be soaked in water at the surgery, but it is preferable for it to be performed at home in a large bucket or container (the bath is suitable) (Fig. 15.7a). The POP bandage can then be easily teased out and unrolled (Fig. 15.7b), or cut with a knife or scalpel. This method saves time and the unpleasant experience of a plaster cutter or saws.

Note: Making the initial plaster: a fun thing is to add a food dye to children's plaster when smoothing it out, or the dye can be put in the bucket of water.

Cutting plaster with an electric saw

Children will be more reassured if a wooden tongue depressor or similar object is inserted under the plaster in the sawing line.

THE CRYING INFANT
Checklist of common causes

- Hunger (underfeeding is the main feeding problem causing crying)
- Wet or soiled nappy
- Loneliness
- Infant 'colic': typically 2 to 16 weeks
- Teething (more likely after 12 months)
- Reflux oesophagitis

Unusual causes to consider

- Corneal scratch from infant's nail (fluorescein helps diagnose)
- Hair 'ring' wrapped around digit (particularly toe)
- Testicular torsion, irreducible hernia
- Otitis media
- Shaken baby

The role of 5 Ss to comfort the infant

1. Swaddling—firm clothing, not too loose
2. Lie baby on side or stomach
3. Shush (i.e. 'sshusshhing' as loudly as the child)

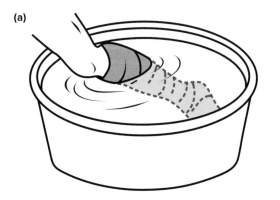
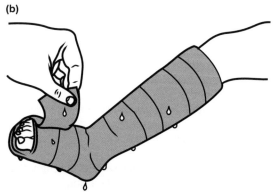

Fig. 15.7 Removal of plaster cast: **(a)** soak in warm water to soften; **(b)** unroll bandage

4. Swing—sway from side to side
5. Suckling—nipple, teat or dummy

Infant colic (period of infant distress or period of 'purple' crying)

Consider cow's milk intolerance, lactose intolerance and oesophagitis from reflux, although these labels are probably dished out too liberally.

Recommend the pacifying methods above. Avoid medications if possible. Some parents are desperate and buy OTC preparations from pharmacists (e.g. Hartley's Gripe Water, Infants' Friend, Brauer Colic Relief). These may contain naturopathic oils, baking soda or ethanol and tend to cause loose bowels and nappy rash.

A safe preparation to consider is Infacol Wind Drops (simethicone).

Reflux with oesophagitis

Peaks at 4 months of age and can cause great distress. Avoid diagnosing it without significant vomiting/regurgitation. Discourage switching from breastmilk to formula.[5]

If basic methods such as thickening of feeds and antacids are ineffective, specific medication can be effective—check with your paediatrician about prescribing safely.

CLEANING A CHILD'S 'SNOTTY' NOSE

A child's blocked nose can be cleaned with sodium chloride (normal saline) including Narium mist spray or FLO Saline Plus. A simpler way to remove lumps of mucus is to use the firmer tissue 'spears' described in the section 'The ear and hearing' in Chapter 13. Insert the 'spear' adjacent to and then behind the snot to dislodge it.

Another method is to use an all-rubber 30 mL ear syringe (usually stocked by pharmacies). Insert the lubricated tip in the infant's nostril and use the suction effect to clear the nares.

TEST FOR LACTOSE INTOLERANCE

Theory

If lactose intolerance is suspected in a child with diarrhoea, especially if frothy fluid diarrhoea follows milk feeds, a simple test can be performed with a Clinitest tablet. This test detects reducing sugars such as lactose and glucose but not sucrose. Specific glucose oxidase reagents such as Tes-Tape and Glucostix detect glucose only and will not detect lactose or sucrose. Primary lactose intolerance is extremely rare; more common is functional lactose overload or malabsorption secondary to GIT infection or allergy.[6]

Method

1. Line a napkin with plastic and collect faecal fluid (Fig. 15.8a).
2. Pour some of the stool into a test tube and add two parts of water.
3. Place 15 drops into another test tube.
4. Add a Clinitest tablet and note the reaction.

Alternatively, put 5 drops of the faecal fluid directly into a test tube and add 10 drops of water.

Interpretation

A reading of 0.75 to 2 indicates lactose intolerance. A reading of 0 or 0.25 is probably negative (Fig. 15.8b).

BREATH-HOLDING ATTACKS

Diagnosis

- Precipitating event (minor emotional or physical).
- Children emit a long loud cry, then hold their breath.
- They become pale and then blue.
- If severe, may result in unconsciousness or a fit.
- Lasts between 10 to 60 seconds.
- Age group usually 6 months to 6 years (peak 2 to 3 years).

Management

- Reassure the parents that attacks are self-limiting and are not associated with epilepsy or mental retardation.

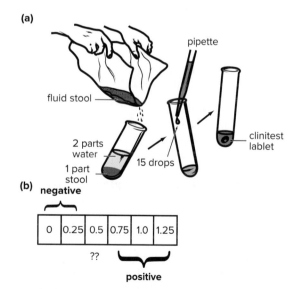

Fig. 15.8 Test for lactose intolerance: **(a)** test method; **(b)** interpreting reading

- Encourage parents to set consistent behavioural limits and to resist spoiling the child.
- Try to avoid incidents known to frustrate the child or to precipitate a tantrum.

ITCHING AND SWOLLEN SKIN RASHES

An ice pack is an excellent method of giving relief to an acute itchy or swollen skin lesion such as an insect bite in a child (or adult). A simple method is to place a few ice cubes in a handkerchief or small cloth and complete the pack with a string tie or rubber band. It soothes and prevents excessive scratching.

TRAUMATIC FOREHEAD LUMP

If a child develops a forehead lump, such as after a fall onto the edge of a table, apply a cold flannel. Repeat twice a day for 3 days.

SUPRAPUBIC ASPIRATION OF URINE

This is the most accurate way of collecting urine in children less than 2 years old. It is very suitable in the toxic and ill child.[7]

Contraindications

- Age greater than 12 months (unless the bladder is palpable or percussable).
- Coagulopathy.

Preparation

- Best performed when the child has not voided for at least 1 hour. Give the child a drink, e.g. bottle over the preceding hour or so.
- Select a 23-gauge needle attached to a 5 mL syringe.
- Local anaesthetic is not necessary but a topical anaesthetic is recommended.

Position of patient

- The patient's legs should be straight (preferable) or bent in the frog-leg position.

Method

1. Check the bladder position by gentle percussion.
2. Prepare the skin in the suprapubic area with povidone-iodine solution.
3. Ask an assistant to hold the child supine with the legs extended.
4. Insert the needle attached to the syringe directly through the abdomen wall in the midline 1-2 cm above the symphysis pubis (this usually corresponds to the skin crease above the pubis) (Fig. 15.9).

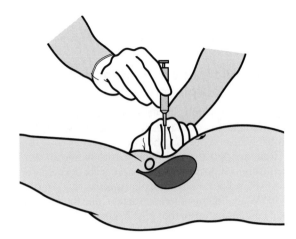

Fig. 15.9 Suprapubic aspiration of urine in a child

5. Insert it to a depth of about 2-3 cm in infants or deeper according to the child's age. Have a bottle on stand-by for a midstream clean catch in case the child voids.
6. Apply steady suction until urine is obtained.
7. Aspirate the urine while slowly withdrawing the needle.
8. Take the needle from the syringe and express the sample into a sterile microurine container.
9. Forward the urine for microscopy and culture.

Note: If unsuccessful, the bladder is probably empty so try at another time.

Tip: Hold the tip of the penis in males to prevent voiding but have a sterile bottle on standby for a clean catch should voiding occur.

CLEAN CATCH MIDSTREAM SPECIMEN

Although prone to contamination, this is a good method in skilled hands. It is best collected by a person trained in the method such as a practice nurse or a nurse in the emergency department of your local hospital or pathology laboratory. The parent holds the child over a sterile bowl placed under a cleansed genitalia.

THE 'DRAW A DREAM' TECHNIQUE

A useful interview technique for children with behavioural disorders is to ask them to 'draw a dream', especially if bad dreams are a feature of their problem. It is an excellent avenue to help children effectively communicate their understanding of the stressful events in their lives.

Chapter 15 | TIPS ON TREATING CHILDREN **219**

Professor Tonge believes that 'it is the royal road to the child's mental processes and the doctor is ideally placed to use the technique'.[8]

Method

1. Make a simple drawing of someone in bed and add a large cartoon balloon (Fig. 15.10).
2. If the child's name is John, for example, say as you draw the dream balloon, 'Here is a boy named John having a bad dream; perhaps it is even you. I wonder if you could draw that dream for me'.
3. Then ask the child to help you interpret the significance of the drawing.

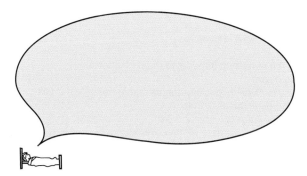

Fig. 15.10 The 'draw a dream' technique

ASSESSING ANXIOUS CHILDREN AND SCHOOL REFUSAL

Assessment of the degree and nature of the child's anxiety and possible contributing factors to school refusal is an essential first step in management and provides a baseline against which to monitor progress. The following two useful measures of school refusal assist in the assessment of such children.

Fear thermometer

The fear thermometer (Fig. 15.11) is an easily administered measure that provides a global rating of the child's fear about school attendance. In relation to their worst day in the past few weeks of school, the child is asked: 'How afraid were you of going to school on that day?' They are asked to nominate their level of fear, from 0 'not scared' to 100 'very scared', on the pictorial thermometer. This global rating may reflect fear related to (a) separation from significant others; or (b) a dreadful aspect of the school setting.

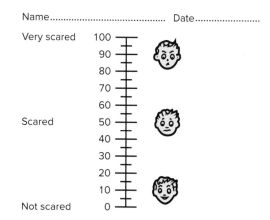

Think about your worst day over the past 2 school weeks. How afraid were you of going to school on that day?

Fig. 15.11 The fear thermometer

Date: _____
Child: _____
Interviewer: _____
Tell me what thoughts you have about...
(a) going off to school _____
(b) being separated from mum and/or dad _____
(c) school work _____
(d) how clever you are _____
(e) other kids at school _____
 (f) teachers _____
(g) the principal _____
(h) (anything the child would like to nominate regarding why he/ she doesn't want to go school)_____

Fig. 15.12 Self-statements: child form

Self-statement questionnaire

The self-statement questionnaire (Fig. 15.12) allows for a more detailed understanding of the sorts of things that may be contributing to school refusal. It taps the child's thoughts about seven aspects of school attendance (including such things as the other children at school, and the process of actually going to school in the morning). In addition, it allows the child to nominate any other issues that may lead to a reluctance to attend.

The clinician can use the information elicited during administration of the questionnaire to help in the development of a treatment program that addresses the specific anxiety-provoking thoughts of the child.

In an older child whose parent is at home during the day, consider the possibility of unconscious 'secondary gain' for the lonely or depressed parent.

SURGERY

Table 15.2 Optimal times for surgery/intervention in children's disorders

Disorder	Surgery/intervention
Squint (fixed or alternating)	12–24 months Absolutely before 7 years
Deafness (in children born with hearing)	Screen at or before 8 months hearing aids required by 12 months
Outer ear deformity	After 6 years
Tongue tie	3–4 months or 2–6 years
Cleft lip	Less than 3 months
Cleft palate	6–12 months
Inguinoscrotal lumps • Undescended testes	best assessed before 6 months surgery best at 6–18 months
• Umbilical hernia	leave to age 4 surgery at 4 if persistent (tend to strangulate after 4) never tape down!
• Inguinal hernia	general rule is ASAP, especially infants and irreducible hernias reducible herniae: the '6–2' rule birth–6 weeks: surgery within 2 days 6 weeks–6 months: surgery within 2 weeks over 6 months: surgery within 2 months
• Femoral hernia	ASAP
• Torsion of testicle	surgery within 4 hours (absolutely within 6 hours)
• Hydrocele	leave to 12 months then review (often resolve)
• Varicocele	leave and review
Leg and foot development problems Developmental dysplasia of hip • Bowed legs (genu varum)	most treated successfully by abductor bracing with a Pavlic harness normal up to 3 years usually improve with age: refer if ICS > 6 cm
• Knock knees	normal 3–8 years then refer if IMS > 8 cm
• Flat feet	no treatment unless stiff and painful
• Internal tibial torsion	refer 6 months after presentation if not resolved
• Medial tibial torsion	leave for 8 years then refer if not resolved
• Metatarsus varus	refer 3 months after presentation if not resolved

CARDIOPULMONARY RESUSCITATION IN CHILDREN

Sudden primary cardiac arrest is rare in children. Mostly due to hypoxia. Asystole or severe bradycardia is the usual rhythm at the time of arrest.

The basic life support plan of DRSABCD should be followed:

- Check for any dangers.
- Check response of child.
- Send for help.
- Check breathing and pulse.
- Open airway: Inspect oropharynx and clear any debris.

- Basic life support outside the hospital setting is 30:2 compression ventilation ratio, including two initial rescue breaths. The ratio of 30:2 is recommended for all ages regardless of the number of revivers present <www.resus.org.au/policy/guidelines/index.asp>.
- Tilt head backwards, lift chin and thrust jaw forwards (the sniffing position).
- Ventilate lungs at about 20 inflations/min with bag-valve-mask or mouth to mask or mouth to mouth. An Air-viva using 8–10 L/min of oxygen is ideal if available.
- Intubate via mouth and secure, if necessary (must pre-oxygenate).

- If intubation not possible, use a needle cricothyroidotomy as an emergency.
- Start external cardiac compression if pulseless or < 60 beats/min.

  Infant < 1 year:
  - on centre of sternum
  - use two fingers or thumb
  - depth of compression 2–3 cm

Children 1–8 years:
- on centre of sternum
- use heel of one hand
- depth 3–4 cm

- If > 8 years use a two-handed technique. Avoid pressure over ribs and abdominal viscera. The compression ratio for children is 100 to 120 per minute (one per 0.5 to 0.6 seconds).
- Defibrillation—if required.

References

1. Carbajel, Paupe A et al. *Randomised trial of analgesic effects of sucrose, glucose and pacifiers in term neonates.* BMJ, 1999; 319: 1393–97.
2. Harrison D, Stevens B, Bueno M, Yamada J, Adams-Webber T, Beyene J, et al. *Efficacy of sweet solutions for analgesia in infants between 1 and 12 months of age: a systematic review.* Archives of Dis in Childhood, 2010; 95(6): 406–13.
3. Stevens B, Yamada J, Lee GY, Ohisson A. *Sucrose for analgesia in newborn infants undergoing painful procedures.* Cochrane Database Syst Rev, 2013; Issue 1: Article no: CD001069.
4. Gwee A, Rimer R, Marks M (eds). *Paediatric Handbook* (9th edn). Oxford: Wiley Blackwell, 2015: 22–24.
5. Royal Children's Hospital. Gastrooesophageal reflux in infants. Clinical Practice Guidelines. Melbourne: 2019, https://www.rch.org.au/clinicalguide/guideline_index/Gastrooesophageal_reflux_in_infants/
6. Royal Children's Hospital. Unsettled or crying babies (Colic). Clinical Practice Guidelines. Melbourne: 2019, https://www.rch.org.au/clinicalguide/guideline_index/Crying_Baby_Infant_Distress/
7. Gwee A, Rimer R, Marks M (eds). *Paediatric Handbook* (9th edn). Oxford: Wiley Blackwell, 2015: 37–38.
8. Tonge B. *I'm upset, you're upset and so are my mum and dad.* Aust Fam Physician, 1983; 12: 497–99.

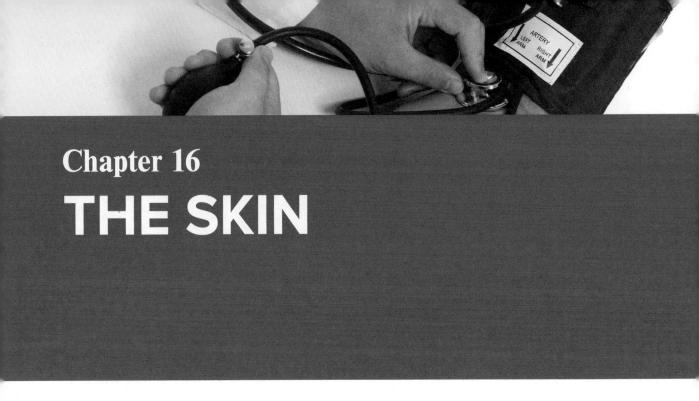

Chapter 16
THE SKIN

RULES FOR PRESCRIBING CREAMS AND OINTMENTS

How much cream?

On average, 30 g of cream will cover the body surface area of an adult. Ointments, despite being of a thicker consistency, do not penetrate into the deeper skin layers so readily, and the requirements are slightly less. Pastes are applied thickly, and the requirements are at least 3 to 4 times as great as for creams.

The 'rule of nines', used routinely to determine the percentage of body surface area affected by burns (Fig. 16.1), may be used also to calculate the amount of a topical preparation that needs to be prescribed.

For example:
• If 9% of the body surface area is affected by eczema, approximately 3 g of cream is required to cover it.
• Nine grams of cream is used per day if prescribed 3 times daily.
• A 50 g tube will last 5 or 6 days.

One gram of cream will cover an area approximately 10 cm × 10 cm, and this formula may be used for smaller lesions.

Some general rules

1. Use creams or lotions for acute rashes.
2. Use ointments for chronic scaling rashes.
3. A thin smear only is necessary.
4. On average, 30 g:
   • will cover an adult body once
   • will cover hands twice daily for 2 weeks
   • will cover a patchy rash twice daily for 1 week.

On average, 200 g will cover a quite severe rash twice daily for 2 weeks.

SUNBURN

Sunburn is usually caused by UV–B radiation and it can vary from mild erythema (minimal discomfort for about 3 days) to severe redness, heat, pain and swelling, and even general constitutional signs with fever, headache and delirium.

First-line treatment includes oral aspirin or ibuprofen for pain and cool compresses. Topical agents, depending on the severity of the burn, include corticosteroid ointment or cream to unblistered skin, Solugel, bicarbonate of soda paste or oily calamine lotion.

Topical corticosteroids for sunburn

When a patient with severe sunburn presents early, the application of 1% hydrocortisone ointment or cream can reduce significantly the eventual severity of the burn. This has been proved experimentally by covering one-half of the burnt area with hydrocortisone and comparing the outcome with the untreated area.

The application can be repeated 2 to 3 hours after the initial application and then the next morning. The earlier the treatment is applied the better, as it may not be useful after 24 hours.

Hydrocortisone should be used for unblistered erythematous skin, and not used on broken skin.

SKIN EXPOSURE TO THE SUN

There is evidence that our skin needs exposure to sunlight to provide a substantial dose of vitamin D. This is a preventive for osteoporosis. Hats and sunscreens reduce the natural synthesis of vitamin D in the body.

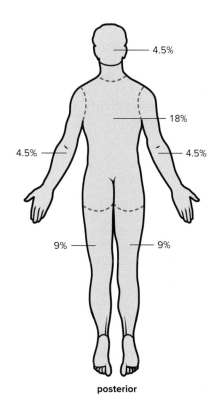

Fig. 16.1 Rule of nines' for body surface areas

There should be a balance between receiving enough sunlight exposure to prevent vitamin D deficiency on one hand and receiving too much, predisposing to skin cancer, on the other (see Table 16.1). A simpler guideline for most geographical areas is to recommend exposure (for those at risk of deficiency) to the face, bare arms and hands of 5 to 6 minutes mid-morning or mid-afternoon in summer and in winter 5 to 6 minutes a day in hotter climates, 15–30 minutes a day in all other climates and up to 50 minutes a day in winter in milder temperate areas. In Australia, check exposure times with local authorities (see Table 16.1 for a guide).

Table 16.1 Recommended sunlight exposure to the head and hands per day (minutes) in Australia

Australian city	Summer	Winter
Darwin	5	5
Brisbane	5	5
Perth	5	12
Sydney	5	15
Adelaide	6	20
Melbourne	8	25
Hobart	10	65

Ocular protection from UV light

The best protection from the harmful effects of strong UV light is from wraparound UV-absorbing sunglasses (Australian Standard AS/NZS 1067:2003 for sunglasses and fashion spectacles).

ACNE

Some topical treatment regimens

Start with a topical retinoid in combination with an anti-inflammatory such as benzoyl peroxide.

Mild to moderate acne

1. Apply isotretinoin 0.05% gel or tretinoin 0.025% cream or adapalene 0.1% cream or gel each night (especially if comedones).
2. If inadequate response after 6 weeks, add benzoyl peroxide 2.5% or 5% gel or cream once daily (in the morning). That is, after 6 weeks, maintenance treatment is:
   - isotretinoin 0.05% gel at night
   - benzoyl peroxide 2.5% or 5% mane.

   In more severe cases, add clindamycin 1% topically to benzoyl peroxide.
3. Maintain for 3 months and review.

   For a large area of mild truncal acne, consider topical salicylic acid 3% in ethanol 70% once daily.

Clindamycin use

Use clindamycin HCl in alcohol. Apply to each comedone with fingertips twice daily.

- A ready clindamycin preparation is Clindatech.
- Clindamycin is particularly useful for pregnant women and those who cannot tolerate antibiotics or exfoliants. Other topical alternatives are:
- erythromycin 2% gel
- azelaic acid lotion, apply bd
- adapalene 0.1% cream or gel, apply nocte
- tazarotene 0.1% cream, once nocte.

Oral antibiotics

Use if acne is resistant to topical agents. Doxycycline 100 mg day or minocycline 50–100 mg nocte for 4 weeks (or up to 10 weeks if slow response), then reduce according to response (e.g. doxycycline 50 mg for 6 weeks).

If tetracyclines not tolerated or contraindicated (e.g. in pregnancy), use erythromycin 250–500 mg (o) bd.

Facial scars

Injections of collagen can be used for the depressed facial scars from cystic acne.

Common mistakes with acne

- Not treating comedones with a comedolytic
- Monotherapy (e.g. antibiotics only)
- Not using recommended combinations
- Not using oral isotretinoin for cystic acne

NAPPY RASH

- Keep the area dry.
- Change wet or soiled napkins often—highly absorbable disposable ones are good.
- Wash area gently with warm water and pat dry (do not rub).
- Avoid excessive bathing and soap.
- Avoid powders and plastic pants.
- Use emollients to keep skin lubricated, e.g. zinc oxide and castor oil cream, or petroleum jelly with each change.
- A mild topical corticosteroid ointment is the treatment of choice. Standard treatment for persistent or widespread rash is 1% hydrocortisone with nystatin or clotrimazole cream, e.g. Hydrozole (qid after changes)—you can get separate steroid and antifungal creams and mix before application. Avoid stronger steroid preparations. Consider continuing the antifungal cream for another 7 days. If nappy rash is severe, apply a stronger topical steroid for up to 7 days, e.g. methylprednisolone aceponate 0.1% fatty ointment once daily. If infection is suspected, confirm by a swab or skin scraping.

If seborrhoeic dermatitis: 1% hydrocortisone and ketoconazole ointment.

Tip: If rash is resistant and ulcerated, add Orabase (benzocaine) ointment bd or tds. Another tip is to add petroleum jelly to the above medication in equal parts—this can be used for a 'normal' nappy rash since it promotes longer action. Another strategy is to give oral zinc.

ATOPIC DERMATITIS (ECZEMA)

Note importance of good education.

Medication

Mild atopic dermatitis

- Avoid soap. Use soap substitutes, such as emulsifying ointment or a bland bath oil in the bath and a cleansing bar, e.g. DermaVeen.
- General rules for strength of topical corticosteroids:
  - face, axillae and groin—mild potency
  - trunk and limbs—moderately potent, potent if severe
  - hands and feet—potent.
- Emollients (choose from):
  - emulsifying ointment with 1% glycerol
  - sorbolene or sorbolene with 10% glycerol, e.g. Hydraderm
  - paraffin creams (e.g. Dermeze) (good in infants)
  - bath oils, e.g. Alpha-Keri, QV, DermaVeen
  - moisturising lotions (e.g. QV) in dry conditions.
- 1% hydrocortisone (if not responding to above). Use twice daily (if poor response).

Moderate atopic dermatitis

- As for mild eczema.
- Topical corticosteroids (twice daily):
  - vital when condition is active
  - moderate strength (e.g. fluorinated) to trunk, scalp and limbs
  - weaker strength (e.g. 1% hydrocortisone) to face and flexures
  - use in cyclic fashion for chronic cases (e.g. 10 days on, 4 days off).
- Non-steroidal alternative: pimecrolimus (Elidel) cream bd; best used when eczema flares, then cease.
- Oral antihistamines at night for itch.

Severe dermatitis

- As for mild and moderate eczema.
- Potent topical corticosteroids to worst areas (consider occlusive dressings).
- Consider hospitalisation.
- Systemic corticosteroids (may be necessary but rarely used).
- Allergy assessment if unresponsive.

Weeping dermatitis (an acute phase)

This often has crusts due to exudate. Burrow's solution diluted to 1:20 or 1:10 can be used to soak the affected areas.

Tip for children

If severe eczema is not responding to topical treatment, try oral evening primrose oil and/or oral zinc.

General tips

- Skin rehydration is the single most important treatment strategy. Avoid soaps.
- Favour ointments over creams (creams tend to sting and are less potent).
- Topical steroids:
  - potent steroids safe for short periods
  - intermittent rather than continuous use
  - replace with emollients when skin clears.
- Lotions rather than creams are best for moisturising.
- For dry scaly lesions, use ointments with or without occlusion.

PSORIASIS

General adjunctive therapy

- Tar baths, e.g. Pinetarsol or Polytar.
- Tar shampoo (e.g. Polytar, Ionil-T).
- Sunlight (in moderation).

For chronic stable plaques on limbs or trunks

- Coal tar 1% emulsion or gel, once or twice daily for 1 month, or
- LPC 6% + salicylic acid 3% cream or ointment twice daily for 1 month.
  If insufficient or flare, add:
- moderately potent to potent topical corticosteroid ointment, daily until skin is clear (usually 2–6 weeks) or, if inadequate response:
- calcipotriol + betamethasone dipropionate (50 + 500 mcg/g) ointment, daily until skin is clear (usually about 6 weeks).

Once psoriasis is controlled, reduce the potency of steroid and withdraw if possible. Continue tar as maintenance therapy.

Palmoplantar psoriasis

Treat as for trunk and limb psoriasis; however, higher dose of salicylic acid is required if hyperkeratotic, i.e. LPC 6% + salicylic acid 6%. Also consider earlier use of calcipotriol, given common resistance to topical therapy.

For milder stabilised plaques

- EgoPsoryl TA—apply bd or tds, or
- topical fluorinated corticosteroids.

For resistant plaques

- Topical fluorinated corticosteroids (II–III class) with occlusion.
- Intralesional injection of triamcinolone mixed (50:50) with LA or normal saline (see Fig. 3.21).

For failed topical therapy (options)—specialist case

- Refer for PUVA or other effective therapy.
- Acitretin—often used with UVB.
- Methotrexate—can have dramatic results.
- Biologicals, e.g. infliximab, etanercept.

SKIN SCRAPINGS FOR DERMATOPHYTE DIAGNOSIS

Equipment

You will need:
- a scalpel blade
- glass slide and cover slip
- 20% potassium hydroxide (preferably in dimethyl sulfoxide)
- a microscope.

Method

1. Scrape skin from the active edge.
2. Scoop the scrapings onto the glass microscope slide.
3. Cover the sample with a drop of potassium hydroxide.
4. Cover this with a cover slip and press down gently.
5. Warm the slide and wait at least 5 minutes for 'clearing'.

Microscopic examination

1. Examine at first under low power with reduced light.
2. When fungal hyphae are located, change to high power.
3. Use the fine focus to highlight the hyphae (Fig. 16.2).
   Note: Some practice is necessary to recognise hyphae.

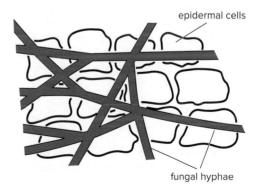

epidermal cells

fungal hyphae

Fig. 16.2 Diagrammatic representation of microscopic appearance of fungal hyphae

SPIDER NAEVI

The most effective treatment of spider naevi for cosmetic reasons is to insert the fine tip of the electrocautery or the hyfrecator (diathermy) needle into the central papule and cauterise the vascular lesion.

No local anaesthetic is required.

WOOD'S LIGHT EXAMINATION

Wood's light examination is an important diagnostic aid for skin problems in general practice. It has other uses, such as examination of the eye after fluorescein staining. Low-cost, small LED ultraviolet light units called 'the black light' are available in many stores and online.

Method

Simply hold the ultraviolet light unit above the area for investigation in a dark room.

Limitations of Wood's light in diagnosis

Not all cases of tinea capitis fluoresce, because some species that cause the condition do not produce porphyrins as a by-product. See Table 16.2 for a list of the skin conditions that do fluoresce.

Table 16.2 Skin conditions that produce fluorescence in Wood's light

Tinea capitis	green
Erythrasma	coral pink
Tinea versicolor	pink
Pseudomonas pyocyanea	yellowish green
Porphyria	red (urine)
Squamous cell carcinoma	bright red

Porphyrins wash off with soap and water, and a negative result may occur in a patient who has shampooed the hair within 20 hours of presentation. Consequently, a negative Wood's light reading may be misleading. The appropriate way of confirming the clinical diagnosis is to send specimens of hair and skin for microscopy and culture.

APPLYING TOPICALS WITH A 'DISH MOP'

The self-application of creams or ointments to relatively inaccessible areas such as the back, especially in the elderly, can be difficult. One method is to acquire an old-fashioned dish mop, give it a 'crew cut' and use this to apply the preparations.

ENHANCING TOPICAL EFFICACY WITH OCCLUSION

- Patients with florid hand dermatitis handicapped by a slow response to topical corticosteroids can be boosted by the application of a surgical glove to wear for 60 minutes after applying the cream or ointment or even overnight if tolerated. This leads to less frequent application.
- Cut out plastic cling wrap on a firm board to the size of the area for treatment—apply the steroid cream or ointment, then the plastic film. Cover with a supportive bandage or a sock with the end cut off.

WATCH BASE ALLERGY

For the common problem of patients prone to nickel sensitivity from a watch, apply clear nail polish to the back of the watch to act as a protective barrier.

CHILBLAINS

Precautions

- Think Raynaud.
- Protect from trauma and secondary infection.
- Do not rub or massage injured tissues.
- Do not apply heat or ice.
- Wear warm gloves and socks.

Physical treatment

- Elevate affected part.
- Warm gradually to room temperature.

Drug Rx

- If severe and recurrent, there is some weak evidence for applying glyceryl trinitrate vasodilator spray or 2% ointment or patch (e.g. Nitro-Bid ointment). Use plastic gloves and wash hands for ointment
  or
- Apply a potent topical corticosteroid.

Other Rx

- Rum at night (worth a try).
- Nifedipine 20 mg bd or CR 30 mg once daily (if very severe)
- UVB therapy weekly for 4 to 6 weeks prior to cold weather.

HERPES SIMPLEX: TREATMENT OPTIONS

Herpes labialis (classical cold sores)

The objective is to limit the size and intensity of the lesions.

Topical treatment

At the first sensation of the development of a cold sore:

- apply an ice cube to the site for up to 5 minutes every 60 minutes (for first 12 hours)

  or

  saturated solution of menthol in SVR.
- topical applications include:
  - idoxuridine 0.5% preparations (Herplex D liquifilm, Stoxil topical, Virasolve) applied hourly

    or
  - povidone-iodine 10% cold sore paint: apply on swab sticks 4 times a day until disappearance

    or
  - acyclovir 5% cream (Zovirax), 5 times daily for 4 days

    or
  - penciclovir 1% cream for 4 days.

  Note: Corticosteroids are contraindicated.

Oral treatment

Acyclovir or famciclovir or valaciclovir for 5 to 10 days or until resolution (reserve for immunocompromised patients and severe cases).

Prevention

If exposure to the sun precipitates the cold sore, use a 30+ or 50+ sun protection lip balm, ointment or solarstick. Zinc sulfate solution can be applied once a week for recurrences. Oral acyclovir 200–400 mg bd or similar agent (6 months) can be used for severe and frequent recurrences (> six per year).

Genital herpes: Antimicrobial therapy

Topical treatment

The proven most effective topical therapy is topical acyclovir (not the ophthalmic preparation).

Alternatives:

- 10% povidone-iodine (Betadine) cold sore paint on swab sticks for several days.

  Pain relief can be provided in some patients with 2% topical lidocaine, but be cautious of hypersensitivity.

  Saline baths and analgesics are advisable.

Oral treatment

Acyclovir for the first episode of primary genital herpes (preferably within 24 hours of onset).

Dosage: 400 mg 3 times a day for 5 to 7 days or until resolution of infection.

Famciclovir or valaciclovir can be given bd for 5 to 10 days.

This appears to reduce the duration of the lesions from 14 days to 5 to 7 days. These drugs are not usually used for recurrent episodes, which last only 5 to 7 days. Very frequent recurrences (six or more attacks in 6 months) benefit from low doses of these agents for 6 months (200 mg 2 to 3 times per day).

HERPES ZOSTER (SHINGLES)

Topical treatment

For the rash, use a drying lotion such as menthol in flexible collodion. Acyclovir ointment can be used but it tends to sting.

Oral medication

1. Analgesics, e.g. paracetamol, codeine or aspirin.
2. Guanine analogue antiviral therapy for:
   - all immunocompromised patients
   - any patient, provided rash present < 72 hours (especially those over 60 years)
   - ophthalmic zoster (evidence–reduces scarring and pain but not neuralgia)
   - severe acute pain.

Drugs and dosage

- acyclovir 800 mg 5 times daily for 7 days

  or
- famciclovir 250 mg 8 hourly for 7 days

  or
- valaciclovir 1000 mg 8 hourly for 7 days.

Post-herpetic neuralgia

Some treatment options are:

1. Topical capsaicin (Capsig) cream. Apply the cream to the affected area 3 to 4 times a day. Give ice massage 20 minutes beforehand.
2. Oral: paracetamol is first line. Second line is a tricyclic antidepressant, gabapentin or pregabalin.
3. TENS as often as necessary, e.g. 16 hours/day for 2 weeks, plus antidepressants.
4. Excision of painful skin scar. If the neuralgia of 4 months or more is localised to a favourable area of skin, a most effective treatment is to excise the affected area, bearing in mind that the scar tends to follow a linear strip of skin. This method is clearly unsuitable for a large area.

Method

1. Mark out the painful area of the skin.
2. Incise it with its subcutaneous fat, using an elongated elliptical excision (Fig. 16.3).
3. Close the wound with a subcuticular suture or interrupted sutures.

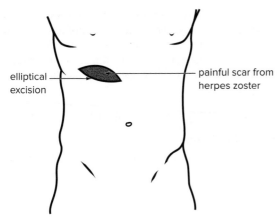

elliptical excision

painful scar from herpes zoster

Fig. 16.3 Example of type of excision for severe post-herpetic neuralgia

UNUSUAL CAUSES OF CONTACT DERMATITIS

Reactions to the following have been reported:

- spirit preparation
- paper-based 'hypoallergenic' tape
- turpentine
- sunscreen (some)
- leather
- cement.

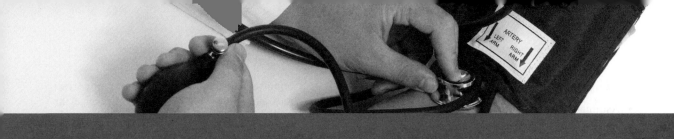

Chapter 17
EMERGENCY PROCEDURES

NORMAL VALUES FOR VITAL SIGNS

Two standard tables (average and normal limits) are shown for comparison.

Table 17.1 Vital signs (average)

	< 6 months	6 months–3 years	3–12 years	Adult
Pulse (beats/min)	120–140	110	80–100	60–100
Respiration rate (breaths/min)	45	30	20	14
BP (mmHg)	90/60	90/60	100/70	≤ 130/85

Source: J. Murtagh, *General Practice Companion Handbook* (7th Edn), 2019, p. xxxix

Table 17.2 Paediatric vital signs: American College of Surgeons

Age (years)	Wt (kg)	Heart rate (bpm)	Blood pressure (mmHg)	Respiratory (/min)	Urine output (mL/kg/hr)
0–1	0–10	< 160	> 60	< 60	2.0
1–3	10–14	< 150	> 70	< 40	1.5
3–5	14–18	< 140	> 75	< 35	1.0
6–12	18–36	< 120	> 80	< 30	1.0
>12	36–70	< 100	> 90	< 30	0.5

PULSE OXIMETRY

The pulse oximeter measures oxygen saturation of arterial blood (SpO_2).

Facts and figures

In a healthy young person the O_2 saturation should be 95-99%. It varies with age, the degree of fitness, current altitude and oxygen therapy. Studies show that Caucasian race, obesity and male sex but not smoking are associated with lower SpO_2 readings.[1]

The ideal value is 97-100%.

The median value in neonates is 97%, in young children 98% and adults 98%.

Target oxygen saturation

- Asthma—the aim is to maintain $SpO_2 > 94\%$
- Acute coronary syndromes $\geq 94\%$
- Opioid effect $\geq 94\%$
- Type 1 (hypoxemic) respiratory failure (e.g. interstitial lung disease, pneumonia, pulmonary oedema) $\geq 94\%$
- Severe COPD with hypercapnoeic respiratory failure 88–92%
- Critical illness (e.g. major trauma, shock) 94–98%
- Children $> 94\%$ ($< 94\%$ is a concern)

Indications for oxygen therapy to be beneficial

- Australian guideline to improve quality of life $> 88\%$
- UK: adults < 50 years 90%, asthma 92.3%

Availability and cost

Pulse oximeters are readily available from medical and surgical suppliers with a range in cost from about $30 to $2000. A good-quality unit is available for about $200 to $400.

ACUTE CORONARY SYNDROMES

In the author's rural practice, over a period of 10 years, the most common cause of sudden death was myocardial infarction, which was responsible for 67% of deaths in the emergency situation. The importance of confirming early diagnosis with the use of the electrocardiogram (ECG) and serum markers, especially troponin, is obvious. A summary of acute coronary syndromes is presented in Table 17.3.

THE ELECTROCARDIOGRAM

Recording a 12-lead ECG

Interesting tips

- The 12-lead ECG uses 10 wires (also known as leads) attached to electrodes.
- There are four limb leads and six chest leads.

- It is important that the leads are placed in correct positions since incorrect positions will change the proper signal and may lead to an incorrect diagnosis.
- The right and left arms are active recording leads.
- The 'standard leads' (I, II, III, aVR, aVL and aVF) are recorded from the limb electrodes.
- The electrodes can be placed far down the limb or close to the hips and shoulders (e.g. in case of an amputee or heavily clothed patient) *but* they must be evenly placed on corresponding sides.
- The right leg lead is used as an electrical ground or reference lead and not used for measurement.
- The leads work effectively through stockings, including pantyhose.

The label of each of the 10 electrodes and their placement is as follows (Fig. 17.1):

- RA: on right arm (avoid thick muscles)
- LA: same location to RA but on left arm
- RL: on right leg, lateral calf muscle
- LL: same location as RL but on left leg
- V1: in 4th intercostal space—between ribs 4 and 5, just to right of sternum
- V2: as above but just to left of the sternum
- V3: between leads V2 and V4
- V4: in 5th intercostal space in mid-clavicular line
- V5: at the same level with V4 and V5 in anterior-axillary line
- V6: at the same level with V4 and V5 in mid-axillary line.

Areas 'looked at' by the standard leads are shown in Figure 17.2.

Interpreting rate and rhythm

Rate

- R to R interval (i.e. from the pointy tip of one QRS to the next): $300 \div$ number of big squares between the QRS complexes.
- For an irregular rhythm use the 6-second method: 5 big squares = 1 second; 30 big squares = 6 seconds.
- Count QRS complexes in 6 seconds and multiply by 10.

Table 17.3 Types of acute coronary syndromes

	Serum markers		ECG at evaluation
	Creatinine kinase	Troponin	
Unstable angina			
• low risk	normal	not raised	normal
• high risk	normal	raised	ST depression
Myocardial infarction			
• non-ST elevation	elevated	raised	ST depression no Q wave
• ST elevation (STEMI)	elevated	raised	± Q wave

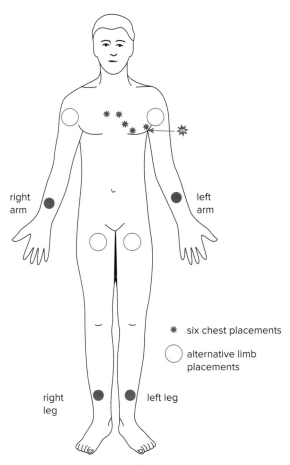

Fig. 17.1 The 12-lead ECG

Table 17.4 Which lead looks at which part of the heart?[2]

Area of the heart	Leads
Inferior wall	II, III, aVF
Anterior wall	V1 to V5
Lateral wall	V5, V6, I, aVL
Posterior wall	V1 to V3 (maybe)

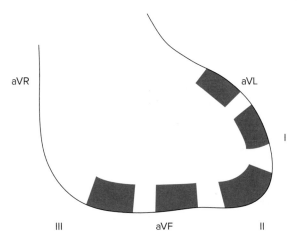

Fig. 17.2 Areas of the heart 'looked at' by the standard leads

Rhythm

Based on QRS complexes, use a piece of paper to mark the spaces between the QRS complexes and move the paper along the rhythm strip to assess their regularity (e.g. Fig. 17.3). Is it regular or irregular? If it is irregular, is there a regular pattern or are they irregularly irregular?

The ECG and myocardial infarction

From Figure 17.4 it is apparent that:

- the leads overlying the anterior surface of the left ventricle will be V2-5 and these will be the leads giving evidence of anterior infarction
- the leads overlying the lateral surface will be the lateral chest leads V5-6
- no leads directly overlie the inferior or diaphragmatic surfaces. However, the left leg leads, although distant, are in line with this surface and will show evidence of infarction in this area
- no leads directly overlie the posterior surface.

Typical acute inferior infarction

The typical ECG changes of acute myocardial infarction (AMI) with pathological Q waves, S-T segment elevation

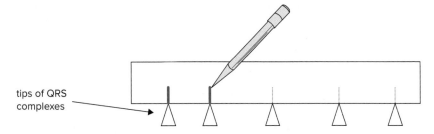

Fig. 17.3 Method of assessing the rate and rhythm from the ECG

left lateral view

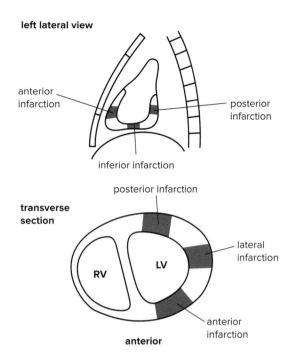

Fig. 17.4 Areas of heart wall affected by myocardial infarction

Reproduced from J. Murtagh, *GP Companion Handbook* (5th Edn), McGraw-Hill, Sydney, 2010.[3]

and T wave inversion are highlighted in leads III and aVL of acute inferior infarction (Fig. 17.5). Lead aVL facing the opposite side of the heart shows reciprocal S-T depression.

Atypical acute anterior infarction pattern is demonstrated in Figure 17.6. This ECG strip shows sinus rhythm with a rate of 75 ($300 \div 4$).

URGENT INTRAVENOUS CUTDOWN

In emergencies, especially those due to acute blood loss, intravenous cannulation for the infusion of fluids or transfusion of blood can be difficult. For the short-term situation, a surgical cutdown into the long saphenous vein at the ankle or the cephalic vein at the wrist can be lifesaving. Ideally, use the long saphenous vein in children.

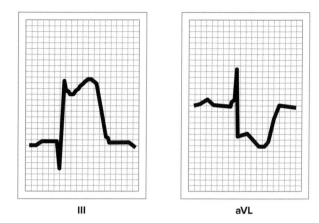

Fig. 17.5 Two leads from ECG of AMI (inferior infarction)

Reproduced from J. Murtagh, *General Practice Companion Handbook* (5th Edn), McGraw-Hill, Sydney, 2019.[3]

Surface anatomy

Long saphenous vein: The vein lies at the anterior tip of the medial malleolus. The best site for incision is centred about 2 cm proximal to and 2 cm anterior to the most prominent medial bony eminence (Fig. 17.7a).

Cephalic vein: The cephalic vein 'bisects' the bony eminences of the distal end of the radius as it winds around the radius from the dorsum of the hand to the anterior surface of the forearm. The incision site is about 2–3 cm proximal to the tip of the radial styloid (Fig. 17.7b).

Equipment

You will need:
- scalpel and blade (disposable)
- small curved artery forceps
- aneurysm needle (optional—a blunt metal hook for lifting vein)
- vein scissors (small, sharp surgical scissors)
- absorbable suture material
- vein elevator (optional—a blunt right-angled probe to slide into vein)
- intravenous catheter.

A dedicated 'cutdown kit' would be ideal.

Table 17.5 Region of heart wall assessed by ECG

Region of heart wall	Artery occluded	Leads showing ECG changes (ST elevation)
Anterior	L anterior descending (LAD)	V2–V5, I, aVL
Lateral	Circumflex, branch of LAD	V5–V6, (occ'y I, aVL)
Anteroseptal	LAD	V1–V4
Inferior	R coronary	II, III, aVF, aVL (reciprocal)
Posterior	RCA or circumflex	V1–V2 (unclear, reciprocal)
Subendocardial	Non specific	Any lead

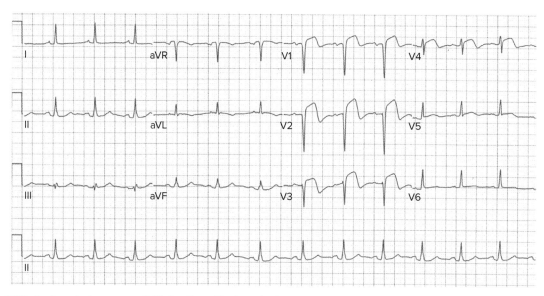

Fig. 17.6 Acute anterior myocardial infarction with sinus rhythm

Reproduced from Duncan Guy, *Pocket Guide to ECGs* (2nd Edn), McGraw-Hill, Sydney, 2010.[4]

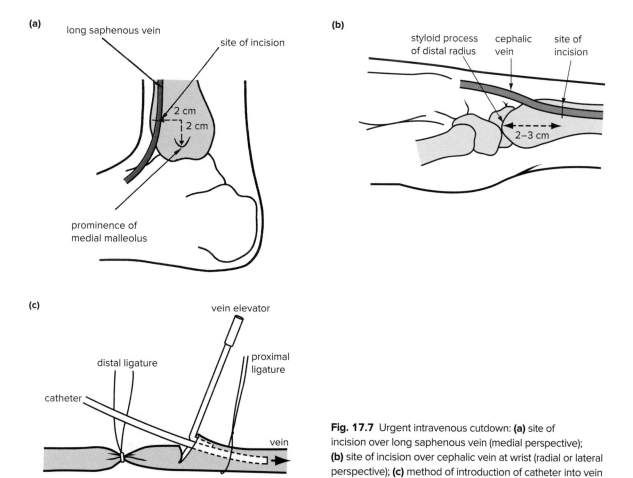

Fig. 17.7 Urgent intravenous cutdown: **(a)** site of incision over long saphenous vein (medial perspective); **(b)** site of incision over cephalic vein at wrist (radial or lateral perspective); **(c)** method of introduction of catheter into vein

Method of cutdown

After fitting gloves and using a skin preparation:

1. Make a 1.5–2 cm transverse skin incision over the vein.
2. Locate the vein by blunt dissection. (Do not confuse the vein with the pearly white tendons.)
3. Loop an aneurysm needle or fine curved artery forceps under and around the vein.
4. Place a ligature around the distal vein and use this to steady the vein.
5. Place a loose-knotted ligature over the proximal end of the vein, ready for later use.
6. Incise the vein transversely with a small lancet or scissors or by a carefully controlled stab with a scalpel.
7. Use a vein elevator (if available) for the best possible access to the vein.
8. Insert the catheter (Fig. 17.7c).
9. Gently tie the proximal vein to the catheter.
10. After connecting to the intravenous set and checking the flow of fluid, close the wound with a suitable suture material.

INTRAOSSEOUS INFUSION

In an emergency situation where intravenous access in a collapsed person (especially children) is difficult, parenteral fluid can be infused into the bone marrow (an intravascular space). Intraosseous infusion is preferred to a cutdown in children under 5 years. It is useful to practise the technique on a chicken bone.

Site of infusion:

- adults and children over 5: distal end of tibia (2–3 cm proximal to medial malleolus)
- infants and children under 5: proximal end of tibia
- the distal femur: 2–3 cm above condyles in midline is an alternative (angle needle upwards).

Avoid growth plates, midshafts (which can fracture) and the sternum. Complications include tibial fracture and compartment syndrome.

Note: Any fluid or drug that can be given by IV can be given by intraosseous infusion.

Method for proximal tibia

Note: Strict asepsis is essential (skin preparation and sterile gloves).

1. Inject local anaesthetic (if necessary).
2. Choose a 16-gauge intraosseous needle (Dieckmann modification) or a 16- to 18-gauge lumbar puncture needle (less expensive).
3. Hold it at right angles to the anteromedial surface of the proximal tibia about 2 cm below the tibial tuberosity (Fig. 17.8). Point the needle slightly downwards, away from the joint space.

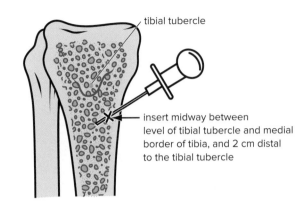

tibial tubercle

insert midway between level of tibial tubercle and medial border of tibia, and 2 cm distal to the tibial tubercle

Fig. 17.8 Intraosseous infusion

4. Carefully twist the needle to penetrate the bone cortex; it enters bone marrow (medulla) with a sensation of giving way (considerable pressure usually required).
5. Remove the trocar, aspirate a small amount of marrow (blood and fat) or test with an 'easy' injection of 5 mL saline to ensure its position.
6. Hold the needle in place with a small POP splint. A temporary splint can be fashioned out of a polystyrene cup split down one side, heavily taped to the limb.
7. Fluid can be infused with a normal IV infusion—rapidly or slowly. If the initial flow rate is slow, flush out with 5–10 mL of saline.
8. The infusion rate can be markedly increased by using a pressure bag at 300 mmHg pressure (up to 1000 mL in 5 minutes).

ACUTE PARAPHIMOSIS

In paraphimosis the penile foreskin is retracted, swollen and painful. Manual reduction should be attempted first. This can be done without anaesthesia, but a penile block with local anaesthetic (never use adrenaline in LA) can easily be injected in a ring around the base of the penis. The two dorsal nerves lie on either side of the midline dorsal vessels.

Method 1

Manual reduction can be performed by trying to advance the prepuce over the engorged glans with the index fingers while compressing the glans with the thumb (Fig. 17.9a).

Method 2

1. Take hold of the oedematous part of the glans in the fist of one hand and squeeze firmly. A gauze swab or warm towelette will help to achieve a firm grip (Fig. 17.9b).
2. Exert continuous pressure until the oedema passes under the constricting collar to the shaft of the penis.
3. The foreskin can then usually be pulled over the glans.

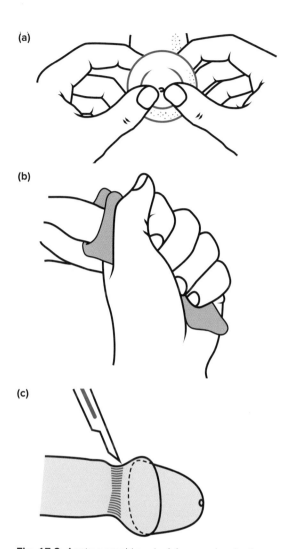

Fig. 17.9 Acute paraphimosis: **(a)** manual reduction; **(b)** squeezing with swab; **(c)** dorsal slit incision in the constricting collar of skin

Method 3

If manual reduction methods fail, a dorsal slit incision should be made in the constricting collar of skin proximal to the glans under local or light general anaesthesia (Fig. 17.9c). The incision allows the foreskin to be advanced and reduces the swelling. Follow-up circumcision should be performed.

Method 4

Cover the swollen oedematous prepuce with fine crystalline sugar and wrap a cut rubber glove over it to exert continuous pressure. Leave for 1 to 2 hours. The foreskin can then be readily retracted.

DIAGNOSING THE HYSTERICAL 'UNCONSCIOUS' PATIENT

One of the most puzzling problems in emergency medicine is how to diagnose the unconscious patient caused by a conversion reaction. These patients really experience their symptoms (as opposed to the pretending patient) and resist most normal stimuli, including painful stimuli.

Method

1. Hold the patient's eye or eyes open with your fingers and note the reaction to light.
2. Now hold a mirror over the eye and watch closely for pupillary reaction (Fig. 17.10). The pupil should constrict with accommodation from the patient looking at his or her own image.
3. Hold the patient's hand above their face and let go. Observe if the falling hand is pulled away from the face.

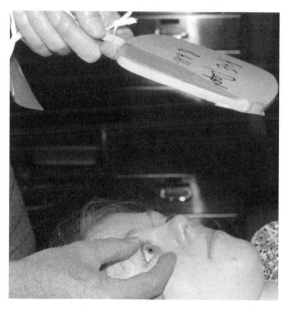

Fig. 17.10 Testing for pupillary reaction

ELECTRIC SHOCK

Household shocks tend to cause cardiac arrest due to ventricular fibrillation (Fig. 17.11).

Principles of management

- Make the site safe: switch off the electricity. Use dry wool to insulate the rescuers.
- 'Treat the clinically dead.'
- Attend to the ABC of resuscitation.
- Give a praecordial thump in a witnessed arrest.
- Consider a cervical collar (? cervical fracture).
- Provide basic cardiopulmonary resuscitation, including defibrillation (as required).

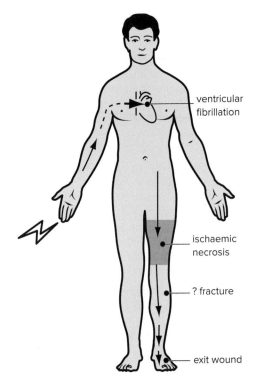

ventricular fibrillation

ischaemic necrosis

? fracture

exit wound

Fig. 17.11 Effect of electric shock passing through the body

- Give a lidocaine infusion (100 mg IV) after cardiac arrest.
- Investigate and consider:
  - careful examination of all limbs
  - X-ray of limbs or spine as appropriate
  - check for myoglobinuria and renal failure
  - give tetanus and clostridial prophylaxis.
- Get expert help—intensive care unit, burns unit.

HEAD INJURY

Head injury is the main cause of death in major trauma. The Glasgow coma scale (Table 17.6) can be used to assess a patient's cerebral status. A useful simplified method of recording the conscious state is the AVPU system below. Assess the *A* first and, if that fails, work down the list to record the best response.

A alert (still applies even if confused)

V verbal (e.g. responds by opening eyes to the verbal 'Are you okay?')

P pain (e.g. winces or groans to the pain of a sternal rub or finger squeeze)

U unresponsive (unconscious)

Glasgow coma scale

The Glasgow coma scale (GCS) is frequently used as an objective guide to the conscious state (Table 17.6).

If the GCS score is:
- 8 or less: severe head injury
- 9 to 10: serious
- 11 to 12: moderate
- 13 to 15: minor.

Arrange urgent referral if the score is less than 12. If the score is 12 to 15, keep under observation for at least 6 hours.

Table 17.6 Glasgow coma scale

	Score
Eye opening (E)	
• Spontaneous opening	4
• To verbal command	3
• To pain	2
• No response	1
Motor response (M)	
• Obeys verbal command	6
Response to painful stimuli	
• Localises pain	5
• Withdraws from pain stimuli	4
• Abnormal flexion	3
• Extensor response	2
• No response	1
Verbal response (V)	
• Orientated and converses	5
• Disorientated and converses	4
• Inappropriate words	3
• Incomprehensible sounds	2
• No response	1
Coma score E + M +	
• Minimum 3	
• Maximum 15	

Emergency exploratory burr hole

After a head injury, a rapidly developing mass lesion (classically extradural) is heralded by a deteriorating conscious level (e.g. Glasgow coma scale drops from 13–15 to 3–6); a rising blood pressure (e.g. rises from 140/70 to 160/100 mmHg); slowing respirations (from 16 to 10); a slowing pulse (from 70 to 55) and a dilating pupil. In such conditions an urgent burr hole is indicated, even in the absence of a plain X-ray and a CT scan of the head. Even elevating a depressed fracture may be sufficient to alleviate the pressure. The relative sites of extradural and subdural haematomas are shown in Figure 17.12 and the classic development of the extradural haematoma in Figure 17.13. This procedure may be life-saving in a rural or remote location.

Method (in absence of neurosurgical facilities)

- This is ideally performed in an operating theatre.[5]
- The patient is induced, paralysed, intubated and ventilated (100% oxygen). Dehydrating dose of 20% mannitol (1 g/kg IV in 1 hour) administered.

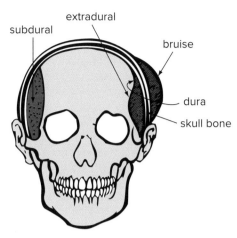

Fig. 17.12 The sites of subdural and extradural haematomas in relation to the dura, skull and brain

- After shaving the scalp, a mark is made over the site of external bruising, especially if a clinical fracture is obvious. A 5 cm long incision is made over the site of external bruising or swelling. Otherwise the burr hole is made in the low temporal area. A vertical incision is made above the zygoma 2.5 cm in front of the external auditory meatus and extending down to the zygoma, and the skull is trephined 2–3 cm above it (Fig. 17.14). This is the site of the classic middle meningeal haemorrhage.
- The clot is gently aspirated and the skin is loosely sutured around the drain.
- If there are difficulties controlling the bleeding, the intracranial area is packed with wet balls of Gelfoam or similar material.
- Other areas that can be explored in the presence of subdural haematoma include:
  - frontal region: a suspicion of an anterior fossa haematoma (e.g. a black eye)

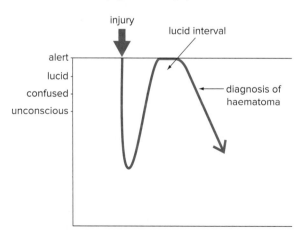

Fig. 17.13 Classic conscious states characteristic of extradural haematoma after injury

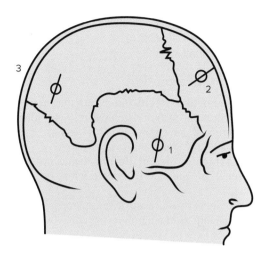

Fig. 17.14 Three sites suggested for burr holes: **(1)** low in the temporal region will disclose a classic middle meningeal artery bleed; on division of the muscle, haematoma should be found between the muscle and the fracture line; **(2)** frontal region; **(3)** parietal region

  - parietal region: haematoma from the posterior branch of the middle meningeal artery (Fig. 17.14).

ASSESSING SEXUAL ASSAULT

Your first offer should be to provide privacy, confidentiality and emotional support.

Four important things to say initially to any victim

- 'You are safe now.'
- 'I am sorry this happened to you.'
- 'It was not your fault.'
- 'It's good that you are seeing me.'

Initial advice to the victim

- If victim reporting to police
  1. Notify the police at once.
  2. Take along a witness to the alleged assault (if there was a witness).
  3. Do not wash or tidy yourself or change your clothing.
  4. Do not take any alcohol or drugs.
  5. Don't drink or wash out your mouth if there was oral assault.
  6. Take a change of warm clothing.
- If not reporting to police or unsure
  Contact any of the following:
  1. a friend or other responsible person
  2. 1800RESPECT (national sexual assault and domestic family violence service), or 'Lifeline'

3. a state-based sexual assault service (searchable on 1800RESPECT website)
4. a counselling service.

Obtaining information

1. Obtain consent to record and release information.
2. Take a careful history and copious relevant notes.
3. Keep a record, have a protocol.
4. Obtain a kit for examination.
5. Have someone present during the examination (especially in the case of male doctors examining women).
6. Air-dry swabs (media destroy spermatozoa).
7. Hand specimens to the police immediately.
8. Work with (not for) the police.

Examination

If possible, the victim should be dressed when seen. When the victim is undressing for examination, get them to stand on a white sheet. This helps to identify small foreign objects that fall to the floor.

Note any injuries as each item of clothing is removed. Each part of the body should be examined under good illumination, and all injuries measured and recorded carefully on a diagram.

Injuries should be photographed professionally. Perform a careful speculum examination in women. Palpate the scalp for hidden trauma. Collect appropriate swabs.

Making reports

Remember that as a doctor you are impartial. Never make inappropriate judgements to authorities (e.g. 'This patient was raped' or 'Incest was committed').

Rather, say: 'There is evidence (or no evidence) to support penetration of the vagina/anus' or 'There is evidence of trauma to _____'.

Handy tips

- Remember that some experienced perpetrators carry lubricants or amyl nitrate to dilate the anal sphincter.
- Urine examination in female children may show sperm. (If the child is uncharacteristically passing urine at night, get the mother to collect a specimen.)
- Vaginal and rectal swabs should be air-dried.
- For suspected abuse of children, you cannot work in isolation: refer to a sexual assault centre or share the complex problem.

Post-examination

After the medical examination a discussion of medical problems should take place with the patient. This should be done in private and kept totally confidential.

A management plan for physical injuries and emotional problems is discussed.

Consider the possibility of STI and possible referral. Consider also the possibility of pregnancy and the need for postcoital hormone tablets. Organise follow-up counselling and STI screening.

Management issues

- Take swabs and/or first-void specimen for testing gonococcus and chlamydia (PCR).
- Take blood for HIV, syphilis.
- Collect specimens—swab aspirate of any fluid and keep for DNA analysis.
- Give prophylactic antibiotics—depends on type of assault and assailant.
- Emergency contraception.
- Review in 3 weeks—check tests.
- Screen for syphilis and HIV in about 3 months.
- Refer to rape crisis centre.

Drug-facilitated sexual assault

Consider this when patient has no memory of events and time or other suspicious circumstances. Urine or blood testing may be appropriate.

MIGRAINE TIPS

At first symptoms of common or classic migraine:
- start drinking 1 litre of water over 20 minutes
- aspirin or paracetamol + anti-emetic, e.g.
  - soluble aspirin 600–900 mg (o) and
  - metoclopramide 10 mg (o)
  - if vomiting: metoclopramide 10 mg dissolved sublingually.

For established migraine:
- IV metoclopramide 10 mg, then 10 to 15 minutes later give 2 to 3 soluble aspirin and/or codeine tablets

  or
- IM metoclopramide 10 mg, then 20 minutes later IM dihydroergotamine 0.5–1 mg

  or
- lidocaine 4% topical solution—as spray 2.5 mL per nares

  or
- serotonin receptor agonist, such as:
  - sumatriptan (o), SC injection or nasal spray

    or
  - zolmitriptan (o), repeat in 2 hours if necessary

    or
  - naratriptan (o), repeat in 4 hours if necessary. If very severe (and other preparations are unsuccessful):
- haloperidol 5 mg IM or IV.

  Note: Avoid pethidine.

The IV fluid load method

Many practitioners claim to obtain rapid relief of migraine by giving 1 L of intravenous fluid over 20 to 30 minutes, supplemented by oral paracetamol. However, trials demonstrate no or minimal benefit over treatments listed above, so it should probably be reserved for the vomiting, dehydrated patient.[6]

Intravenous lidocaine

Lidocaine (1% solution intravenously) can give rapid relief to many people with classic or common migraine.

The dose is 1 mg lidocaine per kg (maximum) (a 70 kg adult would have a maximum dose of 7 mL of 1% solution). The IV injection is given slowly over about 90 seconds with monitoring of pulse and blood pressure.

HYPERVENTILATION

Improvised methods to help alleviate the distress of anxiety-provoked hyperventilation include:
- Breathe in and out of a paper bag.
- Breathe in and out slowly and deeply into cupped hands.
- Suck ice blocks slowly (a good distractor).

PNEUMOTHORAX

Pneumothoraces can be graded according to the degree of collapse:
- small: up to 15% (of pleural cavity)
- moderate: 15–60%
- large: > 60%.

A small pneumothorax is usually treated conservatively and undergoes spontaneous resolution.

Simple aspiration can be used for a small to moderate pneumothorax—usually 15–20%.

Traumatic and tension pneumothoraces represent potential life-threatening disorders.

Tension pneumothorax requires immediate management.

Intercostal catheter

A life-saving procedure for a tension pneumothorax is the insertion of an intercostal catheter (a 14-gauge intravenous cannula is ideal) or even a needle as small as 19-gauge (if necessary) into the second intercostal space in the midclavicular line along the upper edge of the third rib. The site should be at least two finger-breadths from the edge of the sternum, so that damage to the internal mammary artery is avoided. The catheter is connected to an underwater seal.

An alternative site, which is preferable in females for cosmetic reasons, is in the mid-axillary line of the fourth or fifth intercostal space (Fig. 17.15).

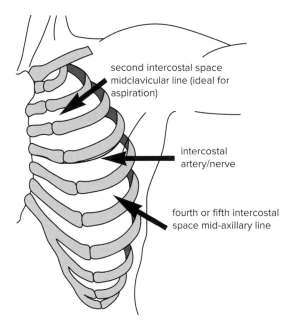

second intercostal space midclavicular line (ideal for aspiration)

intercostal artery/nerve

fourth or fifth intercostal space mid-axillary line

Fig. 17.15 Positioning of intercostal catheter

Simple aspiration for pneumothorax

For patients presenting with pneumothorax, the traditional method of insertion of an intercostal catheter connected to underwater seal drainage may be avoided with simpler measures. Patients with a small pneumothorax (less than 15% lung collapse) can be managed conservatively.[7] Larger uncomplicated cases can be managed by simple aspiration using a 16-gauge polyethylene intravenous catheter.

Method

1. The patient lies propped up to 30–40°.
2. Infiltrate LA in the skin over the second intercostal space in the midclavicular line on the affected site.
3. Insert a 16-gauge polyethylene intravenous catheter into the pleural space under strict asepsis.
4. Aspirate air into a 20 mL syringe to confirm entry into this space, and then remove the stilette.
5. Connect a flexible extension tube to this catheter, and then connect this tube to a three-way tap and a 50 mL syringe.
6. Aspirate and expel air via the three-way tap until resistance indicates lung re-expansion.

Obtain a follow-up X-ray. Repeat aspiration may be necessary, but most patients do not require inpatient admission.

CRICOTHYROIDOTOMY

This procedure may be life-saving when endotracheal intubation is either contraindicated or impossible. It may have to be improvised or performed with commercially available kits such as the Surgitech Rapitrac kit or the Portex Mini-Trach II kit. Cricothyroidotomy can be performed using a standard endotracheal tube, from which the excess portion may be excised after insertion.

Method for adults

1. The patient should be supine, with the head, neck and chin fully extended (Fig. 17.16a).
2. Operate from behind the patient's head.
3. Palpate the groove between the cricoid and thyroid cartilage.
4. Make a short (2 cm) transverse incision (or longitudinal) through the skin and a smaller incision through the cricothyroid membrane (Fig. 17.16b).
   • Ensure the incision is not made above the thyroid cartilage.
   • Local anaesthesia (1–2 mL of 1% lidocaine) will be necessary in some patients.
     An artery clip or tracheal spreader may be inserted into the opening to enlarge it sufficiently to admit a cuffed endotracheal or tracheostomy tube.
5. Use an introducer to guide the cannula into the trachea.
6. Insert an endotracheal or tracheostomy tube if available.
   Since damage to the cricoid cartilage is a concern in children, surgical cricothyroidotomy is not recommended for children under 12 years of age.

Method for children

1. Do not perform a stab wound in children because of poor healing.
2. Use a 14- to 15-gauge intravenous cannula attached to a 5 mL syringe.
3. Pierce the cricothyroid membrane at an angle of 45°, aiming distally. Free aspiration of air confirms correct placement.
4. Fit a 3 mm endotracheal tube connector into the end of the cannula or a 7 mm connector into a 2 mL or 5 mL syringe barrel connected to the cannula.
5. Attach the connector to the oxygen circuit; this system 'buys time' by allowing oxygenation for about 30 minutes but carbon dioxide retention will occur. Ideally, the oxygen enriched air should be humidified.

Improvisation tips

1. Any piece of plastic tubing, or even the 'shell' of a ballpoint pen, will suffice as a makeshift airway.
2. A 2 mL or 5 mL syringe barrel will suffice as a connector between the cannula and the oxygen source.

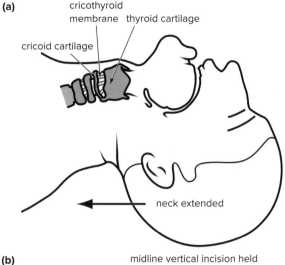

(a)

cricothyroid membrane thyroid cartilage
cricoid cartilage
neck extended

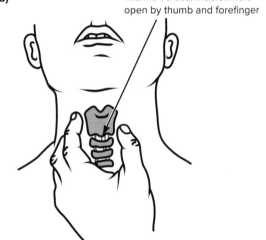

(b)

midline vertical incision held open by thumb and forefinger

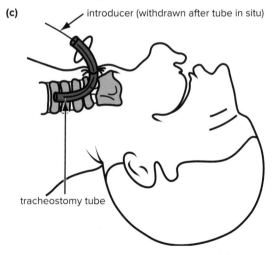

(c)

introducer (withdrawn after tube in situ)
tracheostomy tube

Fig. 17.16 Cricothyroidotomy

CHOKING

Children: Encourage coughing. If unsuccessful, place the child over your knees with head down and give hard blows with the heel of your hand to the upper back (5 to 10 blows). Also chest compression to depress the chest by one-third of its diameter can be used. In older children, get them to lean over you as you deliver blows to the back.

Adults: Encourage coughing. If unsuccessful, first-line treatment is to give 5 firm blows to the upper back followed by 5 chest thrusts or 5 abdominal thrusts (not in child < 8 years) if necessary.

The Heimlich manoeuvre

This procedure is most useful for an adult with an impacted foreign body in the pharynx.

Method

1. Remove any dentures and try hooking out the bolus with a finger. Ask them to cough.
2. Standing behind the patient, the rescuer links both arms firmly to make a fist over the epigastrium 2 finger breaths below the xiphisternum (keep the elbows out).
3. Following one of the patient's gasps, a firm squeeze is given to the upper abdomen. If necessary, this is repeated every 10 seconds for half a minute.

Problems with procedure

- Wrong position
- Damage to underlying organs and structures
- May precipitate regurgitation of stomach contents

SUPRA VENTRICULAR TACHYCARDIA (SVT)

The older, simple methods used to treat SVT, including carotid sinus massage, are now regarded as unsafe, especially in the elderly. A method that is now used routinely in emergency departments is to ask the patient to blow into a plastic syringe.

Method

Slightly loosen the plunger of a 20 mL syringe and ask the patient to blow into the tip of the syringe, attempting to move the plunger. This type of Valsalva manoeuvre may abort the tachycardia. Another method is to briefly immerse the patient's face in cold water.

For failed procedure

Give IV adenosine or verapamil.

BITE WOUNDS

Snake bites

Most bites do not result in envenomation, which tends to occur in snake handlers, inebriated subjects or in circumstances where the snake has a clear bite of the skin.

First aid

1. Keep the patient as still as possible.
2. Do not wash, cut or manipulate the wound, or apply ice or use a tourniquet.
3. Immediately bandage the bite site firmly (similar pressure to sprained ankle bandage—not too tight). A crepe bandage is ideal: it should extend above the bite site for 15 cm, e.g. if bitten around the ankle, the bandage should cover the leg to the knee.
4. Splint the limb to immobilise it: a firm stick or slab of wood would be ideal.
5. Transport to a medical facility for definite treatment. Do not give alcoholic beverages or stimulants.
6. If the snake is dead, bring it along.

Note: A venom detection kit can be used to examine a swab of the bitten area or a fresh urine specimen (the best) or blood.

The bandage can be removed when the patient is safely under medical observation. Observe for symptoms such as vomiting, abdominal pain, excessive perspiration, severe headache and blurred vision.

Treatment of envenomation

1. Set up a slow IV infusion of N saline.
2. Give IV antihistamine cover (15 minutes beforehand) and 0.3 mL of adrenaline 1:1000 SC (0.1 mL for a child).
3. Dilute the specific antivenom (1:10 in N saline) and infuse slowly over 30 minutes via the tubing of the saline solution.
4. Have adrenaline on standby.
5. Monitor vital signs.

Spider bites

First aid

Sydney funnel-web: as for snake bites.
Other spiders: apply ice pack, do not bandage.

Treatment of envenomation

- Sydney funnel-web:
  - specific antivenom
  - resuscitation and other supportive measures.

- Red-back spider:
  - give oral antihistamines and analgesia, as well as ice pack to bite site
  - antivenom IM (IV if severe) is controversial—seek expert advice.

Human bites and clenched fist injuries

Human bites, including clenched fist injuries, often become infected by organisms such as *Staphylococcus aureus,* streptococcus species and beta-lactamase producing anaerobic bacteria.

Principles of treatment

- Clean and debride the wound carefully, e.g. aqueous antiseptic solution or hydrogen peroxide.
- Give prophylactic penicillin if a severe or deep bite.
- Avoid suturing if possible.
- Tetanus toxoid.
- Consider rare possibility of HIV, hepatitis B or C, or infections.

For wound infection

- Take swab.
- Procaine penicillin 1 g IM, plus Augmentin 500 mg, 8 hourly for 5 days.

For severe penetrating injuries (e.g. joints, tendons)

- IV antibiotics for 7 days.

Dog bites (non-rabid)

Animal bites are also prone to infection by the same organisms as for humans, plus *Pasteurella multocida.*

Principles of treatment

- Clean and debride the wound with aqueous antiseptic, allowing it to soak for 10 to 20 minutes.
- Aim for open healing—avoid suturing if possible (except in 'privileged' sites with an excellent blood supply, such as the face and scalp).
- Apply non-adherent, absorbent dressings (paraffin gauze and Melolin) to absorb the discharge from the wound.
- Tetanus prophylaxis: immunoglobulin or tetanus toxoid.
- Give prophylactic penicillin for a severe or deep bite: 1.5 g of procaine penicillin IM statim, then orally for 5 days. Tetracycline or flucloxacillin are alternatives.
- Inform the patient that slow healing and scarring are possible.

Cat bites

Cat bites have the most potential for suppurative infection. The same principles apply as for management of human or dog bites, but use flucloxacillin. It is important to clean a deep and penetrating wound. Another problem is cat-scratch disease, presumably caused by a Gram-negative bacterium.

Sandfly (biting midges) bites

These blood sucking insects are a problem in sandy areas such as beaches by day, and mangroves and dense forests at night. Cover skin with clothing and insect repellant.

Oral thiamine (100 mg daily) has long been purported to prevent sandfly bites, although no credible academic evidence supports this.[8]

For relief of itching apply an anti-itch cream and consider oral anti-histamines if severe.

Bed bug bites

The common bed bug (*Cimex lectularis,* Fig. 17.17) is now a major problem related to international travel. It travels in baggage and is widely distributed in hotels, motels and backpacker accommodation. Clinically, bites are usually seen in children and teenagers. The presentation is a linear group of three or more bites (along the line of superficial blood vessels), which are extremely itchy. They appear as maculopapular red lesions with possible wheals. The lesions are commonly found on the neck, shoulders, arms, torso and legs. A bed bug infestation can be diagnosed by identification of specimens collected from the infested residence. Look for red- or rust-coloured specks about 5 mm long on mattresses.

Management

- Clean the lesions.
- Apply a corticosteroid ointment.
- A simple anti-pruritic agent may suffice.
- Call in a licensed pest controller.

Control treatment is basically directed towards applying insecticides to the crevices in walls and furniture. *Tip:* If a backpack is thought to harbour the bugs, put it in the freezer overnight.

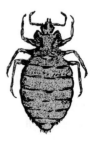

Fig. 17.17 Bed bug

STINGS

Bee stings

First aid

1. Scrape the sting off sideways with a fingernail or knife blade. Do not squeeze it with the fingertips.
2. Apply 20% aluminium sulfate solution (Stingose).
3. Apply ice to the site.
4. Rest and elevate the limb that has been stung.
   If anaphylaxis occurs, treat accordingly.

Centipede and scorpion bites

The main symptom is pain, which can be very severe and prolonged. Australian scorpion species rarely cause significant systemic symptoms.

First aid

1. Apply local heat, e.g. hot water with ammonia (household bleach).
2. Clean site.
3. Local anaesthetic, e.g. 1–2 mL of 1% lidocaine infiltrated around the site.
4. Check tetanus immunisation status.

Other bites and stings

This includes bites from ants, wasps, fleas and mosquitoes.

First aid

1. Wash the site with large quantities of cool water. Consider soapy water for mosquito bites.
2. Apply vinegar (liberal amount) or 20% aluminium sulfate solution (Stingose) to the wound for about 30 seconds.
3. Apply ice for several minutes.
4. Use soothing anti-itch cream e.g. hydrocortisone 0.5 or 1% cream or 5% lidocaine cream or ointment if very painful.
   Medication is not usually necessary, although for a jellyfish sting the direct application of Antistine-Privine drops onto the sting (after washing the site) is effective.
   Special tip: A cost-effective and antipruritic agent for insect stings is topical Mylanta or similar antacid, containing aluminium sulfate or hydroxide.

Bluebottle and other stinging jellyfish

(excludes box jellyfish and *Carukia barnesi*)

- Wash sting site with sea water.
- Remove any tentacles with sea water or gloved hands.
- Immerse affected part in tolerably hot water—ideally 45° for 20 minutes (test tolerance on other limbs).
- Give oral paracetamol ASAP.

Box jellyfish (*Chironex fleckeri:* the sea wasp)

Treatment

1. The victim should be removed from the water to prevent drowning.
2. Inactivate the tentacles by pouring vinegar over them for 30 seconds (do not use alcohol)—use up to 2 L of vinegar at a time. Gently remove the tentacles.
3. Check respiration and the pulse.
4. Start immediate cardiopulmonary resuscitation (if necessary).
5. Give box jellyfish antivenom by IV injection.
6. Provide pain relief if required (ice, lidocaine and analgesics).

Stinging fish and stingrays

The sharp spines of stinging fish and stingrays have venom glands that can produce severe pain if they spike or even graze the skin. The best known of these is the stonefish. The toxin is usually heat sensitive.

Treatment

1. Bathe or immerse the affected part in very warm to hot water (not scalding; test on other limbs. Aim at 45°C[9] (measured with a thermometer) for 20 minutes). This may give instant relief. If immersion or hot water is not available, heat packs are suitable.
2. If pain persists, give a local injection/infiltration of lidocaine 1% or even a regional block. If still persisting, try pyroxidine 50 mg intralesional injection.
3. A specific antivenom is available for the sting of the stonefish.
Note: Heat immersion is worth trying for other marine 'stingers' such as the bluebottle jellyfish.

CORAL CUTS

Treatment

1. Carefully debride the wound.
2. If infected, phenoxymethyl penicillin 500 mg (o), 6-hourly.

USE OF THE ADRENALINE AUTOINJECTOR FOR ANAPHYLAXIS

Dose

- Adult and child > 30 kg: 300 mcg
- Child 15–30 kg (usually 1–5 years): 125 mcg

Types

- EpiPen

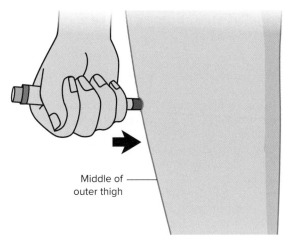

Middle of —— outer thigh

Fig. 17.18 Method of using autoinjector

Method

- Hold the pen tightly in the palm of the hand with the needle tip down.
- Place the needle tip gently against the mid-outer thigh in the 'fleshiest' part of the muscle (with or without clothing). It should be perpendicular to the thigh.
- Push down *hard* against the thigh until you hear or feel a 'CLICK' (in case of the EpiPen) or for the Anapen press the red button until it clicks (Fig. 17.18).
- Hold in place for 10 seconds.
- Remove and massage the injection site for 10–20 seconds.
- Call 000 for an ambulance.
  Note: Do not inject into the buttock.

Major trauma

BLOOD LOSS: CIRCULATION AND HAEMORRHAGE CONTROL

A rapid assessment is made of the circulation and possible blood loss. Haemostasis should be achieved with direct pressure rather than the use of tourniquets. Multiple packs into wounds should be avoided. Two important monitors are a cardiac monitor and a central venous line.

To replace blood loss two peripheral lines should be inserted into the cubital fossa, if possible. The larger the needle gauge, the better; for example, the rate of flow for a 14-gauge cannula is 175–220 mL/min and for a 16-gauge cannula is 100–150 mL/min. Flow rates are improved by using pressure bags to 300 mmHg.

Cutdown can be used and if problems occur, an interosseous infusion is a suitable alternative or addition. A colloid solution (e.g. Gelofusine or Haemaccel) can be used initially with 1 L infused rapidly. If there are two lines, a crystalloid solution such as normal saline

or Hartmann's solution can be used on one side and the plasma volume expander on the other line.

Consider the rapid intravenous infusion catheter (Chapter 4). Blood is required after a major injury or where there has been a limited response to 2 L of colloid. Blood should be warmed before use. Beware of those suspected of having fractures of the pelvis and legs. Massive amounts of blood loss can be associated with these fractures (Table 17.7).

It must be remembered that young patients can compensate well for surprising degrees of blood loss and maintain normal vital signs simply by increasing the cardiac stroke volume. Such patients can collapse dramatically.

SERIOUS INJURIES AND CLUES FROM ASSOCIATION

When certain injuries, especially bony fractures, are found it is important to consider associated soft-tissue injuries.

Table 17.7 General rules for acute blood loss with trauma (after Rogers)

Normal circulating volume 5000 mL	
< 10% (500 mL) loss	no significant change in vital signs
10–20% (500–1000 mL) loss	tachycardia, postural hypotension, slightly anxious
20–40% (1000–2000 mL) loss	progressive hypotension, anxious, confused, pale, weak pulse
> 40% (2000 mL) loss	circulatory failure, ashen, confused, lethargic
Potential concealed loss with fractures	
Tibia and fibula	750 mL
Neck of femur	1000–1500 mL
Shaft of femur	1500–2000 mL
Pelvis	up to 3000 mL[10]

Note: Blood donation is 450 mL

Table 17.8 presents possible associated injuries with various fractures, while Table 17.9 outlines possible associated injuries with various physical signs or symptoms.

Table 17.8 Associated injuries related to specific fractures

Fracture	Associated injuries to consider
Ribs	Pneumothorax Haemothorax Ruptured spleen (lower left 10–11) Ruptured diaphragm (lower 10–11, especially left)
Sternum	Ruptured base of heart with tamponade Ruptured aorta
Lumbar vertebra	Ruptured kidney (L1, L2) and other viscera (e.g. pancreas–L2)
Pelvis	Heavy blood loss Ruptured bladder Ruptured urethra Fractured femur
Temporal bone of skull	Cerebral contusion Extradural haematoma Subdural haematoma
Femur	Blood loss, possible > 1 L

Table 17.9 Associated serious injuries and typical clinical features

Physical sign or symptom	Associated serious injury
Subconjunctival haematoma with no posterior limit	Fractured base of skull
Sublingual haematoma	Fracture of mandible
Surgical emphysema	Pneumothorax with pleural tear Ruptured trachea
Unequal pupils	Cerebral compression (e.g. extradural haematoma) Trauma to cranial nerves II and III Eye injuries, including traumatic mydriasis Brain-stem injuries
Shoulder tip pain without local injury	Intra-abdominal bleeding (e.g. ruptured spleen) Intra-abdominal perforation or rupture (e.g. perforated bowel)
Bluish-coloured umbilicus	Intra-abdominal bleeding (e.g. ruptured ectopic pregnancy)

ROADSIDE EMERGENCIES

The first two hours after injury can be vital: proper care can be life-saving, inappropriate care can be damaging. The first step is for someone to notify the police and ambulance or appropriate emergency service. The site of an accident should be rendered safe by eliminating as many hazards as possible, e.g. turning off the ignition of a vehicle, warning people not to smoke, moving victims and workers out of danger of other traffic. Avoiding subsequent second accidents is paramount.

Attention should be given to:
- the airway and breathing
- the cervical spine: protect the spine
- circulation: arrest bleeding
- fractured limbs (gentle manipulation and splintage)
- open wounds, especially open chest wounds, should be covered by a firm dressing.

Major haemorrhage is a common cause of death in the first few hours. Lacerated organs and multiple fractures can lose 250 mL of blood a minute; pressure should be applied to control haemorrhage where possible. Colloids that can be administered intravenously for blood loss include Haemaccel and Gelofusine.

Intramuscular narcotic injections (morphine, pethidine) and alcohol 'to settle the victim's nerves' must be avoided. Consider inhalational analgesia with the Penthrox Inhaler. It can be used with oxygen or air, providing pain relief after 8 to 10 breaths, continuing for several minutes. When the patient is under control (with no cervical injury), he or she should be shifted into the coma position (Fig. 17.19).

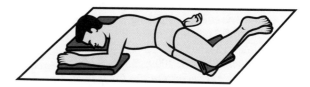

Fig. 17.19 The coma position

Administration of first aid to the injured at the roadside

A simple guide is as follows:
1. Check airway and breathing (being mindful of cervical spine)
   a. Check oral cavity
      - tongue fallen back
      - dentures or other foreign matter in mouth.
      Clear with finger and insert oral airway if available, or hold chin forward.
   b. Check breathing
      If absent, commence artificial respiration if feasible.

2. Check circulation
   If pulse absent, commence external cardiac massage if possible.
3. Check for haemorrhage, especially bleeding from superficial wounds. Apply a pressure bandage directly to the site.
4. Check for fractures, especially those of the cervical spine. Rules to remember:
   - Immobilise all serious fractures and large wounds before shifting.
   - Always apply traction to the suspected fracture site.
   - Splint any fractured limbs with an air splint, wooden splint or to body, e.g. arm to chest, leg to leg.
   - For a suspected or actual fractured neck, apply a cervical collar, even if made out of newspaper; or keep the head held firmly in a neutral position with gentle traction (avoid flexion and torsion).
   - Lay the patient on his or her back with head supported on either side.
5. Shifting the patient
   - Immobilise all fractures.
   - Lift the casualty without any movement taking place at the fracture site, using as much help as possible.
   - Always support the natural curves of the spine.
   - Protect all numb areas of skin (e.g. remove objects such as keys from the pockets).
6. The unconscious patient
   - Transport the casualty lying on the back if a clear airway can be maintained.
   - If not, gently move into the coma position.
7. Reassure the patient (if possible)
   - Reassurance of the casualty is most important.
   - Conduct yourself with calmness and efficiency.
   - Assign tasks to bystanders as appropriate—traffic safety, preparing the scene for ambulance access, supportive companion for less-injured victims, recording notes.
8. Take notes of your observations at the accident, e.g. record times, colour of casualty, conscious level, respiration, pulse, blood pressure.

Roadside emergency 'tricks of the trade'

- Emergency split towel: The inner sterile paper envelope of sterile surgical gloves can be used as a split towel to cover the wound and the inner sterile side of the outer paper envelope as a sterile sheet for instruments.
- Emergency sterilisation: The tip of forceps, knives, needles and other instruments can be sterilised by passing through the flame of a gas lighter.
- Emergency flushing fluid: One can use the water from an unopened water bottle.

References

1. Witting MD, Scharf SM. Diagnostic room-air pulse oximetry: effects of smoking, race and sex. AmJEM, 2008; 26(2): 131-6.
2. Kumar P, Clark M. *Clinical medicine.* London: Saunders Elsevier, 2009: 755-6.
3. Murtagh J. *General Practice Companion Handbook* (7th Edn). Sydney: McGraw-Hill, 2019.
4. Guy D. *Pocket Guide to ECGs* (2nd Edn). Sydney: McGraw-Hill, 2010.
5. Hayes JA, Burdon JEW. The management of spontaneous pneumothorax by simple aspiration. Aust Fam Physician, 1988; 17: 458-62.
6. Jones CW, Remboski LB, Freeze B, Braz VA, Gaughan JP, McLean SA. Intravenous fluid for the treatment of emergency department patients with migraine headache: a randomized controlled trial. *Ann Emerg Med,* 2019, 73(2): 150-156. doi: 10.1016/j.annemergmed.2018.09.004.
7. Webster V. Trauma. Melbourne RACGP CHECK Programme, 1986; Unit 176: 3-14.
8. Ask The Expert: Thiamine as a prevention of insect bites. American Academy of Allergy Asthma & Immunology, 2013, https://www.aaaai.org/ask-the-expert/thiamine-insect-bites.
9. Loten C, Stokes B, Worsley D, Seymour JE, Jiang S, Isbister GK. A randomised controlled trial of hot water (45°C) immersion versus ice packs for pain relief in bluebottle stings. Med J Aust, 2006; 184: 329-33.
10. Veith NT, Klein M, Köhler D, Tschernig T, Holstein J, Mörsdorf P, Pohlemann T, Braun BJ. Blood loss in pelvic ring fractures: CT-based estimation. Ann Trans Med, 2016, 4(19): 366.

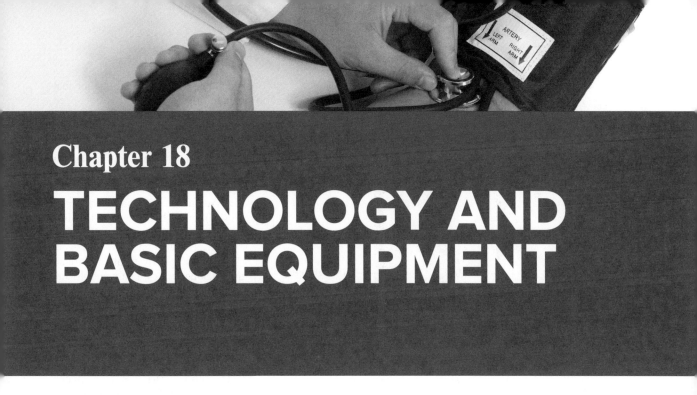

Chapter 18

TECHNOLOGY AND BASIC EQUIPMENT

NOTE OF CAUTION

The use of technology in medicine is rapidly expanding. This new chapter highlights a few technological tools that are either low-tech or relatively inexpensive. For tools not specifically designed for medical use, the clinician should judge the appropriateness and reliability of the technology in each situation.

Brand names and phone apps change quickly, so generic descriptions are used wherever possible. Specific names are provided as examples rather than recommendations, to facilitate searching for further information. Web links are not provided in this printed version, but all names can be rapidly found online. The authors do not recommend or endorse any named brand over any other equivalent brand.

Tips involving smart phone and social media should take into account guidelines around using personal devices for clinical images (e.g. RACGP, Sept 2019).[1]

TECHNOLOGY

The phone as a medical tool

Phones are an almost ubiquitous fixture carried everywhere by both doctors and patients. Standard functions on most smart phones can be used in the medical context (Fig. 18.1).

Alarms

A phone alarm set on permanent repeat (silent vibration if preferred) can serve as a reminder to take medication, whether daily for the oral contraceptive pill or more complex regimens of multiple medications throughout the day.

Medical alerts

Purchasing a 'medical alert' has the advantage of being a single-press button that connects to an operator without too much cognitive or manual effort. However, a phone may be preferred as a free or budget-priced option. Emergency contact details (triple-zero and family/neighbours) can be programmed to appear at the very top of the contacts list, which may also be used by onlookers or medical services to contact next-of-kin if the phone is readily unlocked with a swipe.

Various commercial phone apps attempt to reproduce the 'single big button' functionality of a traditional medical alert system. Pressing the button may result in auto-dialling an operator (for a monthly subscription), sending an emergency SMS text message to a group of contacts, sending the location via the phone's GPS tracking system or sounding an alarm to attract attention. Some apps place the button on the lock screen, reducing complexity for the user.

Neurology

The phone's LED light can be used as an eye torch and the vibration function as a 'tuning fork' for testing proprioception. Some apps integrate these functions onto a single screen, and at least one packages this with 60 neurological calculators and scoring systems (e.g. Neuro Toolkit, under $10).

Audiological screening

A phone with soundproofed headphones can provide single-tone audiological screening that is not as diagnostic as formal audiometry, but is a more accurate screening test than traditional office methods such as the whisper

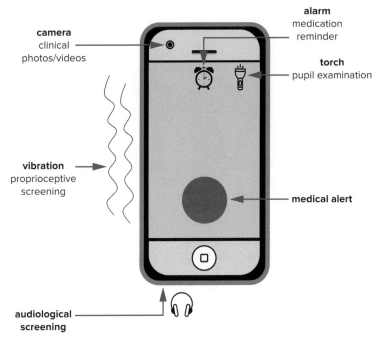

camera
clinical
photos/videos

alarm
medication
reminder

torch
pupil examination

vibration
proprioceptive
screening

medical alert

audiological
screening

Fig. 18.1 Mobile phones have many medical uses

accompanying clinical information may be identifiable.

- Once a photo is sent, it can be shared by the receiver, who may judge confidentiality differently to the sender. A social media closed group markedly multiplies this risk, while an open group is the modern equivalent of newspaper publication.
- The Australian Medical Association (AMA) publishes a guide 'Clinical images and the use of personal mobile devices', available online.

There are fewer privacy pitfalls around patients taking their own photographs and videos for medical purposes. Examples include:

- recording progression or regression of a skin lesion over time (e.g. burns healing)
- video of a child's cough and dyspnoea overnight
- video/audio of partner's sleep apnoea
- photographing the cause of trauma (e.g. work machinery, snake species)
- mental health—a photo 'diary' to record a pleasurable activity (e.g. countryside walk).

test. A disconnected second-hand phone can be set up for screening by the doctor or nurse, or self-directed in a quiet room. uHear (free) is one of a number of validated apps for initial screening.

The World Health Organization has developed the free hearWHO app to screen adults for hearing loss using speech over background noise.

Phone camera

Increasingly, many doctors use the convenience and high quality of their phone cameras for clinical use. Photos of skin lesions, rashes, joints and wounds are sent for specialist opinion or for group-consensus opinion on doctors' closed social media groups.

Photos can be electronically filed in the medical record, as can short videos of gait and mobility. A video phone link can substitute for real-time telehealth consultations.

The emerging medicolegal and privacy implications are complex, and various cautions need addressing:

- Patient permission with meaningful explanation and informed consent is a must. Document this in the notes.
- Once the image has been uploaded to the medical records or sent to the intended recipient, delete it from the phone.
- End-to-end message encryption is the de facto standard for medical communication.
- De-identification means more than just pixelating the face—a tattoo, unusual body appearance or

Plug-ins

Various medical tools plug into the phone's headphone jack via a wire or, more expensively, connect wirelessly:

- **Thermometer.** Current smart phones do not have a reliable external temperature sensor, despite various apps claiming to turn the fingerprint sensor or camera into a body thermometer. Plug-in thermometers are plentiful and inexpensive, although the benefit of connecting to a phone is questionable.
- **Digital stethoscope.** A good quality stethoscope bell will give similar results whether connected by traditional rubber tubing to the ears or electronically to speakers. Advantages of digitalising the sound waves include volume amplification, remote transmission during telehealth consultations, and easier access to hard-to-reach body areas. Higher-tech possibilities, probably of less value in primary care, include software analysis of heart sounds, real-time monitoring and clinical teaching.
- **Receiving biochemical results.** Glucose monitors adhered to the skin can transmit data from a subcutaneous probe to a nearby smart phone (Fig. 18.2). The phone can not only display results for the user, but installed software can analyse this and relay immediate instructions to an insulin pump—a 'closed loop' system. The requisite software was initially the domain of 'hackers' and shared freely online, but not TGA-approved. Commercial, TGA-approved options are fast moving into this space.

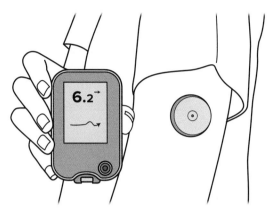

Fig. 18.2 Phone wireless connection to glucose sensor

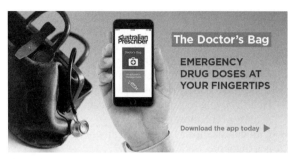

Fig. 18.3 Apps with updated drug information are useful in emergencies away from the clinic

Source: The Doctor's Bag, *Australian Prescriber*, www.nps.org.au/australian-prescriber/the-doctors-bag-app

- **Dipstick readers.** Although at the time of writing there is no app readily available for purchase, a number of recent studies have demonstrated the impressive accuracy of using a phone camera to read the colours on a urine dipstick—a task often currently assigned to an automated reflectance analyser.

MEDICAL PHONE APPS

Apps for doctors

Plenty of apps collate medical information in a readily accessible format, with a user-friendly interface that beats searching the internet, and much of the information remains available while offline. The following are useful apps downloadable for free from the main app stores.

The Doctor's Bag

Released by the *Australian Prescriber* journal, The Doctor's Bag app lists every drug provided by the PBS for use in the doctor's emergency bag, and is continuously updated (Fig. 18.3). Selecting any drug gives specific emergency uses, dosages and tips on administration.

Red Cross First Aid app

This pocket guide to first aid and CPR is easy to use. Selecting the type of emergency from the main screen takes the user through an intuitive, step-wise approach to management. It is aimed at the level of a trained first aider, but would also provide useful backup for a less experienced doctor caught outside the surgery in an emergency.

Palliative care

palliMEDS is an app designed by NPS MedicineWise in collaboration with caring@home. It is particularly handy during home visits, where detailed information about dose, route and frequency of palliative medications may be difficult to access. It also contains PBS drug data and ethico-legal information related to end-of-life care.

A handy companion app would be the Opioid Calculator produced by the Faculty of Pain Medicine of the Australian and New Zealand College of Anaesthetists. This covers opioid prescribing (regardless of palliative status), allowing rapid calculation of total oral morphine equivalent daily dose (oMEDD) for all opiates available in Australia.

Medical score calculator

The Calculate by QxMD app has rapidly expanded to include most medical scores you have ever heard of and another 400 besides. Whether it's depression, CV risk, anticoagulation or coma, if someone has invented a validated scoring tool, this app will guide you through a series of questions to arrive at the score and its interpretation. US-centric but accepts metric measurements.

Evidence-based medicine

The TRIP Database has been around since 1997 but launched its first phone app in 2019. Type in a question about medical evidence using normal language (no need to do a formal 'PICO' search) and its search function instantly produces a list of evidence-based guidelines and research findings relevant to answering your query. The hits are more relevant than Google Scholar and it's far quicker than wading through PubMed article lists.

Medicare item numbers

The MBS Search app searches all up-to-date Australian MBS item numbers and calculates the rebate, including for multiple claimed items.

Apps for patients

Health apps number in the hundreds of thousands, and many fare poorly when it comes to accuracy of information. Look for referenced sources of evidence, positive user reviews and, best of all, reliable third-party recommendations (e.g. Vic Health 'Healthy living apps guide' or 'NHS Apps Library')

The RACGP's 'Recommending Health Apps' webpage lists five broad categories of apps for use by patients:

- Healthy living (e.g. mental health, smoking, physical activity). The most popular.
- Clinical diagnosis (e.g. symptom checkers). Quality is a big issue.
- Remote monitoring (e.g. blood glucose, cardiac telehealth).
- Personal health records. Privacy and security are issues.
- Reminders (esp. medication adherence).

COMPUTER

Google

The world's most popular search engine is increasingly good at guessing what you need quickly, even mid-consultation, without having to open a specific website.

- Type the word 'translate' followed by any sentence followed by the name of a language and you can instantly show the patient the translated sentence on the screen, or click on the audio button to let them hear it spoken.
- Bad at drawing? No need to remember websites for anatomical or pathological images. Type the name of the organ or condition and click on 'images'. If the first 30 aren't to your liking, synonyms and related terms are suggested at the top of the page, or use the 'tools' function to choose between photos and diagrams.
- Typing the name of a hospital, pharmacy, radiology or specialist rooms automatically opens a Google map option to explain how to get there ('directions') and the opening hours, and you can check the photos to ensure you and the patient are talking about the same place.

Messages within the practice

While medical records software is a secure way of sending messages to other practice staff regarding a specific patient, it is not designed for general office conversations. For quick notes that don't require password-level security ('Running late', 'Tearoom needs milk', 'Who has cryo spray?') several free messaging services designed for general use can be admirably adapted for communication between rooms in a medical practice.

Most can be set up as a small box on each computer (and phone, if mobility is desired) that pops up or 'blinks' unobtrusively when a new message arrives. Messages can be sent to everyone, to an individual or to a defined group of computers such as 'front desk' or 'practice nurses' (Fig. 18.4).

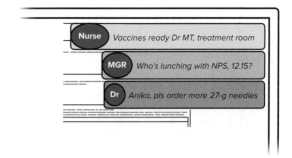

Fig. 18.4 User-friendly and discreet message pop-up boxes can be set up on every practice computer

Free messaging software, each with pros and cons, includes Facebook Messenger, Slack and Skype (better known for video calls, but use the chat function). Skype for Business has more functionality than Skype, but requires a monthly subscription.

Word

Microsoft Word contains more functions than you could poke a stick at, although most doctors won't need to go much beyond setting up document templates, using 'Insert Symbol' for mathematical notation ($\geq$, $\uparrow$, $^\circ$) and learning to click on 'Styles' rather than repeatedly changing fonts and spacing for each heading. Other tips include:

- When doing home visits or if the practice software crashes, rather than writing medical notes on paper, open a blank Word document on a laptop and type notes, inserting a couple of line spaces between each new patient. Upon return to a functioning computer medical records system, a cut-and-paste is far quicker than typing up handwritten notes from scratch.
- Patients with hearing impairment sometimes bring in a notepad for the doctor to write on. Instead, set a Word document to a large font (say, 48-point) and type away. Delete the document when you're done.
- Official prescription paper has two tear-off redundant squares at the bottom, which doctors frequently recycle for writing messages for the patient, nurse or receptionist. To make this faster (and to allow cut-and-pasted information to be printed), set up a template in Word that is already perfectly aligned for printing on those two squares. First create a document with a 'table' of one row and two columns. Expand the two squares and adjust the printing margins so the square edges align with the tear-off perforations. Select 'no border' to make the lines disappear. Save the document as a template and add a shortcut to the desktop. When needed, type what you want inside the table and, after printing and tearing off the squares, the untouched prescription area can still be used for scripts.

- When patients bring in crumpled paper forms for filling in, use the rollers on the printer as a de facto ironing board. Insert the paper smoothest edge first, then open a blank Word document and click 'print'.

MEDICAL RECORDS

Each medical record software system has its own tips and tricks, but some features are universal.

- The electronic 'patient recall' system can be borrowed for non-clinical use. In similar fashion to a library, create a recall system for lent objects such as home BP monitors, crutches and, indeed, books. Set a default number of weeks for a pop-up reminder to appear on their notes. Instead of keeping a ledger elsewhere, these recalls are readily searchable and can be marked as complete when the object is returned.
- For consultations that are likely to need a medical report in the future (assaults, work injuries, etc.), type the initial progress notes in the past tense, using full sentences rather than abbreviations. Use report-friendly phrases like 'complained of' and 'was noted to have'. This allows for a simple cut-and-paste if a report is eventually requested.

BASIC EQUIPMENT
Magnification and illumination

Plenty of diagnoses and procedures benefit from magnification and good lighting. Inexpensive technology can help.

- Vision magnifier loupes with an adjustable headband can be found online for under $20. Powerful LED lights on elastic headbands cost about the same, and can be worn over the top of the loupe.
- But why not treat yourself to a combined unit? Often sold as jeweller's magnifiers, they lack the sophistication of medical-grade loupes, but also lack the last zero on the price tag (Fig. 18.5a). The SE LED Head Magnifier sells for under $20 and the Carson Optical Pro with its bright, removable light costs around $50.
- The traditional Wood's lamp was a filtered mercury arc, later replaced by a fluorescent ultraviolet light tube, but now there is little reason to look beyond LED ultraviolet lights, which are smaller, cheaper and far more energy efficient—to the point where keyring-sized ones require only button batteries (Fig. 18.5b).

(a)

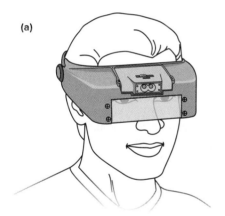

(b)

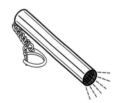

(c)

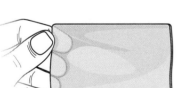

(d)

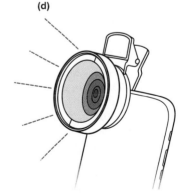

Fig. 18.5 Magnifying lenses and light sources come in all shapes and sizes

Use them to examine the eyes with fluorescein and the skin (see 'Wood's light examination', p. 226).

- Pocket magnifiers are flat plastic lenses the size of a credit card (Fig.18.5c). At around $5 they are a handy wallet accessory for people with visual impairment and for doctors on home visits.
- When no other magnifier is available, remember that an ophthalmoscope is really just a fancy magnifier with a light source. Turn the diopter to +20 (or the maximum black number setting) and it will focus at about three centimetres. An even lower-tech (and rather desperate) alternative is to use a circular pinhole occluder, normally used for testing refractive error. It doesn't magnify per se, but allows the eye to focus on an object (such as a suspected louse or tick) from just a few centimeters away.
- The ever-present phone camera can double as a magnifier, with the phone flashlight as the illuminator. At maximum zoom, the only magnification limitation is the distance at which the phone needs to be held to maintain focus. Taking a photo for the records is optional–simply turning on the camera function may be enough to help diagnosis.
- For even further magnification, purchase a macro-lens that clips on to the edge of the phone (Fig.18.5d). Many good quality clip-ons are available for under $20 (e.g. ZoeTouch Professional 12.5× macro lens). Far higher magnification can be achieved when the lens actually touches the phone camera glass. Blips are tiny 1 mm thick flexible plastic strips that adhere to the phone camera when needed, giving up to 150× magnification. Foldscopes make a similar product out of paper with a tiny glass bead as the lens. However, these setups are more akin to a microscope than a zoom, so lighting issues and hand vibration preclude most practical uses on skin.
- When illumination is required for viewing an X-ray and no viewer box is available, open a full-screen blank document on the computer and crank up the screen brightness for an even, white light source.

GADGETS
Ear camera

The leading medical brand of video otoscope retails for around $1000, but if high-definition isn't important, far cheaper toys are available. Called 'Video Ear Cleaners', various makes of these cameras sell for under $20 on eBay. Throw away the dubious cleaning attachment and what remains is quite a reasonable knitting-needle-thin camera with LED lighting and a USB connection to a real-time video on the computer (Fig. 18.6). Useful for patient education about how their grommet or glue ear compares to an image of a normal eardrum.

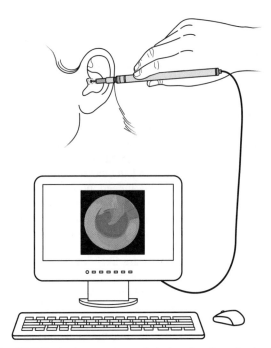

Fig. 18.6 Budget cameras can help to educate patients about the ear condition

Spirometer

Bulky spirometers with paper printouts are fast being supplanted by small handheld versions with USB or wireless connections (Fig. 18.7). The smarter ones (e.g. MiniSpir 2) are now compatible with the major medical record software, allowing data insertion directly into the patient record–although that added convenience is reflected in the cost. Cheap (around $200) versions have entered the home market without meeting professional medical standards, but the gap is fast closing. Beware expensive disposable mouthpieces.

Tips for spirometry recording (adapted from National Asthma Council Australia):
- Particularly for women, suggest they empty their bladder before spirometry–the threat of stress incontinence may impede effort.
- Sitting rather than standing reduces the risk of dizziness or fainting.
- Spirometry is a team sport and needs a coach. Preparation and verbal encouragement is key.
- Inadequate readings are common. Aim for three similarly good blows . . . this may take up to eight attempts.
- Of those three, take the largest FEV1 and the largest FVC, even if they come from different blows.

Point-of-care ultrasound (POCUS)

The miniaturisation and substantial price reduction in ultrasound equipment has brought this tool to the

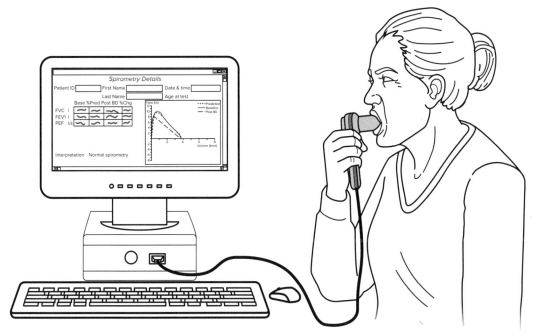

Fig. 18.7 Small handheld spirometers work excellently, as long as the blowing technique is sound

bedside in emergency departments, obstetric practices and more recently to general practice rooms (Fig. 18.8). Small handheld probes that bring real-time images to a computer or smart phone are a third of the price of their bulky predecessors and will become cheaper every year.

Studies have shown point-of-care ultrasonography to be useful in general practices in diagnosing DVTs, gallstones, shoulder dislocations and assisting in nerve blocks, venesection and joint injections (although whether

large-joint injection benefits from any imaging at all remains doubtful).

Many medical societies around the world have produced guidelines for POCUS. Common themes include:

- POCUS is not a replacement for comprehensive ultrasound, but rather allows clinicians a tool to clarify uncertain examination findings in order to enhance the accuracy of rapid solutions.
- POCUS, like an ECG, is a diagnostic aid that helps clinical decision-making and can reduce delays in treatment.
- The reliability of the findings is very user-dependent. As with all complex clinical skills, accuracy improves with experience.
- POCUS should primarily be used to provide targeted information that helps rule in or rule out a specific diagnosis that is known to be reliably detectable via an operator with substantially less experience than a qualified imaging specialist.
- Examinations should be stopped if a patient complains of discomfort from heat.
- Ideally, the relevant image(s) should be captured and retained in the medical record.

Dermatoscopy

Dermatoscopy has the potential to (modestly) increase the sensitivity and specificity of melanoma diagnosis. In addition to the basic functions of magnification (approx. ×10) and illumination, dermatoscopes have the capacity to contact the skin, use polarised light and some models digitally connect to a computer or phone.

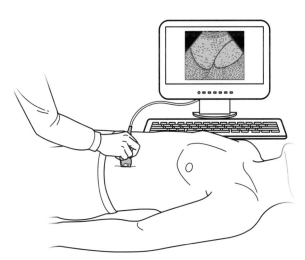

Fig. 18.8 Point-of-care ultrasound (POCUS) is an increasingly popular diagnostic screening tool, particularly in rural areas

- Skin visualisation is improved (particularly for non-polarised light) by using a thin layer of oil or alcohol. Commercial sprays or drops may be substituted by ultrasound gel, cooking oil, an alcohol wipe or simply water.
- Disposable cling wrap under the lens can reduce cross-contamination.
- A 2018 review[2] showed that a number of other skin conditions have a specific, diagnostic dermatoscopic appearances: tinea capitis, trichotillomania, alopecia and onychomycosis.

Pulse oximetry

These fingertip (or toe or ear lobe) gadgets are now cheap enough to afford an oximeter in every clinic room; brand choice depends upon reliability and whether connectivity to a computer or multipurpose gadget is required.

- The absorbance of two wavelengths of light distinguishes oxyhaemoglobin from deoxyhaemoglobin. An algorithm ignores the steadily flowing venous blood to analyse only the pulsing arterial blood, then matches this result to a database originally obtained from research volunteers, which is the number displayed.

- Inaccurate readings can result from: carbon monoxide poisoning, fetal haemoglobin, decreased peripheral perfusion, severe anaemia, nail polish, calloused skin or excessive movement.
- See Chapter 17 regarding the use of oximetry.

Gadgets for children

Keeping a bored child preoccupied with something harmless and quiet in the waiting room or consulting room can be a sanity saver.

- Purchase a wall-mountable 'play panel'. Commercial-grade panels cost quite a few hundred dollars but are safe, easily cleaned and keep toys off the floor. Avoid models with bells and loud clicks.
- Ask around for an old, outdated computer and before disconnecting it from the internet, load a selection of free point-and-click games for both preschool and primary school ages (an online search finds thousands). Select a colourful children's TV or movie character as a screensaver. Set it up in a corner of the waiting area with a mouse—no keyboard and definitely no speakers! Cheap headphones are optional, but may not survive for long.

References

1. RACGP. Using personal mobiles devices for clinical photos in general practice. The Royal Australian College of General Practitioners, 2019, https://www.racgp.org.au/FSDEDEV/media/documents/Running%20a%20practice/Practice%20resources/Using-personal-mobile-devices-for-clinical-photos.pdf

2. Micali G, Verzi A E, Lacarrubba F. Alternative uses of dermoscopy in daily clinical practice: An update. J Am Acad Dermatol, 2018, 79: 1117–32.e1

Chapter 19
MISCELLANEOUS

MEASUREMENT OF TEMPERATURE

Temperature can be measured by many methods. These include the following thermometers:

- mercury thermometer (now superseded)
- digital electronic pacifier
- digital peak thermometer with LED light
- digital infrared aural
- electronic probe
- forehead thermometer (temporal area).

The favoured general instrument for oral and rectal use is the digital peak-hold thermometer.

Table 19.1 gives a basic guide to interpreting the temperature values obtained.

Basic rules of thermometer usage

Oral use

1. Place under the tongue at the junction of the base of the tongue and the floor of the mouth to one side of the frenulum—the 'heat pocket'.

Table 19.1 Interpretation of temperature measurement

Normal values (average)	
Mouth	36.8°C
Axilla	36.4°C
Rectum	37.3°C
Ear	37.4°C
Pyrexia	
Mouth	> 37.2 early morning
	> 37.8°C at other times of day

2. Ensure the mouth is kept shut.
3. Remove dentures.

Note: Unsuitable for children 4 years and under, especially if irritable; use axilla or rectum.

Rectal use

A suitable route for babies and young children under the age of 4.[1]

Method

1. Lubricate the stub with petroleum jelly.
2. Insert for 2–3 cm (1 inch).

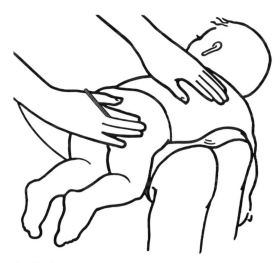

Fig. 19.1 Rectal temperature measurement

3. Keep the thermometer between the flexed fingers with the hand resting on the buttocks.
4. Wipe rectal thermometers with alcohol and store separately from oral.

Don't

- Dig thermometer in too hard.
- Hold it too rigidly.
- Allow the child to move around.

Axillary use[1]

Although unreliable, it is practical for young children and gives a helpful guide. If used it should be placed high in the axilla.

Groin use

This route is not ideal but is more reliable than the axilla. It closely approximates oral temperature.

In infants, the thigh should be flexed against the abdomen.

Vaginal use

Mainly used as an adjunct to the self-assessment of ovulation during the menstrual cycle. Should be placed deeply in the vagina before leaving the bed in the morning.

Infrared aural (ear drum) use[2]

The temperature can be measured in 3 seconds with an infrared device placed in the ear canal. Hold the child's head firmly so that it does not move. There is much debate about its efficacy but it appears to be worthwhile as it is a simple method and in general practice the benefits of convenience outweigh possible lack of accuracy. The normal range is the same as for rectal temperature.

Digital electronic pacifier (dummy) thermometer

This is a popular method in infants and younger children, favoured by many paediatricians in the United States.

MEASUREMENT OF WEIGHT

Addition method

To measure a person whose weight exceeds the upper limit of your clinic scales, borrow identical scales from another room, and place both (almost touching) on non-carpeted floor. Ask the patient to stand with one leg on each, very still. Add the two values.

Subtraction method

The weight of a child equals the weight of the child-plus-parent minus the weight of the parent.

Weight variation

All scales—even expensive digital ones—have some degree of inherent measuring inaccuracy, usually not clinically significant ($+/-$ a fraction of a per cent). Minimise variation by comparing weights measured on the same set of scales.

However, human bodies have natural weight variation diurnally and seasonally, and depending on hydration, on the contents of stomach, bowel and bladder, and on clothing. Measure weight in light clothing, and don't ascribe too much clinical meaning to a gain or loss of 1–2 kg in a large adult.

OBTAINING REFLEXES

Ankle-jerk technique

The method, illustrated in Figure 19.2a, provides a good opportunity to see and feel for a doubtful reflex. It is

(a)

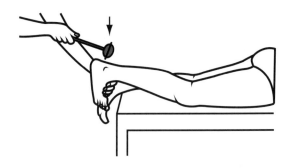

(b)

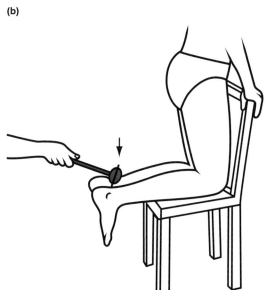

Fig. 19.2 Testing a doubtful reflex: **(a)** while the patient lies prone; **(b)** while the patient kneels on a chair

readily performed on a patient lying prone to allow examination of the back.

Method

1. Lift the foot slightly off the examination couch and hold it so that the Achilles tendon is under slight tension.
2. With the plessor held in the other hand, tap the tendon.

Alternatively, have the patient kneel on a chair with the feet freely suspended over the edge (Fig. 19.2b). Ask him or her to grasp the back of the chair firmly; this adds an element of reinforcement, which tends to increase the reflex. Tap the Achilles tendon in the usual way.

Uncooperative children

Children under 10 years of age have a disturbing tendency to tense their arms and legs at the wrong moment. Give them a squash ball or similar rubber object and instruct them to squeeze the ball as hard as possible on the count of 3.

Test the required reflex during this distraction.

RESTLESS LEGS SYNDROME

This consists of poorly localised aching in the legs (a crawling sensation) and spontaneous, continuous leg movements. Organic causes that need to be excluded include the neuropathies caused by diabetes, uraemia, hypothyroidism and anaemia. However, it is generally a functional disorder affecting the elderly, and results in marked insomnia.

Management

- *Diet:* Eliminate caffeine and follow a healthy diet.
- *Medications* (last resort): Taken before bed time, these include paracetamol, hypnotics, tricyclic antidepressants, clonazepam, levodopa and propranolol. First choice is paracetamol 1000 mg (o) or clonazepam 1 mg, 1 hour before retiring.
- *Exercises:* These involve stretching of the hamstrings and posterior leg muscles for at least 5 minutes before retiring (Fig. 19.3). Exercise (a) demonstrates hamstring stretching; (b) illustrates calf muscle stretching; (c) stretches all posterior muscles of the lower limb, especially the hamstrings. The patient lies on his or her back and uses a 1.2 m (4-foot) length of rope or flat tape to lift the leg. This exercise should be repeated to produce effective stretching.

NIGHTMARES

For severe nightmares persistent enough to warrant consideration of medication, give a trial of phenytoin (in recommended dosage) for 4 weeks and review.

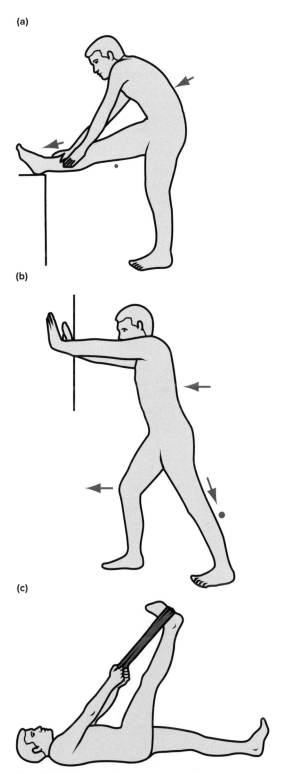

(a)

(b)

(c)

Fig. 19.3 Exercises for restless legs: **(a)** hamstring stretching; **(b)** calf muscle stretching; and **(c)** stretching of all posterior muscles of the lower limb

NOCTURNAL CRAMPS

Consider underlying causes such as drugs and electrolyte disturbances.

Physiological muscle-stretching and relaxation techniques may be effective in the prevention of nocturnal cramps. Other strategies include keeping well hydrated and avoiding caffeine before retiring.

Exercise 1

1. Stand bare-footed approximately 1 m (3 ft) from a wall, leaning forwards with the back straight and outstretched hands against the wall.
2. Lift the heels off the floor and then force the heels to the floor to produce tension in the calf muscles.
3. Hold for 30 seconds and repeat 5 to 6 times.

An alternative is to keep the heels on the floor and climb the hands up the wall.

Do these exercises 2 to 3 times a day for 1 week, then each night before retiring (Fig. 19.4).

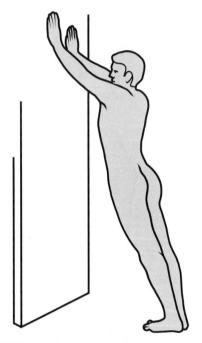

Fig. 19.4 Exercise for leg cramps

Exercise 2

This can follow Exercise 1 before retiring.

The patient should rest in a chair with the feet out horizontally to the floor, with support from a cushion under the Achilles tendon, for 10 minutes.

Drug treatment

The evidence for drug treatments is disappointing.

- Quinine—although this has more evidence of its effectiveness than any other drug, quinine is not recommended because of thrombocytopaenia risks.[3] Consider quinine-containing drinks, e.g. tonic water or bitter lemon or lime, last thing at night.
- Magnesium compound—often marketed for this indication, and relatively harmless, but a Cochrane review of magnesium did not find any benefit for leg cramps.[4]
- Biperiden 2–4 mg nocte—minimal evidence. Baclofen evidence is similar to that for magnesium.
- Baking soda (sodium bicarbonate)—consider a half-teaspoon of baking soda in half a glass of water at the onset of the cramp.

SPECIAL USES FOR VASODILATORS

Venepuncture

Venepuncture, whether for blood collection, the introduction of intravenous drugs or cannulation, can be very difficult in some patients whose veins are not dilated.

Methods

- Rub glyceryl trinitrate (GTN) ointment (e.g. Nitro-Bid) over the vein that you wish to puncture.
  or
- Give the patient one-half of an Anginine tablet (or one GTN spray) sublingually, provided there are no contraindications to glyceryl trinitrate use. The veins will soon appear.
- Warm the area with a hot flannel.

Painful heels

Some patients, particularly elderly people with diabetes and small-vessel disease, develop painful heels. Glyceryl trinitrate ointment or transdermal pads applied to the painful area can provide considerable relief.

The transdermal pads (e.g. Nitro-dur, Minitran, Transderm-Nitro) are applied once daily and the ointment applied twice daily in a small amount under tape.

Apply skin moisturiser and wear closed shoes. A particularly painful crack can benefit from skin glue (e.g. Histoacryl).

Tendinopathy

The use of transdermal GTN patches to treat tendinopathies such as Achilles and lateral epicondyle tendinopathies has been advocated by many therapists. The usual dose is 1.25 mg per day (a quarter of a 5 mg/24 hr patch) over the affected area. A 2005 Australian study[5] by G. Hunte and R. Lloyd-Smith concluded that the method was better than a placebo, but the overall evidence is unclear and the routine treatment cannot be recommended at this point.

NOCTURNAL BLADDER DYSFUNCTION

The woman with the urethral syndrome or bladder dysfunction who constantly wakes during the night with an urge to micturate, yet only produces a small dribble of urine, can be helped by the following.

Method

Instruct the patient to perform the following pelvic lift exercise when she awakes.

Balance on her upper back.

Lift her pelvis, supported by her flexed knees, and hold this position for about 30 seconds.

As she holds the position, squeeze the pelvic floor inward.

Repeat the exercise 2 or 3 times.

FACILITATING A VIEW OF THE CERVIX

Fists under the buttocks

If having difficulty viewing a cervix for the cervical smear test, ask the patient to rest her hands, preferably as fists, under her buttocks. If necessary, she can lift her buttocks slightly higher with her fists.

A small, firm cushion could be placed under the buttocks as an alternative.

If you are still having trouble, have the patient cough (this is very effective).

Note: If using a metal speculum, remember to warm it in warm water and test the comfort of the temperature on the patient's thigh.

CONDOM ON THE SPECULUM

If you are troubled by the vaginal walls collapsing into the gap between the two blades of the bivalved speculum, you can slip a condom over the blades and then cut the tip off the condom. The condom then supports the vaginal walls.

PRIAPISM

Various methods can be attempted to alleviate the acute or subacute onset of priapism, especially that which is drug induced:

- ice cubes, inserted rectally
- pseudoephedrine, especially for alprostadil (Caverject or Muse injection) induced priapism.

If drug-induced priapism lasts longer than 2 hours, give the patient two pseudoephedrine tablets—repeat at 3 hours if necessary.

If all fails and specialist help is remote, aspiration and irrigation should be attempted and is best performed in the first 6 to 8 hours.

Under local anaesthetic and using a 16-gauge needle, aspirate thick blood from the ipsilateral corpora cavernosa through the glans penis. 20 mL of blood is drawn out at a time and the penis is then flushed with saline.

If resolution is incomplete, use a very slow injection of 10 mL of saline containing 1 mg aramine, followed by massage.

Look for any underlying cause, including a blood film for polycythemia or leukaemia.

PREMATURE EJACULATION

It is worth a trial in men 18–64 years (with PE < 2 minutes latency time) of dapoxetine (Priligy) 30 mg 1–3 hours pre sex (max. 30 mg per 24 hours).

Caution: Possible syncope.

INDOMETHACIN FOR RENAL/ URETERIC COLIC

After a patient has received an intramuscular injection of morphine for the severe pain of renal colic, further pain can be alleviated by indomethacin. Suppositories are satisfactory, but limit them to two a day.

Some practitioners have submitted an anecdotal tip of getting the sufferer of ureteric colic to jump up and down vigorously on the leg of the affected side.

An effective alternative treatment is an IM injection of 75 mg diclofenac (if available), then diclofenac 50 mg (o) tds for 1 week.

COOL CABBAGES FOR HOT BREASTS

Cabbage leaves have been used in some cultures for hundreds of years in the treatment of sprains, infections and some breast problems. Recently, they have become popular in many maternity hospitals for managing breast engorgement. They appear to result in decreased oedema and improved milk flow.

Uses

Local breast engorgement:
- blocked ducts or mastitis.
  Generalised breast engorgement:
- when milk supply is greater than demand
  - early postpartum
  - sudden weaning
- when lactation suppression is required
  - after a baby dies
  - after mid-trimester abortion.

Method

1. Wash the cabbage leaves well (beware risk of contamination with dirt or pesticides) and dry. Store the cabbage in a refrigerator.

2. Cut stalks from leaves (to prevent pressure on breast) and apply the crisp leaves to the breast, avoiding the nipple area. (Cut out openings for the nipples.)
3. Remove after 2 hours (or earlier if the leaves are limp) and assess the need for further leaves.
4. Cease using leaves when engorgement settles, as prolonged use can reduce the milk supply.
5. Do not use if the patient has a history of allergy to cabbage.

It is still essential to correctly position the baby on the breast and not restrict the baby's access to the breast.

MAKESHIFT SPACING CHAMBERS FOR ASTHMATICS

An improvised temporary 'aerochamber' can be made by one of three methods:
1. Plunge the end of the puffer through the bottom of a paper or polystyrene (preferable) cup.
2. Cut the end (base) off a plastic soft drink bottle and insert the end of the puffer into the mouth of the bottle.
3. Make a cruciate incision in the base of a plastic bottle to accommodate the end of the puffer and then advise the patient to breathe through the normal bottle opening.

COPING WITH AND SWALLOWING TABLETS

Breaking tablets in half

When a tablet is manufactured with a line down the middle it may be easily broken, especially if it is a big tablet with a deep scored line.

Various methods

1. Place the tablet on a flat surface with the line uppermost. Place one finger on each side of the tablet and press down firmly (Fig. 19.5). The tablet should split easily.

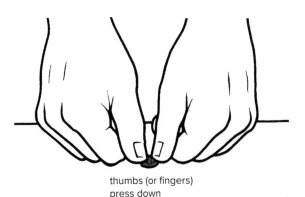

thumbs (or fingers)
press down
simultaneously

Fig. 19.5 Coping with tablets

2. If problematic, press over the shaft of a pen rather than a flat surface.
3. To produce quarters, first start with the score at right angles to the pen, then repeat to break each half along the score.
4. An alternative is to sticky-tape the pill to a chopping board and cut with a sharp knife.
5. Commercial pill cutters: a variety of gadgets are available from pharmacies and online.

Swallowing tablets

These methods are recommended for those who may have trouble swallowing tablets. Drink plenty of water before swallowing to lubricate the throat, then take the tablet or capsule with water.

Method 1

Capsules float and pills don't. Whereas most people extend their neck to swallow pills, for capsules tilt the chin slightly towards the chest.
• Put the capsule on the tongue.
• Take a sip of water but hold on—don't swallow yet.
• Tilt the chin slightly towards the chest.
• Swallow the capsule with the water with the head bent forward.

Method 2

Simply place the tablet on the tongue and drink water through a straw with the head slightly flexed forwards. The stream of water 'hoses' the tablet down the throat. A Medi-Straw® pill swallowing system is available commercially. A similar method is to fill a flexible plastic bottle with water. Place the capsule on the tongue, close the lips tightly around the open bottle and, using a sucking motion, drink from the bottle to swallow water and the pill simultaneously. Don't let air get into the bottle as you suck.

Method 3

Try a lubricant. Water is first line but a medicated lubricant Pill Glide®, which is a flavoured swallowing spray, or Gloup® lube may help children (in particular) to cope with swallowing tablets and capsules.

Method 4

Place the pill, preferably crushed if possible or the contents of a capsule in soft food such as mashed banana or soft chocolate. This is most applicable for children.

Method 5

Pre-teens can prepare for tablet swallowing by practising swallowing whole Smarties or M&M's.

Cost of tablets vs liquid medication

Tablets are usually a fraction of the cost of liquids per milligram. Paracetamol tablets retail at less than 1/20th the cost of baby paracetamol drops. Tablets can be crushed and mixed with honey or jam.

The standard dose of a 500 mg paracetamol tablet is:
- ¼ tab aged 6–12 months (7–9 kg)
- ⅓ tab aged 1–2 years (10–12 kg)
- ½ tab aged 3 years
- 1 tab aged 10 years.

PATIENT EDUCATION TECHNIQUES IN THE CONSULTING ROOM

Organ removal torso model

A colourful model of the human body (head to groin) can be obtained to install in the surgery. The organs can be systematically removed and explained to the patient (Fig. 19.6).

Whiteboard

A small whiteboard can be installed, either portable or fixed to the wall, in the consulting room. A Sanford Expo kit can be installed alongside the board. It consists of a set of coloured whiteboard markers that clip onto slots in the kit and an eraser. This is ideal for explanatory sketches.

Computer education

Your patient can be briefly taken through a patient education information program (e.g. J. Murtagh's *Patient Education,* 8th Edn, McGraw-Hill Australia, Sydney, 2019) on the computer screen and then take home a printout. This can be individualised by including the patient's name on the top of the general sheet.

This visual education can be enhanced by the use of graphics, and plenty of software programs allow the drawing of diagrams on the screen.

Online information is a key health education source for patients; advise them of website clues that help distinguish credible scientific information from uninformed opinion.

IMPROVISED SUPPOSITORY INSERTER

Some people find it difficult or unaesthetic to insert a suppository digitally. An interesting method is to rearrange a disposable plastic syringe so that it is converted into a plunger for ease of insertion of the suppository.

Rearranging the syringe

- Remove the plunger.
- Cut the end off the barrel (at the narrow end).
- Place the plunger through the opposite end at this new opening.

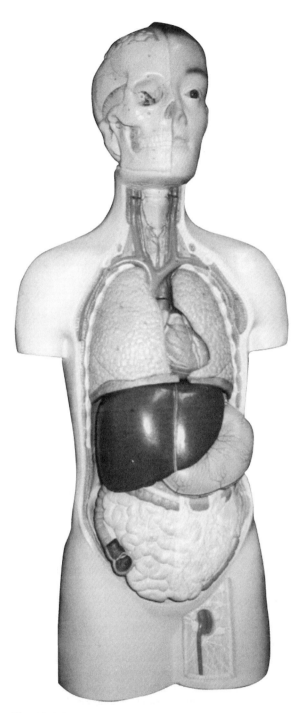

Fig. 19.6 Patient education model

Inserting the suppository

- Place the suppository in the syringe barrel (Fig. 19.7).
- Firmly place the flange up against the anus.
- Press the plunger rapidly.

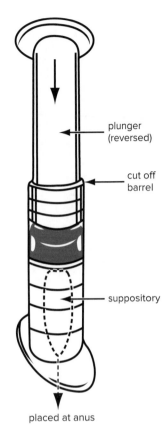

plunger (reversed)

cut off barrel

suppository

placed at anus

Fig. 19.7 Position of suppository

COLLECTING URINE SPECIMENS

The simple transfer of urine from urethra to urine container is not necessarily straightforward; more so in females, older people and babies.

- Tape a tongue depressor to the base of the urine container, for the patient to use like a saucepan handle.
- Instruct the female patient to place the urine container on the shower drain while the shower is off. Stand over it and aim to get at least some urine into the jar. After putting the lid on, turn on the shower to wash away splashes.
- Female urine funnels are marketed for camping and boating, but silicone ones are too expensive for something that shouldn't be shared. Disposable, waterproofed paper versions include Pee Pocket and Pee Buddy (around $1 each in a bulk pack).
- The main risk in collecting bag urines from babies is false positive results from skin contamination, which can lead to overtreatment and false labelling of being at risk of renal tract anomalies. Clean the skin before applying. Instruct the parent to remove the bag as soon as possible, and to avoid pouring the urine through the opening—dangle the bag over the collection jar and snip a corner with clean scissors.

BUNION 'DONUTS'

Those donut-shaped pieces of adherent felt that distribute pressure over bunions can be costly for a regular user. A single piece of thick hydrocolloid dressing (e.g. DuoDERM) can provide a dozen substitutes. Firmly press the large circle of an otoscope tip onto the dressing as many times as it will fit. Punch out the centre of each ring with a 6 mm biopsy punch, then cut out each circle with scissors.

THE MANY USES OF PETROLEUM JELLY (VASELINE)

- To kill lice, e.g. pubic lice or those on the eyelashes, apply petroleum jelly twice daily for 8 days, then pluck off any remaining nits.
- Apply to dry and cracked skin (also useful to prevent cracking), e.g. on heels.
- Apply for the protection of normal skin surrounding lesions such as warts and seborrhoeic keratoses before the application of corrosive substances, e.g. chromic acid or liquid nitrogen.
- Use as a lubricant for rectal examination.
- Use as a lubricant and sealant for the plunger on the metal ear syringe.
- For nappy rash, use it in equal parts with a mixture of hydrocortisone and antifungal creams to promote length of action of the medication.
- Mix with cotton wool balls for ear plugs (see p. 188).

THE MANY USES OF PAPER CLIPS

- Heated clips for subungual haematoma (see p. 99)
- Removal of foreign body from nose and ears (see pp. 121–128)
- Removal of wax hearing aids
- Removal of 'stuck' punch biopsy specimens
- Eyelid eversion (with care)
- Pin back scalp hair during minor repairs

THE USES OF FINE CRYSTALLINE SUGAR

Fine crystalline sugar (common table sugar) can be used to help reduce oedematous swelling, for example:

- paraphimosis
- rectal prolapse
- prolapsed haemorrhoids.

SEA SICKNESS

There are several 'mariner's tips' to prevent sea sickness, especially involving the use of ginger.

- Take a ginger preparation, e.g. drink ginger ale or ginger beer.
- Place a plug in one ear.
- Look to the horizon.
- Lie down on your back for several minutes.

SNAPPING THE TOP OFF A GLASS AMPOULE

Breaking off the top of those stubborn ampoules can cause injury. To reduce the risk of this, it is best to use a small file; however, even these may not be effective. If you are using your hands to complete the snap, try using a gauze swab, the alcohol swab package or an appropriate-sized plastic auriscope earpiece.

MEDICO-LEGAL TIPS

Tips from medical defence

The big six presenting problems requiring extra care and follow up:

- breast lumps
- acute abdominal pain
- acute chest pain
- sick, febrile children < 2 years
- headache
- chronic dyspnoea/cough.

10 deadly sins—resulting in negligence claims

- Poor record keeping.
- No documentation of consent process.
- The altering of records with a problem.
- Failure to follow up referrals.
- Failure to follow up test results.
- Failure to check history with scripts.
- Giving phone diagnosis and treatment.
- Rushing consultations.
- Insufficient time/care to establish sound doctor–patient rapport.
- Not saying anything if something has gone wrong.

Handball tip (for undiagnosed multiple visits problem)

- Three strikes and you're out. It's someone else's turn.

TIPS FOR AGED CARE

(Dr Jill Rosenblatt)

Scalp seborrhoea

An effective treatment is ketoconazole shampoo, e.g. Sebizole or Nizoral. A second lather must be used and this kept on the scalp for 3–5 minutes (with care to protect the eyes). This presents a challenge with the elderly showering themselves or a carer assisting.

Wax in the ears

The most effective drops are carbonide peroxide, e.g. Ear Clear. These may be used twice daily or even hourly during waking hours and with the resultant wax dissolution, syringing can be avoided.

Patients with dementia often do not tolerate ear syringing, but sometimes they don't tolerate ear drops every hour either.

Impaired hearing

Up to 80% of hearing aids become expensive chest-of-drawers ornaments!

Some considerations: If you can converse easily one-to-one, a hearing aid should not be necessary. If a hearing aid is to be used, it should be worn in the ear with the better hearing. When in a crowded room, attempt to stand or sit next to a wall for greater sound concentration. If an audiogram demonstrates R and L hearing disparity, a CT scan should be performed.

Rhinorrhoea

Clear rhinorrhoea in the elderly may be related to lactose intolerance; if so, a dairy-free diet is known to relieve symptoms in 4 weeks. Lactose-free milk and yoghurt may be used as alternatives.

Long-term, intermittent oxymetazoline nasal drops or spray (e.g. Drixine) can be effective but the preferred treatment is lubrication of the nasal passages with an oil-based preparation such as natural sesame seed oil spray, e.g. Nozoil.

Insomnia

Exclude underlying causes of sleep disturbance. Avoid hypnotics if possible and in particular avoid combining them with alcohol. Ideally, the use of benzodiazepines as hypnotics should be short term only.

Sleep hygiene issues need to be discussed; consider caffeine cessation from lunch time onwards and the avoidance of electronic stimulation right before bed time.

Paraphrenia

This is isolated paranoia in the elderly and a sign of early dementia. It can cause havoc with family, neighbours and police, with accusations of theft or property trespass. Auditory hallucinations may also be present.

Low-dose risperidone or olanzapine are very effective medications for this problem. Keep in mind that risperidone can aggravate Lewy body dementia.

Faecal impaction

A useful approach is to use macrogol 3350 (Movicol), up to eight sachets in 6 hours on successive days with subsequent daily Movicol maintenance.

Trochanteric bursalgia

This presents as pain in the affected thigh, laterally, and may radiate to the lateral knee and even into the foot. Localised tenderness over the trochanteric bursa site is confirmatory and an ultrasound (not necessary) may add further evidence. An injection of local anaesthetic (a generous 5 mL of 1% lidocaine) with corticosteroid is very effective in the short term. During this procedure, a gritty end-point may be detected with the needle tip.

Benign senescent forgetfulness

This popular term is also referred to as 'aged related memory loss' or 'delayed recall of ageing' or 'mild cognitive impairment of ageing'.

This is a common sign of ageing and may be an early symptom of dementia, which certainly follows on from this condition in at least 10% of cases.

Dementia prevention strategies

This program is based on the research work of Dr Michael Valenzuela, as found in his book *Maintain Your Brain*.[6]

1. Healthy blood pressure—'a healthy heart means a healthy brain'—the strongest evidence for dementia prevention.
2. The three keys:
   a. physical: walking 30–60 minutes 3 to 4 times a week, plus strength exercises, balance and stretching exercises—reportedly known to enhance brain cell growth, brain cell interconnections and angiogenesis
   b. mentally stimulating activities
   c. social activities in company that are both fun and rewarding.
3. Alcohol control: avoid binge drinking and *always* promote a safe intake, i.e. 1 to 2 standard drinks with a meal for 3 days a week.
4. Diet—Mediterranean in style, oily fish 2 to 3 times a week, 2 fruits and 5 vegetables daily (consider chia seeds).

HOLISTIC TREATMENT OF PATIENTS WITH MINOR PROBLEMS

Minor problems, even trivial to us, are commonplace and sometimes the patient or parent feels 'short changed' with a departing derisive comment 'thanks anyway doc',

especially after the doctor comments, 'it should settle without treatment'. Typical minor problems include minor wounds, minor burns especially sunburn and first degree, abrasions and grazes, musculoskeletal problems including neck and back pain/spasm, upper respiratory infections and referred pain. This issue prompted strategies to improve the therapeutic effect on the patient—physically and psychologically. Strategies include:

- time spent with education, reassurance and counselling
- appropriate limited physical examination
- providing a patient education handout
- use of topical agents especially sprays and powders.

A cupboard containing topical agents could include the following: antiseptics, analgesics, musculoskeletal agents (especially useful for massage), inhalation or other associated therapeutic commercial or OTC items:

- Betadine antiseptic spray or dusting powder
- Savlon dry antiseptic spray (also contains povidone-iodine)
- Tea-tree spray
- Isopropyl alcohol spray (as disinfectant and antiseptic)
- Ego SOOV burns spray (antiseptic and analgesic—contains lidocaine)
- Paxyl Sunburn Relief Spray (also contains lidocaine)
- Friar's Balsam (many uses e.g. inhalation agent, skin/wound/blister protector; sticking agent (e.g. hair suture knots))
- Eucalyptus oil spray—antiseptic and musculoskeletal discomfort relief
- Rubesal spray (contains camphor, menthol and salicylic acid)
- Pain Away Sports Spray (contains multiple naturopathic products)
- Vicks VapoRub
  Precautions:
- deep and clean surgical wounds, eyes and nasal passages
- sprays containing anaesthetic agents and other agents which may cause skin hypersensitisation and antiseptics which may irritate wounds and lead to bacterial resistance.

References

1. Craig JV et al. Temperature measurement at the axilla compared with rectum in children and young people: systematic review. BMJ, 2000; 320: 1174–8.
2. Duce SJ. A systematic review of the literature to determine optimal methods of temperature measurement in neonates, infants and children. The Cochrane Library, 1996; 1–124.
3. El-Tawil S, Al Musa T, Valli H, Lunn MPT, Brassington R, El-Tawil T, Weber M. Quinine for muscle cramps. Cochrane Database of Systematic Reviews, 2015, 4, Art. No.: CD005044.
4. Magnesium, a treatment for leg cramps? NPS Medicinewise, 2014, https://www.nps.org.au/news/magnesium-a-treatment-for-leg-cramps.
5. Hunte G, Lloyd-Smith R. Topical glyceryl trinitrate for chronic Achilles tendinopathy, Clin J Sport Med, 2005, 15(2), p. 116–7.
6. Valenzuela MJ. *Maintain your brain,* Sydney: HarperCollins, 2001.

Index

A

abrasions, 108
abscess
  drainage of breast, 63
  healing cavity of, 23
  perianal, 88
  tooth, 180
Achilles tendon
  complete rupture, 171
  injection for paratendinopathy, 46
  tendinopathy, 170, 258
acne, 223–4
acne cysts, 55
acromioclavicular joint
  injection, 47
  sling, 112, 114
Acticoat™, 117–18
acute coronary syndromes, 230
adhesive gel dressings, 62
adrenaline autoinjector, 243–4
aeroplane exercise, 174
aged care, 263–4
airgun wounds, 126
alcohol swabs, 26, 67
Algerbrush II, 99
allergy, 226
ampoules, topping, 263
amputated finger, 107
anaesthetic infiltration for wounds, 16, 27,
    28, 124
anal dilatation, 87
anal fibro-epithelial polyps, 88–9
anal fissures, 87
anal fistula, 88
AnaPen®, 244
anaphylaxis, 243
ankle
  sprained, 172
  strapping, 172
  wobble board technique, 174
ankle-jerk reflex technique, 256–7
ankyloglossia, 183
ano-rectal disorders, cautionary points
    regarding, 89
anosmia, 198
ant bites, 243
anterior compartment syndrome, 170
anterior directed gliding, 137, 141
antiseptic solutions, skin preparation, 2
antral/nasal washout, 196
anxious children, 219
aphthous ulcers, 182
arm pain, 138
arm sling, 112–13
ascites, tapping, 75–6
aspiration
  of breast lump, 64
  of pleural effusion, 76–7
asthma, makeshift spacing chamber, 260
atopic dermatitis, 224–5

attic perforation, 192
audiological screening, 247–8
auriscope, to view nasal cavity, 197
autoinjector for anaphylaxis, 243–4
avascular field in digit, 19–20
avulsion of toenail, 105
axial loading test, 144
axillary temperature measurement, 256

B

back pain
  disc prolapse, 145
  lower back exercise, 147–8
  sciatica, 145
  slump test, 146
  tests for non-organic, 143–4
  trigger point injections, 39, 40
Baker cyst, 60
Barlow test, 161
Bartholin cyst, 64–5
basal cell carcinoma (BCC), 58
bed bug bites, 242
bee stings, 243
benign paroxysmal positional vertigo,
    198–9
benign senescent forgetfulness, 264
bicipital tendinitis injection, 41
Bier block, 35–6
biopsies, 55–6
'bite the bullet' strategy, 210
bite wounds, 241
bladder dysfunction, nocturnal, 259
blanket stitch suture, 6
blepharitis, 202
bloodless field in a digit, 101–2
blood loss, 244
blurred vision, 206–7
botulinum toxin, 87
boutonnière deformity, 158
box jellyfish stings, 243
brachialgia, 138
breast
  abscess drainage, 63
  cabbage leaves for engorgement, 259–60
  lump aspiration, 64
  mastitis, 63
breath-holding attacks, 217–18
Breathing Wonder®, 197
broad arm sling, 112–13
bubbles, in syringe, 28
Burn 'kneeling on a stool' test, 143–4
burns, 115–18
  dressings, 117
  first aid, 115
  hand, 118
  Lund-Browder chart, 117
  major burns, 117
  safety first rules, 115
burr holes, 236–7
bursitis

ischial, 163
olecranon, 57
pre-patellar, 57
subacromial, 40
trochanteric, 44–5, 263–4
bush suture, 21
button hole deformity, 158

C

cabbage leaves, for breast engorgement,
    259–60
calculus, in Wharton duct, 183
calf squeeze test, 171
calluses, 90, 91, 92
canker sores, 182
cannulation, 70–1
  intravenous, in child, 71, 212
cardiopulmonary resuscitation in
    children, 220–1
carotid sinus massage, 241
carpal tunnel injection, 45–6
carpal tunnel syndrome, 155–6
cat bites, 242
catheter, intercostal, 239
catheterisation, 72–4
caudal epidural, 37
cauliflower ear, 108
centipede bites, 243
cephalic vein, 232
cervical polyps, 65
cervical spine
  mobilisation, 136–7
  referred pain, 138
  spinous processes, 138
  traction, 140
cervix, viewing, 259
chalazion, 205, 206
chemical burns to eye, 208
cherry angioma, 59
chest drain, 76
chilblains, 226
children
  ankyloglossia, 183
  anxious, 219
  arm relaxation, 212
  'bite the bullet' strategy, 210
  with bleeding mouth, 180
  breath-holding attacks, 217–18
  cannulation, 71
  cardiopulmonary resuscitation in, 220–1
  choking, 241
  colic, 216
  cricothyroidotomy, 240
  crying infant, 216–17
  distracting, 209–10
  'draw a dream' technique, 218–19
  dummy (pacifier) use, 209, 210, 217
  eczema, 224–5
  eye drops, instilling, 211–12
  fear thermometer, 219

children continued
   fluid administration, 210
   forehead lump, 218
   foreign bodies, removal from nose/ear,
      126-30
      foreign bodies, swallowed, 212-13
      fractures, 215-16
   gadgets for, 254
   hip disorders, 161, 220
   intravenous cannulation, 212
   lactose intolerance test, 217
   making friends with, 209
   mouth opening, 211
   nappy rash, 224
   nasogastric tube insertion, 72
   nose cleaning, 217
   nose drops, instilling, 211
   oesophagitis, 216
   painful procedures, 210
   plaster cast removal, 216
   pulled elbow, 153
   rectal temperature measurement, 255
   reflex, obtaining, 256-7
   reflux, 216
   scalp lacerations, 213
   school refusal, 219
   self-statement questionnaire, 219
   skin rashes, 218
   spatula sketches, 211
   splints, 216
   surgery, optimal times, 220
   suturing wounds, 215
   swallowing tablets, 210
   taking medicine, 210
   tongue tie, 183-4, 220
   topical local anaesthesia, 214-15
   urine aspiration, suprapubic, 218
   vein cannulation, 212
   weighing, 210
   wound infiltration, 215
   wound repair, 213-15
choking, 241
cholesteatoma, 192
chondrodermatitis nodularis helicus, 59
clavicle, fracture, 111
   bandage for, 111
cleft lip, 220
cleft palate, 220
clenched fist injuries, 242
clindamycin, 223
'closed loop' system, 248
cold sores, 226-7
colic, 216, 259
collar and cuff sling, 112-13
Colles fracture, 159-60
coma scale, Glasgow, 236
compression stocking, applying, 83
computer, 250-1
conjunctivitis, 202
contact dermatitis, 228
convulsions, injection for, 28-9
coral cuts, 243
corneal abrasion and ulceration, 204
corneal foreign bodies, 203-4
corns, 90-3

coronary syndromes, 230
costovertebral gliding, 141
cotton wool, in ear, 131
cracked heels, 93
cramps, nocturnal, 258
creams, prescribing rules, 222
cricothyroidotomy, 240
crocodile forceps, 127
crown excisions, 15, 16
crutches, 177
cryotherapy, 58, 65, 66, 67
cutaneous myiasis, 121
cysts
   acne, 55
   Baker, 60
   Bartholin, 64-5
   breast, 63-4
   dermoid, 54, 55
   deroofing, 54
   dissection, 53
   ear lobe, 192
   epidermoid, 52-4
   epididymal, 61
   healing cavity of, 23
   meibomian, 205
   mucous, 98
   recurrent, 64
   removal of, 52-4
   sebaceous, 52-4
   tarsal, 205

D

deafness, 187, 191, 220
debridement
   in hairy area, 22
   of traumatic wounds, 21-2
   for wound debris, 5
deep venous thrombosis (DVT), 81-2
dementia prevention strategies, 264
dental problems see teeth
de Quervain tenosynovitis
   Finkelstein test, 170
   injection for, 43
   symptoms, 170
dermatitis, 224-6, 228
dermatome chart, 146
dermatophyte diagnosis, 225
dermatoscopy, 253-4
dermoid cysts, 54, 55
diabetic hypoglycaemia injection, 28
digital stethoscope, 248
digits
   avascular field, 19-20
   cut, 106
   see also finger
dipstick readers, 249
dish mop, for applying topicals, 226
dislocations
   elbow, 152-5
   finger, 156-7
   hip, 164-5
   patella, 169
   shoulder, 149-51
dog bites, 242

'dog ears,' 8-9
drain, inserting in chest, 76
'draw a dream' technique, 218-19
dressings, 22, 23
dry eyes, 202-3
dupuytren contracture, 63

E

ear
   camera, 252
   cotton bud problems, 131, 193
   deformity, 220
   discharge, 192
   external, nerve block for, 35
   facial blocks for, 34-5
   foreign body removal, 126-30
   glue ear, 197
   hearing tests, 187-8
   insect in, 130-1
   pain when flying, 192
   piercing, 189
   swimmer's ear, 188
   syringing, 189-91
   tropical ear, 188-9
   'unsafe,' 191-2
   waterproofing, 188
   wax, 189-91, 262
   wax softeners, 189-90
   wedge resection, 17-18
   see also golfer's elbow; tennis elbow
ear drum temperature measurement, 256
earlobe
   cysts, 192
   embedded earring stud, 192-3
   infected, 192
   pricking, 29
ear plugs, 188
ECG see electrocardiogram
ECG recording, 230-2
eczema, 224-5
ejaculation, premature, 259
Elastoplast Scar Reduction Patch, 62
elbow
   dislocations, 152-5
   injection, 48
   pulled, 152-3
   see also golfer's elbow; tennis elbow
electric shock, 235-6
electrocardiogram, 230-2
electrocautery
   ingrowing toenail, 101
   sebaceous cyst, 53
   subungual haematoma, 99
electrodissection of warts, 68
elliptical excisions, 8
embedded earring stud, 192-3
emergency procedures, 229-46
entropion, 203
epicondylitis, injection for, 41-2
epidermoid cysts, 52-4
epididymal cysts, 61
EpiPen®, 243, 244
episiotomy, 5, 10
Epistat catheter, 194

epistaxis, 193–5
Epley manoeuvre, 198
eustachian catheter, 127
everted wounds, 3
evidence-based medicine, 249
excisions, 7
  common mistakes, 2
  crown, 15, 16
  dead space, 3
  'dog ears,' 8–9
  elliptical, 8
  everted wounds, 3
  facial, 7–8
  for ingrowing toenail, 101
  knot tying, 3–4
  lazy S repair, 9
  lipomas, 57
  meibomian cyst, 205
  minimising bleeding, 2
  nail bed, 104–5
  non-melanoma skin cancer, 20–1
  repair principles, 1
  safety measures, 2
  scalpel holding, 5
  skin tumours, 11–13
  sutures, 2, 3
eye
  chemical burns, 208
  conjunctivitis, 202
  corneal abrasion and ulceration, 204
  corneal foreign body, 203–4
  drop application in eyes, 206
  dry eyes, 202–3
  examination, infants, 204–5
  examination kit, 201
  flash burns, 202
  fluorescein, 202, 204
  'glitter' removal, 202
  hyphaema, 208
  infections, 208
  maggot removal, 120
  meibomian cysts, 205
  ocular pain relief, 207
  padding, 207
  recurrent erosive syndrome, 204
  Seidal test, 204
  Snellen eye chart, 206, 207
  styes, 206
  subcutaneous fly larvae removal, 121
eyelashes
  entropion, 203
  ingrowing, 203
eyelid
  blepharitis, 202
  everting, 201–2
  local anaesthetic for, 205
  repair of laceration, 18, 19
  styes, 206
  xanthomas, 67

F

Fabere test, 163
face
  acne scars, 224

nerve block, 33–4
  skin lesion excision, 15
facial excisions, 7–8
facial nerve blocks, 33–4
faecal impaction, 133, 263
fall, from height, 106
fear thermometer, 219
femoral nerve, anatomy, 31–2
femur fracture, 165
finger
  amputated, 107
  boutonnière deformity, 158
  dislocated, 156–7
  dressing for tip, 107–8
  fractures, 111–12
  injecting, 42–3, 48
  lancing, 29
  loss of tip, 107
  mallet finger, 157–8
  nerve block, 29–30
  removal of ring, 122
  skin loss, 107
  strapping, 157
  tourniquet, 106
  trauma, 107–8
finger joint, injection, 47, 48
fingernails see nails
Finkelstein test, 155
fish bone, in throat, 131
fish hook, embedded, 124–5
fish-tail cut, 8
flap repairs, 10–15
flap wounds
  double Y on V advancement, 11
  H double advancement, 12
  on lower leg, 10–11
  rhomboid, 15
  rotation, 14–15
  sliding, 11
  transposition, 14
  triangular, 10–11
  Y on V advancement, 12
flash burns, 202
FLO® sinus care, 196
fluid infusions, subcutaneous, 77
fluorescein, 202, 204
foot
  calluses, 90, 91, 92
  corns, 90–3
  cracked heels, 93
  fractures, 106
  heel pain, 258
  injecting, 32–3
  nerve blocks, 33
  plantar warts, 32, 90–2
  rupture of tibialis posterior tendon, 174
  tibialis posterior tendinopathy
    injection, 46–7
  see also ankle; plantar fasciitis; toenail
foreign bodies
  bent hairpin technique, 127–8
  bent paper clip technique, 128
  buried as result of trauma, 106
  corneal, 203–4
  in ear, 126–31

fish bone in throat, 131
  fish hook, 124–5
  gunshot wounds, 126
  hooked needle technique, 128–9
  insect, in ear, 130–1
  'kiss and blow' technique, 130
  leeches, 121
  maggots, 120, 130
  metal fragments, 124
  in nose, 126–31
  pneumatic otoscopic vacuum, 129
  probe technique, 127, 128
  ring on finger, 122
  rubber catheter suction, 129
  soft, 127
  splinters, 122–3
  swallowed by children, 212–13
  ticks, 121–2
  tissue glue and plastic swab
    technique, 130
  ultrasound or X-ray for, 106, 123
foreign-body remover, 127
fractures
  associated injuries, 245
  calcaneus, 114
  in children, 215–16
  clavicle, 111, 114
  Colles, 114, 159–60
  femur, 114, 165
  greenstick, 216
  healing time, 114
  humerus, 112, 114
  mandible, 110–11
  metacarpal, 160–1
  nasal, 195–6
  phalangeal, 111–12, 114
  Potts, 114
  radius, 114
  rib, 111, 114
  scaphoid, 114, 160
  scapula, 114
  slings for, 112–15, 114
  testing for, 109–10
  wrist, 159–60
free-hanging method, 150–1
free messaging software, 250
frenulotomy, 183–4
Froment's sign, 119
frontal sinuses, 185
fungal hyphae, 225
funnel-web spider bites, 241–2

G

gamekeeper's thumb, 159
ganglions, 56
genital herpes, 227
genu varum, 220
geographic tongue, 182
Glasgow coma scale, 236
glenohumeral joint injection, 47–8
glue ear, 197
gluteus medius tendinopathy
    injection, 44–5
golfer's elbow, 42

gout, in great toe, 50
granny knot, 4
gravel rash, 108
grease gun wounds, 126
greenstick fractures, 216
groin temperature measurement, 256
gunshot wounds, 126

H

haemangioma, of lip, 60
haematoma
    block by local infiltration
        anaesthetic, 36, 37
    nasal septum, 109
    perianal, 84-5
    pinna, 108
    pretibial, 109
    septal, 109
    subungual, 99-100
haemorrhage, 244
haemorrhoids
    injecting, 86-7
    rubber band ligation, 85-6
hairpin for removal of foreign
        bodies, 127-8
hand
    burns, 118
    carpal tunnel syndrome, 155-6
    Colles fracture, 114, 159-60
    dermatitis, 226
    fracture healing time, 114
    fractures caused by falling on, 106
    nerve blocks, 30-1
    nerve injury test, 118-19
    oil injection, 126
    scaphoid fractures, 160
    sling, 114-15
    see also finger; thumb
head injuries
    children, 213
    and conscious state, 236
    exploratory burr hole, 236-7
    Glasgow coma scale, 236
headlight, hands-free, 196
hearing loss
    in the elderly, 263
    tests, 187-8
heart wall, assessed by ECG, 232
heat, to relieve eye pain, 207
heels
    cracked, 93
    painful, 258
Heimlich manoeuvre, 241
herpes labialis, 226-7
herpes simplex, 226-7
herpes zoster, 227
hiccoughs, 196
hip
    developmental dysplasia, 161, 220
    dislocated, 164-5
    injecting, 44-5, 49
    ischial bursitis, 163
    and knee pain, 161-2
    Ortolani and Barlow screening tests, 161

osteoarthritis in, 162
Patrick test, 163
snapping/clicking, 163-4
tendinitis, 44
trochanteric bursitis, 44-5, 263-4
hip and shoulder rotation test, 143-4
hip disorders, age relationship of, 161
'hip pocket nerve' syndrome, 162-3
Hippocratic method, 150
honey, as wound healer, 209
hooked needle technique, 128-9
hormone implants, 38-9
hot spoon bathing, 205, 206
human bites, 242
humerus fracture, 112, 114
hydroceles, 60
hypertrophic scars, 62
hyperventilation, 239
hyphaema, 208
hysterical 'unconscious' patient, 235

I

iliotibial band tendinopathy, 170
Implanon rod removal, 123-4
implantation cysts, 54, 55
incisions, 3
indomethacin, 259
infant colic, 217
infants, eye examination, 204-5
inferior infarction, acute, 231-2
infraorbital nerve block, 33-4
infrared aural temperature
        measurement, 256
ingrowing eyelashes, 203
ingrowing toenail
    central thinning, 100-1
    elliptical block dissection, 103
    excision of ellipse of skin, 101
    phenolisation, 102
    post-operative pain relief, 103
    spiral tape, 100-1
inguinoscrotal lumps, 220
inhalations for URTIs, 186-7
injections
    Achilles paratendinopathy, 46
    basic, 25-39
    bicipital tendinitis, 41
    bubbles in the syringe, 28
    carpal tunnel, 45-6
    caudal (trans-sacral), 37
    diabetic hypoglycaemia, 28
    digital nerve block, 29
    elbow, 41-2, 48
    epicondylitis, 41-2
    gluteus medius tendinopathy, 44-5
    great toe gout, 50
    intramuscular, 26, 27
    into joints, 47-9
    musculoskeletal, 39-50
    needle gauge, 26
    painless, 25-6
    plantar fasciitis, 44
    rectal, 28-9
    rotator cuff lesions, 40

slow, 27
    supraspinatus tendinitis, 41
    tarsal tunnel, 46
    tibialis posterior tendinopathy, 46-7
    trigger finger, 43
    trigger points in back, 39, 40
    trochanteric bursitis, 44-5, 263-4
    see also nerve blocks
injection sclerotherapy, 80-1
insect, in ear, 130-1
insomnia, 263
instrument knot, 4
intercostal catheter, 239
international notation of teeth, 181
intraosseous infusion, 234
intravenous cannulation, 71
intravenous cutdown, 232-4
intravenous iron infusion, 77
intravenous regional anaesthesia, 35-6
inverted mattress suture, 10
iron, intravenous infusion, 77
ischial bursitis, 163
isolated vein see leg veins

J

jaw, mandible fracture, 110
jellyfish stings, 243
jogger's knee, 167, 168
joint injections, 47-9
jumper's knee, 167-8

K

keloids, 62, 63
keratoacanthomas, 58
keratoses, 59
'kiss and blow' technique, 130
knee
    anterior pain, 168
    common causes of pain, 165-6
    dislocated patella, 169
    injecting, 49
    jogger's, 167, 168
    jumper's, 167-8
    'kneeling on a stool' test, 143-4
    knock knees, 220
    Lachman test, 167
    meniscal injuries, 166-7
    overuse syndromes, 167
    pain referred from hip, 161-2
    synovial plinca syndrome, 166, 167
knock knees, 220
knot tying, 3-4
Kocher method, 149

L

lacerations
    eyelid, 18, 19
    lip, 16
    ragged, 13
    scalp, 213
Lachman test, 167
lactose intolerance test, 217
lancing finger, 29

laser energy ablation, 80
lateral cutaneous nerve of thigh
    (LCNT), 32
lateral epicondylitis, 41–2
lateral sphincterotomy, 87
lazy S repair, 9
leech removal, 121
leg
    bowed, 220
    crutches, prescription of, 177
    lower leg problems, 171
    nerve roots, pressure on, 145–6
    nocturnal cramps, 258
    overuse syndromes, 170
    pain from disc prolapse, 145–6
    restless legs syndrome, 257
    tennis leg, 169
    torn 'monkey muscle,' 169–71
    triangular flap wounds, 9, 10–11, 15
    ulcers, 82–3
    walking stick, 177
    see also ankle; knee; varicose vein
leg veins
    avulsion, 79–80
    compression stocking, applying, 83
    deep venous thrombosis, 81–2
    endovascular treatment, 80–1
    percutaneous ligation, 79
    ruptured, 82
    thrombophlebitis, 81
    venous ulcers, 82–3
ligatures, on vessels, 4, 13–14
Limberg flap, 15
lip
    cleft, 220
    haemangioma, 60
    repair of cut, 16–17
    wedge excision, 17
lipomas, 57
liquid nitrogen
    plantar wart treatment, 91
    to remove skin tags, 52
    skin lesion therapy, 65–7
Little's area, cautery of, 193
local anaesthetic
    infiltration for wounds, 124
    injection technique, 37–8
longitudinal traumatic nail
    laceration, 105
lumbar epidural, 37, 143
lumbar puncture, 74–5
lumbar spine
    dermatome chart, 146
    movements of, 144–5
    reference points, 143
    stretching and manipulation, 147–8
lumbosacral spine
    bony landmarks, 143
    disc prolapse, 145
    leg nerve roots, 145–6
    lower back exercise, 147–8
    posterior view, 145
    rotation mobilisation, 146–7
    slump test, 146
Lund-Browder chart for burns, 117

M

maggots, removing, 120
Magnuson method, 143
mallet finger, 157–8
mandible
    fracture of, 110–11
    spatula test, 110
manual disimpaction, 133
marsupialisation, 64–5
mastitis, acute bacterial, 63
matchstick tamponade, 193
maxillary sinuses, 186
medial epicondylitis, 42
medial plantar nerve block, 33
median nerve block, 30
medical alerts, 247
medical defence, 263
medical phone apps, 249–50
medical records, 251
medical score calculator, 249
medicare item numbers, 249
meibomian cysts, 205
meniscal injuries, 166–7
mental nerve block, 34
meralgia paraesthetica of thigh, 32
metacarpal fractures, 160–1
metal fragments, 124
mid-thoracic spine manipulation, 141–2
migraine, 138, 238–9
migratory pointing test, 143
Milch method, 150
milker's nodules, 59
minor problems, holistic treatment, 264
molluscum contagiosum, 68–9
'monkey muscle,' torn, 169–71
morphine, subcutaneous infusion of, 77
Morton's interdigital neuroma, 96
moth, in ear, 130–1
mouth
    aphthous ulcers, 182
    calculus in Wharton duct, 183
    opening a child's, 211
    see also teeth; tongue
M-plasty, 9
Mt Beauty method, 151–2
mucous cysts, 98
musculoskeletal injections, 39–50
myocardial infarction, 231–2
myxoid pseudocyst, 98–9

N

nail bed
    ablation, 98
    excisions, 104–5
nails
    avulsion by chemolysis, 105
    onychogryphosis, 98
    paronychia, 103–4
    splinter under, 97–8
    subungual haematoma, 99–100
    see also toenail
nappy rash, 224
nasal fractures, 195–6
nasal polyps, 187

nasal septum haematoma, 109
nasogastric intubation, 71–2
neck
    muscle energy therapy, 139, 140
    palpating, 138
    rolls and stretches, 140
    torticollis, 139
    traction, 139–40
neck movement grid, 136
needles
    disposal, 27–8
    gauge, 26
    recapping, 28
negligence claims, avoiding, 263
nerve blocks
    digital, 29–30
    elbow, 31
    external ear, 35
    facial, 33–4
    femoral, 31–2
    foot, 44
    hand, 30–1
    infraorbital, 33–4
    medial plantar, 33
    median, 30
    mental, 34
    penile, 35
    radial, 31
    supraorbital, 33, 34
    sural, 33
    tibial, 32–3
    ulnar, 30
nerve injury, quick hand test, 118–19
neurology, 247
nightmares, 257
nose
    auriscope, use of, 197
    cleaning child's, 217
    epistaxis, 193–5
    foreign bodies in, 126–31
    fractured, 195–6
    instilling drops, 195
    nasal washout, 196
    offensive smell from, 195
    polyps, 187
    senile rhinorrhoea, 195, 263
    septal haematoma, 109
    severe posterior epistaxis, 194
    'snotty,' 217
    stuffy/running, 195
Nozoil®, 195
Nozovent®, 197

O

ocular pain relief, 207
oesophagitis, 216
oil injections into hand, 126
ointment, prescribing rules, 222
olecranon bursitis, 57
onychocryptosis, 100–1
onychogryphosis, 98
onychomycosis, 98
oral temperature measurement, 255
orf, 59

Ortolani test, 161
osteoarthritis in hip joint, 162
otitis externa
    preventing swimmer's ear, 188
    suppurative, 188
    tissue 'spears' for cleaning, 188
    tropical ear, 188–9
otitis media
    suppurative, 188
    tissue 'spears' for cleaning, 188
Otovent®, 197
oxygen therapy, 230

P

paint gun wounds, 126
palliative care, 249
palmar nodule, 63
Palmer notation of teeth, 181–2
paper clip
    bent, for removal of foreign bodies, 128
    hot, for subungual haematoma, 99
    uses, 262
papillomas, 67–8
paraphimosis, 234–5
paraphrenia, 263
paronychia, 103–4
patella, dislocated, 169
patellar tendinopathy, 167–8
patellofemoral joint pain, 168–9
patient education in consulting room, 261
Patrick test, 163
penile nerve block, 35
penis
    acute paraphimosis, 234–5
    extricating from zipper, 131–2
perianal
    abscess, 88
    haematoma, 84–5
    skin tags, 85
    warts, 88
perineal skin repair, 10
petroleum jelly, uses, 262
phalangeal fractures, 111–12
Phalen test, 156
phenolisation, for ingrowing toenail, 102
phone camera, 248
pilonidal cyst ± abscess, 88
pinhole test, for blurred vision, 206–7
pinna, haematoma, 108
plantar fasciitis, 93–5, 170
    exercises, 93–5
    hydrotherapy, 93
    injecting, 44, 95
    strapping, 95
plantar warts, 32, 90–2
plastering
    leg support for plaster application, 176
    plaster of Paris, 174–5
    plaster walking heel, 176
    removal of cast from child, 216
    silicone filler, 176–7
    supporting shoe, 176
    volar arm plaster splint, 175–6
    waterproofing, 176

pleural effusion, 76–7
pneumothorax, 239
point-of-care ultrasound
        (POCUS), 252–3
polymyalgia rheumatica, 138
polyps
    anal fibro-epithelial, 88–9
    cervical, 65
    nasal, 187
post-cryotherapy, 67
post-herpetic neuralgia, 227
premature ejaculation, 259
pre-patellar bursitis, 57
pressure gun injuries, 126
pretibial haematoma, 109
priapism, 259
prickles, removal of, 123
probe technique, 127, 128
proctalgia fugax, 87
prolapsed disc, 145–6
prolapse, rectal, 89
proprioception exercises, 173
pruritis ani, 89
psoriasis, 225
    steroid injections, 61–2, 225
pulley suture, 6–7
pulse oximetry, 229–30, 254
punch biopsy, 53, 57
pupillary reaction test, 235
purse-string suture, 7
pyogenic granuloma, 59

Q

quadriceps exercise, 169

R

radial nerve block, 31
radiofrequency ablation, 80
rape victims, 237–8
rapid intravenous infusion
        catheter (RIC), 71
rashes, 218
recapping needles, 28
rectal 'injection,' 28–9
rectal prolapse, 89
recurrent erosive syndrome, 204
red-back spider bite, 242
Red Cross First Aid app, 249
reef knot, 3–4, 112, 213
reflexes, 256–7
reflux with oesophagitis, 216
renal colic, 259
restless legs syndrome, 257
resuscitation of child, 220–1
rhomboid flap, 15
rib belt, universal, 111
rib fracture, 111, 114
ring, removing from finger, 122
roadside emergency, 245–6
roller injuries to limbs, 109
rotation flaps, 14–15
rotator cuff lesions, injecting, 40
rule of nines, 223

S

sacral hiatus, identifying, 37
salivary calculus, 183
sandfly bites, 242
saphenous vein, long, 232
scalpel
    holding, 5
    insertion and removal of blade, 5
scalp lacerations, 213
scalp seborrhoea, 263
scaphoid fractures, 160
scapula pressure method, 150
sciatica
    in buttock, 163
    disc prolapse, 145
    epidural to treat, 37
    'hip pocket nerve' syndrome, 162–3
scorpion bites, 243
scrotum, hydroceles, 60
sea sickness, 262
sea wasp stings, 243
sebaceous cysts, 52–4
sebaceous hyperplasia, 54
seborrhoea, scalp, 263
seborrhoeic keratoses, 59, 67
Seidal test, 204
Semont manoeuvre, 199
senile rhinorrhoea, 195, 263
septal haematoma, 109
serious injuries, clues from
        association, 244–5
sexual assault, 237–8
shave biopsy, 55
shaved area, clearing, 22
shingles, 227
shin splints, 170
shoulder
    dislocated, 149–51
    injecting, 47–8
    recurrent dislocation, 152
    referred pain, 138
silicone filler in plaster cast, 176
single big button, 247
sinusitis, unilateral, 185–6
sinus tenderness, 185
skier's thumb, 159
skin cancer, excision, 20–1, 58–9
skin creams and ointments, 222
skin glues, 213–14
skin grafts, 10
skin lesions
    biopsies, 55–6
    liquid nitrogen therapy, 65–7
    steroid injections, 61
skin preparation, for antiseptic
        solutions, 2
skin scrapings, 225
skin tags
    perianal, 85
    removal of, 52
skin tears, avoiding, 13
skin tumours
    excising, 11–13
    primary suture, 13

slings, 112–15
makeshift, 115
slump test, 146
snake bite, 241
Snellen eye chart, 206, 207
snoring, 196–7
'snotty' nose, 217
soft foreign bodies, 127
sore throat, swallowing with, 197
spacing chamber, makeshift, 260
spatula sketches, 211
spectacles, protective, 208
spider bites, 241–2
spider naevi, 226
spine
anterior directed gliding, 137, 141
manipulation, 136–7
mobilisation, 136–7
recording movements of, 136
thoracic, 141–3
see also cervical spine; lumbar spine;
lumbosacral spine
spirometer, 252
splinters
detecting, 123
under nails, 97–8
under skin, 122–3
splints
finger, 158
minor fractures, 216
split skin injuries, 21
squamous cell carcinoma (SCC), 58–9
squint, 220
stab wounds, 106
Steri-Strips, 1–2
sternal thrust, 213
steroid injections
ganglions, 56
hypertrophic scars, 62
psoriasis plaques, 61–2
skin lesions, 61
stingray stings, 243
stings, 243
St John sling, 112, 114
stucco keratoses, 59
styes, 206
subacromial space injections
for rotator cuff lesions, 40
for subacromial bursitis, 40
subcutaneous fluid infusions, 77
subcutaneous fly larvae, removal of, 121
subtalar joint mobilisation, 173
subungual haematoma, 99–100
sugar, uses, 262
sunburn, 222, 264
sunglasses, 223
sunlight exposure, 222–3
suppository inserter, 261
supraorbital nerve block, 33, 34
suprapubic aspiration of urine, 218
supraspinatus tendinitis,
injection for, 41
supra ventricular tachycardia, 241
sural nerve block, 33
surgeon's knot, 4

surgery, optimal times for children's
disorders, 220
sutures
blanket stitch, 6
bush, 21
continuous, 5–6
cross-stitch, 7
inverted mattress, 10
material, 2
non-absorbable, 5, 23–4
number of, 3
over-and-over, 6
primary, 13
pulley, 6–7
purse-string, 7
removal of, 20, 23–4
subcuticular, 5–6
three-point, 9, 12, 13
vertical mattress, 3
suturing
cut tendon, 115
'dog ears,' 8–9
holding the needle, 3
knot tying, 3–4
lip repair, 16–17
painless, 27
practising, 1
skin preparation, 2
taping wounds, 1–2
tongue wound, 19
swallowing, 260–1
with sore throat, 197
swimmer's ear, 188
synovial plinca syndrome, 166, 167
syringing, ear, 189–91

T

tablets, halving, 260
Tailor's bottom, 163
tamponade, 193
tampons, removal of impacted, 132–3
tarsal cysts, 205
tarsal tunnel injection, 46
teeth
abscess, 180
bleeding socket, 180
chipped, 180
dry socket, 180–1
knocked-out, 179
loosened, 179
lost crown, 180
lost filling, 180
notation, 181–2
wisdom teeth, 180, 182
temperature measurement, 255–6
temporomandibular joint
dysfunction, 134–5
injection, 49
TMJ rest program, 135
tendinopathy
Achilles, 46, 170
bicipital, 41
gluteus medius, 44–5
iliotibial band, 170

special uses, 258
supraspinatus, 41
vasodilator use, 258
tendon, severed, 115
tendon sheath injection, 39, 43
tennis elbow
exercises, 154–5
injection for, 41–2
wringing exercise, 154–5
tennis leg, 169
tenosynovitis of the wrist
injection for, 43
see also de Quervain tenosynovitis
tenpin bowler's thumb, 158–9
testicle
torsion of, 61
tumours, 61
therapeutic venesection, 78
thermometers, 248, 255–6
thigh
lateral cutaneous nerve, 32
meralgia paraesthetica, 32
thoracic spine
anterior directed costovertebral gliding,
137, 141
manipulation, 141–2
mobilisation, 136–7
thoracolumbar stretching/manipulation,
142–3
three-point suture, 9, 12, 13
throat
fish bone in, 131
swallowing when sore, 197
ticklish, 198
thrombophlebitis, 81
thumb
injecting, 30, 43, 48
joint, 48
lancing, 29
skier's/gamekeeper's, 159
tenpin bowler's, 158–9
trigger, 43
tibialis anterior tenosynovitis, 170
tibialis posterior tendinopathy, 46–7
tibialis posterior tendon rupture, 174
tibial nerve block, 32–3
tibial stress fracture, 170
tibial stress syndrome, 170
tick removal, 121–2
Tinel test, 156
tinnitus, 197
tissue glue and plastic swab
technique, 130
toenail
dystrophic, 105
ingrowing, 100–1
onychogryphosis, 100–1
paronychia, 103–4
subungual haematoma, 99–100
traumatic avulsed, 105
tongue
black, 182–3
geographic, 182
hairy, 182–3
repairing, 19

tongue tie, 183–4
'too many toes' test, 174
topical anaesthesia for wound repair, 27
torticollis, 139
traction
    for cervical spine, 140
    for dislocated shoulder, 152
    to neck, 139–40
transposition flaps, 14
trauma, 106, 244–6
traumatic avulsed toenail, 105
'triangle of safety,' 76
trichiasis, 203
trichloroacetic acid, 67
trigger finger injection, 42–3
trochanteric bursalgia injection, 44–5,
    263–4
tropical ear, 188–9

U

ulcers
    aphthous, 182
    corneal, 204
    venous, 82–3
ulnar nerve block, 30
ultrasound
    for detecting foreign bodies, 123
    detecting splinters, 123
'unconscious' hysterical patient, 235
upper respiratory tract infections *see* URTIs
Upton's paste, 91
ureteric colic, 259
urethral catheterisation
    children, 74
    female, 73–4
    male, 72–3
urine aspiration, suprapubic, 218
URTIs

anosmia following, 198
inhalations for, 186–7
UV light protection, 223

V

vaccination, needle gauge, 26
vaginal temperature measurement, 256
Varicose vein
    ruptured, 82
    see also leg veins
Vaseline®, uses, 262
veins
    cephalic, 232
    dilating, 70–1
    long saphenous, 232
venepuncture, 70–1, 258
venesection, 78
venous ulcers, 82–3
vertical mattress suture, 3
vertigo, positional, 198–9
vessel ligation, 4, 13–14
vibrator, removal from vagina/rectum, 133
vision, blurred, 206–7
vital signs, normal values, 229
vitamin D, 222–3
volar arm plaster splint, 175–6

W

walking stick, 177
warts
    electrodissection, 68
    perianal, 88
    plantar, 32, 90–2
    treatment options, 68
washout, antral/nasal, 196
wasp stings, 243
wax removal, 189–91
weaver's bottom, 163

wedge excision of lip, 17
wedge resection
    ear, 17–18
    ingrown toenail, 102
wisdom teeth, 180, 182
wobble board technique, 173–4
Wood's light examination, 202, 226, 251
wounds
    debridement, 5, 21–2
    dressings, 22, 23
    everted, 3
    healing cyst/abscess cavities, 23
    honey as healer, 209
    injecting analgesia, 215
    keeping hair out of, 22
    local anaesthetic infiltration, 27, 28, 124
    maggot removal, 120
    painless suturing, 215
    post-operative care, 23
    skin glue, use of, 213–14
    topical anaesthesia for, 27
    traumatic, 22
    Z-plasty, 15–16
    see also sutures; suturing
W-plasty, 21
wrist
    injection, 43, 48
    nerve block, 30–1
    tenosynovitis, 43

X

xanthelasmas, 67
xanthomas, 67
X-ray, detecting splinters, 123

Z

zipper, extricating penis from, 131–2
Z-plasty, 15–16